Health Communication Models and Practices in Interpersonal and Media Contexts:

Emerging Research and Opportunities

Célia Belim
ISCSP, University of Lisbon, Portugal

Cristina Vaz de Almeida
ISCSP, University of Lisbon, Portugal

A volume in the Advances in
Human Services and Public Health
(AHSPH) Book Series

IGI Global
PUBLISHER of TIMELY KNOWLEDGE

Published in the United States of America by
IGI Global
Medical Information Science Reference (an imprint of IGI Global)
701 E. Chocolate Avenue
Hershey PA, USA 17033
Tel: 717-533-8845
Fax: 717-533-8661
E-mail: cust@igi-global.com
Web site: http://www.igi-global.com

Library of Congress Cataloging-in-Publication Data

Names: Belim, Célia, author. | Vaz de Almeida, Cristina, author.
Title: Health communication models and practices in interpersonal and media contexts : emerging research and opportunities / by Célia Belim, Cristina Vaz de Almeida.
Description: Hershey, PA : Medical Information Science Reference, [2021] | Includes bibliographical references and index. | Summary: "The authored book explores the two dimensions of health communication: --interpersonal communication and media communication-- and analyzes the practices of these two dimensions of communication and offers practical solutions for better communication with direct results in the optimization of citizens' health literacy"-- Provided by publisher.
Identifiers: LCCN 2021013281 (print) | LCCN 2021013282 (ebook) | ISBN 9781799843962 (hardcover) | ISBN 9781799843979 (ebook)
Subjects: MESH: Health Communication--methods | Professional-Patient Relations | Communications Media | Models, Psychological
Classification: LCC R118 (print) | LCC R118 (ebook) | NLM WA 590 | DDC 610.1/4--dc23
LC record available at https://lccn.loc.gov/2021013281
LC ebook record available at https://lccn.loc.gov/2021013282

This book is published in the IGI Global book series Advances in Human Services and Public Health (AHSPH) (ISSN: 2475-6571; eISSN: 2475-658X)

British Cataloguing in Publication Data
A Cataloguing in Publication record for this book is available from the British Library.

All work contributed to this book is new, previously-unpublished material.
The views expressed in this book are those of the authors, but not necessarily of the publisher.

For electronic access to this publication, please contact: eresources@igi-global.com.

Advances in Human Services and Public Health (AHSPH) Book Series

ISSN:2475-6571
EISSN:2475-658X

MISSION

The well-being of the general public should be a primary concern for any modern civilization. Ongoing research in the field of human services and public healthcare is necessary to evaluate, manage, and respond to the health and social needs of the global population.

The **Advances in Human Services and Public Health (AHSPH)** book series aims to publish high-quality reference publications focused on the latest methodologies, tools, issues, and strategies for managing the health and social welfare of the public. The AHSPH book series will be especially relevant for healthcare professionals, policy makers, government officials, and students seeking the latest research in this field.

COVERAGE

- Social Welfare Policy
- Public Welfare
- Healthcare Reform
- Domestic Violence
- Poverty
- Social Work
- Public Funding
- Assistance Programs
- Medicare and Medicaid
- Access to Healthcare Services

The Advances in Human Services and Public Health (AHSPH) Book Series (ISSN 2475-6571) is published by IGI Global, 701 E. Chocolate Avenue, Hershey, PA 17033-1240, USA, www.igi-global.com. This series is composed of titles available for purchase individually; each title is edited to be contextually exclusive from any other title within the series. For pricing and ordering information please visit http://www.igi-global.com/book-series/advances-human-services-public-health/102256. Postmaster: Send all address changes to above address.

Titles in this Series

For a list of additional titles in this series, please visit: http://www.igi-global.com/book-series/

Handbook of Research on Economic and Social Impacts of Population Aging
Yilmaz Bayar (Bandirma Onyedi Eylul University, Turkey)
Information Science Reference • © 2021 • 383pp • H/C (ISBN: 9781799873273) • US $245.00

Stakeholder Strategies for Reducing the Impact of Global Health Crises
Vikas Kumar (Chaudhary Bansi Lal University, India) and Geetika Malhotra (Indira Gandhi University, India)
Information Science Reference • © 2021 • 304pp • H/C (ISBN: 9781799874959) • US $195.00

Examining and Solving Health Disparities in the United States Emerging Research and Opportunities
Cheryl Green (Southern Connecticut State University, USA)
Medical Information Science Reference • © 2021 • 177pp • H/C (ISBN: 9781799838746) • US $265.00

Transitioning Healthcare Support in Developing Countries From the US to China Emerging Research and Opportunities
Leo Eyombo (Howard University, USA) and Renee Murray-Bachmann (Northwell Hospital, USA)
Medical Information Science Reference • © 2021 • 135pp • H/C (ISBN: 9781799844501) • US $245.00

Examining Gun Regulations, Warning Behaviors, and Policies to Prevent Mass Shootings
Selina E.M. Kerr (Independent Researcher, UK)
Information Science Reference • © 2021 • 196pp • H/C (ISBN: 9781799839163) • US $195.00

IGI Global
PUBLISHER of TIMELY KNOWLEDGE

701 East Chocolate Avenue, Hershey, PA 17033, USA
Tel: 717-533-8845 x100 • Fax: 717-533-8661
E-Mail: cust@igi-global.com • www.igi-global.com

Table of Contents

Preface

WHEN COMMUNICATION AND HEALTH MEET

Communication is inscribed in human nature, constituting "a fundamental feature of humanity" (McLeod, 2017, p. 3). Plato, for example, described the human being as "the animal that speaks" (*zoon logon echon*) and Tammelo (1966) defined man as a "communicating being" (p. 503). This is the feature that differentiates humans from animals, being the *visceral* essence of the humankind. Tammelo (1966) explains that "man's communication, like his breathing, smiling, sulking, and thinking takes place regardless of whether or not he understands what he is doing" (p. 503). So, the signification that communication expresses and available to the receiver is the raw material that generates the communicative process. Communication requires full understanding of behaviors associated with the sender, independently of his conscience of the potential signification that his behaviors can generate, the receiver and the possible obstacles that probably exist (Munodawafa, 2008).

Communication is very complex and communications experts have difficulty agreeing on one definition to cover every situation (Fielding, 2006, p. 10). Communication can be defined as a process whereby people assign meanings to stimuli in order to make sense of the world, including both unintentional and intentional behaviors (Trenholm, 2001), or a transaction whereby participants together create meaning through the exchange of symbols (Fielding, 2006, p. 10). Blakar (1979) clarifies that the sender, in his encoding, must try to anticipate and determine how the receiver, based on his background and his perspective, will decode and interpret the message transmitted. Through this, the receiver indirectly influences the sender's linguistic and communication structuring. In this alternation, or this interaction between sender and receiver, "that there is the basis for a 'power struggle', that is to say, a battle about which (whose) premises, which (whose) perspective, which (whose) use of language and, thus, which (whose) structuring of social reality shall be fundamental" (Blakar, 1979, p. 161).

On the other hand, health was, pertinently understood by ancient Greece, Indian and Chinese, as a balance between a person and the environment, the unity of soul and body, and the natural origin of disease (Svalastog, Donev, Kristoffersen & Gajović, 2017, p. 431). Plato, in his *Dialogues*, highlighted that a perfect human society, submitted to the ideal of ancient Greek philosophy "a healthy mind in a healthy body", could be achieved by harmonizing the interests of the individual and the social body. Health is the pivotal wealth of an individual, due to without health the individual does not have a balance, faces fragilities to perform his/her objectives and prejudices the other dimensions of his/her life.

The encounter between communication and health is promising and fruitful. For example, Rimal and Lapinski (2009) highlight that the health communication "has much to celebrate and contribute" (p. 247) and that the field is gaining recognition in part because of its emphasis on combining theory and practice in understanding communication processes and changing human behavior. The authors explain that, by bringing together researchers and practitioners from various disciplines and adopting multilevel theoretical approaches, health communicators "have a unique opportunity to provide meaningful input in improving and saving lives" (p. 247). Being a stable concept by consensus, health communication can be understood as "the art and technique of informing, influencing and motivating individuals, institutions and public audiences about important health issues" (U.S. Department of Health and Human Services, 2000).

The formal application of health communication has come a long way (Thomas, 2006, p. 40). In the early twentieth century, there was no dominant medical paradigm. However, medical historians report that the doctors with effective communication skills had the best chance of affecting a cure (Thomas, 2006, p. 40). This evidence shows the potential of the relation between communication and health outcomes.

During the early days of medicine in America, health communication, in a formal sense, was poorly developed and was not recognized as a distinct discipline, associating itself with "common sense" (Thomas, 2006, p. 40). Health communication is a young but rapidly growing interdisciplinary area of study (Kreps, 2014), "an exciting applied social scientific research and application field of study" (Kreps, 2012, p. 11) and it is recognized as a scientific area in the 1970s (Kreps, 2012, p. 11; Kreps & Bonaguro, 2009). However, there are traces that go back to its origin of ancient Greece and

Hippocrates (Kreps, 2014, p. 567). The research and writing on the topic have grown tremendously since the early 1980s, generating increasing numbers of important research findings and publications (CENGAGE, 2019). One reason that justifies this growth is the importance of the research area of health communication "for addressing complex and challenging healthcare demands in society and guiding the promotion of public health" (CENGAGE, 2019).

Hicks (2017), referring that news organizations mirror the growth and diversity in healthcare communications, highlights the role of news organizations in illustrating health/disease stories of patients (pp. 3-4). Diseases "come out of the closet" thanks to the "stunning advances in medical science", societal trends that brought an openness to once whispered diseases and a move from sick care to wellness, ads and news organizations that put the issues on the public agenda (p. 4). The online revolution in health care has had also profound implications (p. 8).

According to Kreps (2012), there is so much more that can be done by health communication scholars to improve public health and wellness (p. 13). The author mentions that while health communication scholarship has already made relevant contributions to improve health care and health promotion, health communication inquiry has the ability to make even more significant and wide-ranging contributions to optimize public health (p. 13). Kreps (2012) recognizes the virtues of the health communication scholarship, that has grown in institutional credibility (within academia, government agencies, and health care systems), and can build exciting new collaborations and partnerships and influence public health policies and practices. For instance, the health communication scholars can focus on conducting serious large-scale studies that can provide compelling results, with large real-world health system populations. They can also develop new and improved research methods and innovative theoretical frameworks for guiding health communication research and inquiry (p. 19).

It cannot be denied that "communication is at the very center of healthcare and health-promotion efforts" (CENGAGE, 2019). Health communication, being in the front and center of today's issues, has become indispensable to the world we live in (Hicks, 2017, p. 11). In the therapeutic, media, consumerist, social contexts and in a broader system-wide level, communication performs an essential role. The communication is also important to design campaigns, conceived to prevent health risks and to foment the adoption of healthy actions and lifestyles. In all these contexts, the communication style, performance, skills have to be adjusted and to be considered, in order to achieve optimized outcomes.

PROBLEMS AND CHALLENGES

Communication can prevent health problems, can be fruitful to promote a healthy behavior and lifestyle, and can help to overcome health challenges. Expressions such as "healthy thanks to communication" (Belim & Vaz de Almeida, 2018a), "open the door of communication for better results" in health (Vaz de Almeida & Belim, 2019), communication "as a light on the patient pathway" (Vaz de Almeida & Belim, 2021) and the "communication competences as the key" to optimize health literacy (Belim & Vaz de Almeida, 2018b) show the value of communication for health.

There is a tendency for literature to emphasize communication as a catalyst for results (Levinson, Roter & Mullooly, 1997; Ong, Haes, Hoos & Lammes, 1995, p. 903; Stewart 1995), as an effective bridge for the construction the therapeutic relationship (Ha & Longnecker, 2010) and as a lever, in the media context, for the massive dissemination of messages with low cost (Wakefield, Loken & Hornik, 2010).

Communication is a *sine qua non* condition for human life and for the social order (Watzlawick, Beavin & Jackson, 1967, p. 13) and all communication affects human behavior (Watzlawick et al., 1967), including health. For example, the practice of good communication competences in health professions influences a significant and trustworthy relationship between practitioners and patients (Ranjan, Kumari & Chakrawarty, 2015, p. 1), with effects on the patients' health outcomes. Communication has been assumed to be the "need of the hour" (Ranjan et al., 2015, p. 1) and the "key to a healthier tomorrow" (Ratzan, 1994), enabling answers to face and solve problems in the context of communication in the health context:

1. The low health literacy: about 50% of Europeans, including Portuguese, have low levels of health literacy (HLS-EU, 2012) and more than a third of adults in the United States of America (USA) (77 million people) would have difficulties with common health tasks, such as following the instructions on a prescription drug label or adhering to a childhood immunization schedule using a standard chart (U.S. Department of Health and Human Services-HHS, 2008). Limited health literacy affects American adults across all racial ethnic groups (U.S. Department of Health and Human Services-HHS, 2008);
2. The overestimation by health professionals of their patients' health literacy: this is the case of nurses (Johnson, 2014, p. 43). This overestimation may contribute to the general problem of poor health outcomes and rates

of hospital readmission (Dickens, Lambert, Cromwell & Piano, 2013; Macabasco-O'Connell & Fry-Bowers, 2011);

3. The patients' reluctance to admit a lack of understanding and the inclination to follow the recommendations as they understand them, instead of asking for clarification (e.g. Baker et al., 1996; Dickens et al., 2013; Martin et al., 2011; Parikh, Parker, Nursers, Baker & Williams, 1996);
4. The scarcity of studies combining communication / interaction and health literacy (e.g. Ishikawa & Kiuchi, 2010);
5. The recommendation to include training in communication skills in the curriculum and practice of doctors (Ranjan et al., 2015) and other health professionals;
6. The lack of effective strategies for a conscious and more permanent change in behaviors oriented towards healthy lifestyles (Vaz de Almeida, 2018);
7. The insufficiency of health literacy tools to generate the organizational changes necessary to improve organizations' health literacy (Lloyd et al., 2018);
8. The tendency towards passivity in exposure to media campaigns, although these can produce positive changes or prevent negative changes in health-related behaviors in large populations. A possible explanation for this behavior of the recipient is the frequent competition between these campaigns and other factors, such as product marketing, powerful social norms and behaviors driven by addiction or habit (Wakefield, Loken & Hornik, 2010);
9. The need for a better understanding of the ideal of a media campaign, given that media campaigns seem to be more effective when intense, long-lasting and well targeted to a population group (Fraser, 2019).

Rimal and Lapinski (2009) clarify that, given the global challenges posed by major threats, health communication scholars and practitioners recognize the pertinence of prevention and, with it, the need to understand human behavior through the prism of theory. The authors identify some challenges, such as the evaluation of communication interventions, especially those adopting national mass media, does not usually lend itself to randomized trials; the difficulties that the behavioral scientists face in designing and testing multilevel and multidisciplinary interventions; the health communication interventions need to make additional efforts to meet their publics at their level of technology use.

Considering the priorization of health in the human life, the health communication has to deal with multiple challenges. One surrounds most of the basic indicators that reflect the well-being of children and vulnerable populations in many parts of the world (Obregon, 2014). The children, placed within some of the various dimensions of poverty and discrimination, are more likely to be affected by disease or by disparities and conditions. The challenge, here, is to guarantee that the intervention program reaches out to the vulnerable children. One recurring challenge is that if the communication is driven by siloed interventions, it has to deal with the possibility to not offer the communities what they need (Hickler, 2014).

Rodrigues, Schulmann and Ilinca (2015) conducted four expert focus groups recruited from different fields (public officials, academics, public health and communication experts, representatives of international organization and of EU advocacy groups), each concentrating on a specific factor risk (smoking, alcohol consumption, unhealthy diet and sedentary lifestyle). The most immediate challenges identified relate to the diversity of epidemiological patterns, cultural underpinnings, social norms, language and communication channels between countries. Similarly relevant is the building of a strong campaign coalition and the consideration of differences in national legislation and of available resources. A set of risk factor-specific challenges is also identified: effective messaging (negative for smoking and alcohol, positive otherwise), message complexity (unhealthy diet), involvement of industry representatives (none for smoking, otherwise desirable to various extents) and the relevance of existing infrastructure (sedentary lifestyles).

The COVID-19 pandemic brings some lessons, to move from the acute phase of the pandemic to the next normal, that are challenges for the health communication: the need for communicators to be proactive and to take preventive actions at times; the relevance of planning ahead while also acknowledging the uncertainty; and the call to focus on people (Ratzan, Sommariva & Rauh, 2020). Among a pandemic context, three questions can constitute challenges to conquer (Finset, 2021): 1. How well do people understand health information? One pivotal aspect of informing people is to use a terminology that can be correctly understood by all; 2. What do people want to know and what do they fear? The information transmitted to the public on COVID-19 should be calibrated to the public's particular information needs; and 3. How is clinical communication affected by COVID-19? A major change in the working day of many clinicians is the transition from face-to-face communication to remote encounters, mediated by online and mobile platforms, for example.

RESEARCH AND OPPORTUNITIES

Health communication scholars have significant opportunities for influencing the landscape of health care globally (Dutta, 2009, p. 88). Having this idea in mind, we propose this book entitled *Health Communication Models and Practices in Interpersonal and Media Contexts: Emerging Research and Opportunities*, that includes both a theoretical and an empirical part, accepting, for example, the challenge launched by Kreps (2012) to explore innovative theoretical frameworks for guiding health communication research (p. 19).

Synnot et al. (2018) conducted an international survey evolving consumers and other stakeholders (n = 151). The participants prioritize, as research topics, structural and cultural challenges in health services (e.g. lack of holistic, patient-centered, culturally safe care) and building health professionals' communication skills (the substance of the Chapters 4 and 5 of this book). The authors emphasize that solutions should be conceived in partnership with consumers, and the focus on the needs of vulnerable groups. Also Dutta (2009), for example, underscores the pertinence of addressing topics of access, culture, quality, and technology in health communication theorization, research, and practice (p. 80).

In spite of the enormous gap between health systems, at the beginning of the 21st century, and the ideals of patient-centered care, the new media landscape, constituting health communication opportunities, brings hope in assisting both developed and developing nations to find creative, "disruptive" solutions and improved health status for their citizens-patients (Parker, Woelfel, Hart & Brown, 2009, p. 19). Media also offers "unprecedented opportunities" to bring to health consumers the information they need in the most effective ways possible (Duffy & Thorson, 2009, p. 111). The chapters 1, 6 and 7 focus on the potential of media campaigns.

Despite being a relevant factor, the doctor–patient communication relation is often ignored (Shukla, Yadav & Kastury, 2010) – is one of the focuses of our book. And there is no standard or consensual core in the health professions concerning the nature of communication competences (Spitzberg, 2013) – the essence of the chapters 4 and 5 of our book. Current health communication models do not specify what concrete and interdependent communication competences are needed in the therapeutic relationship. The assertiveness, clarity of language and positivity-ACP model, composed of these three competences is supposed to fill this gap and is presented in the chapter 5.

Additionally, systematic reviews and meta-analyses show that tailoring health communication is an effective and cost-effective method for promoting health behavior change. For example, Bol, Smit and Lustria (2020), reflecting on opportunities and challenges in the digital area, observe that: while it is important to continue exploring and testing new tailoring strategies, it is also critical to continue building on the science of tailoring and studying the processes and mechanisms that have potential to influence the effectiveness of tailored health communication.

Sharma, Nahak and Kanozia (2019) make a systematic literature review of 20 different research outcomes of health communication. The researchers have discovered that health communication, based on interpersonal, group and mass communication, is considerably a major factor, but missing in campaigns, being this the reason that justifies that it doesn't hit the psychology of human beings (see chapter 1 of this book). They also highlight that human nature, beliefs, behaviors and attitudes could change only through interpersonal communication (see Chapters 1, 4 and 5 of this book). Additionally, the authors detect a gap of theories and models in the context of health communication (see chapters 2 and 3 of this book). Researchers also found while analyzing the data that there is a lack of qualitative and quantitative research (see Chapters 5, 6, 7 and 8 of this book, dedicated to an empirical version).

Living in an online advent, it is evident that digital technologies present "tremendous opportunities for the dissemination of health-related and rehabilitation information" (p. xxxii). Hu (2015) conducted a systematic review, examining research's patterns and trends related to the intersection between technology and health communication, determining possible gaps within the current body of literature, and providing future directions for researchers and practitioners. A sample of peer-reviewed journal articles (n = 348), published from 2008 to 2012, was coded in terms of research focus, health concern, technology, research method, and research agenda development. The most investigated topic were online health information, including search, dissemination, and evaluation, followed by telemedicine/electronic medical records, social support, provider-patient relationship, and health intervention. The less often issues studied were health literacy, technology access, public health emergency preparedness/response, and health policy advocacy. The most examined health concerns were cancer and mental health, followed by HIV/AIDS/STD, general nutrition, diet, exercise/obesity, physical disability, diabetes, and substance/alcohol/tobacco use. Some critical health issues, such as heart disease/stroke, were not highlighted (topic of the chapter 6 of this book). Among the six top global causes of death during 2019, there are cardiovascular diseases (ischaemic heart disease, stroke) and trachea, bronchus and lung cancers (WHO, 2020) – considering these data, we present two chapters (6 and 7) in our book devoted to media campaigns focused on preventing these diseases. The most discussed technology was the Web. Contrarily, the latest technologies, such as mobile phone and 3D virtual world/virtual reality/video game, didn't receive similar attention. In terms of the method used, studies with quantitative methods tripled those that were non-quantitative. Regarding the development of the research agenda, half of the articles concentrated on people's technological uses for health and health care, while one-quarter focused on the technologies' impact.

Knowledge is power. Aiming to provide its readers with knowledge (and thus with power), this book is intended for health professionals (e.g. doctors, nurses, pharmacists, therapists, psychologists), communication professionals, students from both areas, researchers seeking to develop closer, deeper and fruitful relationships between health and communication, whose need for deepening is increasingly evidenced in literature, and for all individuals who care, are interested in and/or cherish what defines them humanly, such as communication, and what provides them with balance, such as health.

ORGANIZATION OF THE BOOK

From the detection of problems and challenges, emerging research and opportunities, identified in the literature, we conceived the book that we present. The benefits of this publication can be: 1. to explore and analyze, theoretically, the fundaments, models, and dimensions of health communication, encompassing the interpersonal, group and media dimensions; 2. to offer practical solutions (checklists and flows) for better communication with direct outcomes in the optimization of citizens' health literacy; 3. to discuss and propose more effective health communication models and practices as a tool for construction of health outcomes more solid and evident.

The book is organized into two parts (theoretical vs. practical) and eight chapters, the first four focused on a theoretical reflection and basis, and the other four endowed with a practical configuration. A brief description of each of the chapters follows:

Being the starting point of the book, the Chapter 1 reviews and (re) constructs the substantive base of health communication, considering two main configurations: interpersonal and media one. It is a reflection and discussion based on the literature review on fundamentals and practices of health communication and on the contributions and implications of informative and persuasive messages and communication practices for health.

The Chapter 2 focuses on the origins of the communication models in health. These models reflect the different perspectives and contextual and environmental variables that influence health and that lead the paths for science to grow and become into structural bases that underlie reasons and justify events. Metaphorically, the theories are the river that allows the sailboat of communication to advance, regardless of the waters can be more or less calm or revolts. Once the theories of communication and health communication project values, actions, results, and ways of dealing with life, this chapter tries to do justice to this busy river, where the theories of health communication live, many disappearing in the foam of the times, and others have consolidated themselves as fortresses for other more robust paths.

The focus of the Chapter 3 is the health communication's models. We have come along the long path of communication since its origin and marking significant positions through the various models that have been thought and applied and that are directly or indirect associated with the universe of health. To fulfill the aim of promoting satisfactory results in health, the health communication and therapeutic relationship can be approached in several ways and based on different models. The literature revision conducted shows that models will be required if they are useful to those who apply them. The authors intend to show a pragmatic view of the models applied to health.

Chapter 4 focuses on the health professional's communication competences and the consequent assessment by patients who, with them, establish a therapeutic relationship. Based on a review of the literature and proposals for good practices to be implemented in health meetings, the chapter shows that a competent communication must pay attention to the verbal and non-verbal dimensions and the expectations of the patient.

Chapter 5 is centered in the specific health communication model - Assertiveness, Clarity and Positivity, called "ACP Model" -, that allows in an aggregated and interdependent way the use of communication competences in the therapeutic relationship. The research conducted is qualitative, based in nine focus groups, consisting of 55 participants, 25 specialists in health literacy and the remaining 30 with no previous knowledge of the ACP Model. The opinion of all participants is unanimous: the ACP Model increases the level of knowledge and understanding of the patient's health, thus promoting better health outcomes.

Chapter 6 makes an effort to provide responses, within the matter of cardiovascular health, to the effectiveness of the relation between the message's content ("what") and form ("how") and explores the cognitive-affective-behavioral effects derived from the message. It is used the mixed method:

the qualitative content analysis, concretely thematic and rhetorical types, was applied to a corpus of five ads from international campaigns (2015-2019) and of three static Portuguese ads (2018-2019); and one online survey to Portuguese university students (n = 55) was conducted.

Chapter 7 concentrates on cancer prevention media campaigns, specifically on the designing of the persuasive message. In terms of method, a qualitative technique is used (semiotic analysis), exploring the verbal and visual dimension of 19 international ads on the five most deadly cancers, in order to understand and deconstruct the message and the communication tactics adopted.

Chapter 8 focuses on the crisis communication motivated by the COVID-19 pandemic, that forced the world to a reflection and globalized intervention. Specifically, the focus is an analysis of the Word International Health (WHO)'s and Centers for Disease Control and Prevention's guidelines in developing countries. The communication crisis demanded the need to elaborate and disseminate a set of key rules and strong efforts between global health authorities (WHO and CDC) and local health authorities. The aim of these partnerships is to provide a robust set of intervention and communication solutions to monitor, address the pandemic and treat people. The key force was the group of health professionals, which followed vaccination.

Célia Belim
ISCSP, University of Lisbon, Portugal

Cristina Vaz de Almeida
ISCSP, University of Lisbon, Portugal

REFERENCES

Almeida, C. V. (2018). Literacia em saúde: Capacitação dos profissionais de saúde: O lado mais forte da balança. In *C. Lopes & C. V. Almeida (Coords.), Literacia em saúde: Modelos, estratégias e intervenção* (pp. 33–42). Edições ISPA.

Baker, D. W., Parker, R. M., Williams, M. V., Pitkin, K., Parikh, N. S., Coates, W., & Imara, M. (1996). The health care experience of patients with low literacy. *Archives of Family Medicine*, *5*(6), 329–334. doi:10.1001/archfami.5.6.329 PMID:8640322

Belim, C., & de Vaz de Almeida, C. (2018b). Communication competences are the key! A model of communication for the health professional to optimize the health literacy – Assertiveness, clear language and positivity. *Journal of Healthcare Communications*, *3*(31). Advance online publication. doi:10.4172/2472-1654.100141

Belim, C., & Vaz de Almeida, C. (2018). Healthy thanks to communication: A model of communication competences to optimize health literacy – Assertiveness, clear language, and positivity. In V. E. Papalois & M. Theodospoulou (Eds.), *Optimizing health literacy for improved clinical practices* (pp. 124–152). IGI Global. doi:10.4018/978-1-5225-4074-8.ch008

Blakar, R. M. (1979). Language as a means of social power theoretical-empirical explorations of language and language use as embedded in a social matrix. *Pragmalinguistics,* 131-169. doi:10.1515/9783110815689-007

Bol, N., Smit, E. S., & Lustria, M. L. A. (2020). Tailored health communication: Opportunities and challenges in the digital era. *Digital Health*, *6*, 1–3. doi:10.1177/2055207620958913 PMID:33029355

CENGAGE. (2019). *Health communication.* Available at: https://www.encyclopedia.com/media/encyclopedias-almanacs-transcripts-and-maps/health-communication

Dickens, D., Lambert, B., Cromwell, T., & Piano, M. (2013). Nurse overestimation of patients' health literacy. *Journal of Health Communication*, *18*(sup1), 62–69. doi:10.1080/10810730.2013.825670 PMID:24093346

Duffy, M. E., & Thorson, E. (2009). Emerging trends in the new media landscape. In J. Parker & E. Thorson (Eds.), *Health communication in the new media landscape* (pp. xxxi–xxxii). Springer Publishing Company, LLC.

Dutta, M. J. (2009). Health communication: Trends and future directions. In J. Parker & E. Thorson (Eds.), *Health communication in the new media landscape* (pp. 59–92). Springer Publishing Company, LLC.

Fielding, M. (2006). *Effective communication in organisations*. Juta & Co.

Finset, A. (2021). Challenges for healthcare communication during the COVID-19 pandemic. *Patient Education and Counseling*, *104*(2), 215–216. doi:10.1016/j.pec.2021.01.006 PMID:33518199

Ha, J. F., & Longnecker, N. (2010). Doctor-patient communication: A review. *The Ochsner Journal*, *10*, 38–43. PMID:21603354

Hicks, N. J. (2017). The growth of health communications: A story of consumer power and medical innovation. In N. J. Hicks & C. M. Nicols (Eds.), *Health industry communication: New media, new methods, new message* (pp. 3–20). Jones & Bartlett.

HLS-EU Consortium. (2012). Comparative report of health literacy in eight EU member states: The European health literacy survey HLS-EU (2nd ed.). Vienna: Ludwig Boltzmann Institute for Health Promotion Research.

Hu, Y. (2015). Health communication research in the digital age: A systematic review. *Journal of Communication in Healthcare*, *8*(4), 260–288. doi:10.1080/17538068.2015.1107308

Ishikawa, H., & Kiuchi, T. (2010). Health literacy and health communication. *BioPsychoSocial Medicine*, *4*(1), 1–5. doi:10.1186/1751-0759-4-18 PMID:21054840

Johnson, A. (2014). Health literacy, does it make a difference? *The Australian Journal of Advanced Nursing*, *31*(3), 39–45.

Kreps, G. L. (2012). Health communication inquiry and health outcomes. *Comunicação e Sociedade*, 11-22.

Kreps, G. L., & Bonaguro, E. (2009). Health communication as applied communication inquiry. In L. Frey & K. Cissna (Eds.), *The Handbook of Applied Communication Research* (pp. 970–993). Lawrence Erlbaum Associates, INC.

Levinson, W., Roter, D. L., Mullooly, J. P., Dull, V. T., & Frankel, R. M. (1997). Physician-patient communication: The relationship with malpractice claims among primary care physicians and surgeons. *Journal of the American Medical Association*, *277*(7), 553–559. doi:10.1001/jama.1997.03540310051034 PMID:9032162

Lloyd, J. E., Song, H. J., Dennis, S. M., Dunbar, N., Harris, E., & Harris, M. F. (2018). A paucity of strategies for developing health literate organisations: A systematic review. *PLoS One*, *13*(4), e0195018. doi:10.1371/journal.pone.0195018 PMID:29641544

Macabasco-O'Connell, A., & Fry-Bowers, E. K. (2011). Knowledge and perceptions of health literacy among nursing professionals. *Journal of Health Communication*, *16*(sup3, Suppl. 3), 295–307. doi:10.1080/10810730.2011.604389 PMID:21951259

Martin, L., Schonlau, M., Hass, A., Derose, K., Rosenfeld, L., Buka, S., & Rudd, R. (2011). Patient activation and advocacy: Which literacy skills mater most? *Journal of Health Communication, 16*(3), 177–190. doi:10.1080/10810730.2011.604705 PMID:21951251

McLeod, S. (2018). Communication rights: Fundamental human rights for all. *International Journal of Speech-Language Pathology, 20*(1), 3–11. doi:10.1080/17549507.2018.1428687 PMID:29466094

Munodawafa, D. (2008). Communication: Concepts, practice and challenges. *Health Education Research, 23*(3), 369–370. doi:10.1093/her/cyn024 PMID:18504296

Obregon, R., & Hickler, B. (2014). Opportunities and challenges for health communication in health disparities settings. *Journal of Communication in Healthcare, 7*(2), 77–79. doi:10.1179/1753806814Z.00000000074

Ong, L., de Haes, J. D., Hoos, A. M., & Lammes, F. B. (1995). Doctor-patient communication: A review of literature. *Social Science & Medicine, 40*(7), 903–918. doi:10.1016/0277-9536(94)00155-M PMID:7792630

Parikh, N., Parker, R., Nurss, J., Baker, D., & Williams, M. (1996). Shame and health literacy: The unspoken connection. *Patient Education and Counseling, 27*(1), 33–39. doi:10.1016/0738-3991(95)00787-3 PMID:8788747

Parker, J., & Thorson, E. (2009). Preface. In J. Parker & E. Thorson (Eds.), *Health communication in the new media landscape* (pp. 93–116). Springer Publishing Company, LLC.

Parker, J. C., Woelfel, R. L., Hart, E. S., & Brown, G. (2009). The challenge of health care and disability. In J. Parker & E. Thorson (Eds.), *Health communication in the new media landscape* (pp. 3–22). Springer Publishing Company, LLC.

Ranjan, P., Kumari, A., & Chakrawarty, A. (2015). How can doctors improve their communication skills? *Journal of Clinical and Diagnostic Research: JCDR, 9*(3), JE01–JE04. doi:10.7860/JCDR/2015/12072.5712 PMID:25954636

Ratzan, S. (1994). Health communication as negotiation. *The American Behavioral Scientist, 38*(2), 224–247. doi:10.1177/0002764294038002005

Ratzan, S. C., Sommariva, S., & Rauh, L. (2020). Enhancing global health communication during a crisis: Lessons from the COVID-19 pandemic. *Public Health Research & Practice*, *30*(2), e3022010. doi:10.17061/phrp3022010 PMID:32601655

Rimal, R. N., & Lapinski, M. K. (2009). Why health communication is important in public health. *Bulletin of the World Health Organization*, *87*(4), 247–248. doi:10.2471/BLT.08.056713 PMID:19551226

Rodrigues, R., Schulmann, K., & Ilinca, S. (2015). Challenges to public health communication campaigns in multinational settings: A European perspective. *European Journal of Public Health*, *25*(suppl_3). Advance online publication. doi:10.1093/eurpub/ckv170.028

Sharma, N., Nahak, F. M., & Kanozia, R. (2019). Identifying the gaps of health communication research: A systematic review. *Journal of Content. Community & Communication*, *10*(9), 122–140. doi:10.31620/JCCC.12.19/13

Shukla, A. K., Yadav, V. S., & Kastury, N. (2010). Doctor-patient communication: An important but often ignored aspect in clinical medicine. *JIACM*, *11*(3), 208–211.

Spitzberg, B. (2013). (Re)Introducing communication competence to the health professions. *Journal of Public Health Research*, *2*(3), e23. doi:10.4081/jphr.2013.e23 PMID:25170494

Stewart, M. A. (1995). Effective physician-patient communication and health outcomes: A review. *CMAJ: Canadian Medical Association Journal*, *152*(9), 1423–1433. PMID:7728691

Svalastog, A. L., Donev, D., Jahren Kristoffersen, N., & Gajović, S. (2017). Concepts and definitions of health and health-related values in the knowledge landscapes of the digital society. *Croatian Medical Journal*, *58*(6), 431–435. doi:10.3325/cmj.2017.58.431 PMID:29308835

Synnot, A., Bragge, P., Lowe, D., Nunn, J. S., O'Sullivan, M., Horvat, L., Tong, A., Kay, D., Ghersi, D., McDonald, S., Poole, N., Bourke, N., Lannin, N., Vadasz, D., Oliver, S., Carey, K., & Hill, S. J. (2018). Research priorities in health communication and participation: International survey of consumers and other stakeholders. *BMJ Open*, *8*(5), e019481. doi:10.1136/bmjopen-2017-019481 PMID:29739780

Tammelo, I. (1966). Analysis of human communication. *ARSP: Archiv Für Rechts-Und Sozialphilosophie / Archives for Philosophy of Law and Social Philosophy, 52*(4), 503-543. Available at: http://www.jstor.org/stable/23678286

Thomas, R. K. (2006). The history of health communication. In *Health Communication* (pp. 39–46). Springer.

Trenholm, S. (2001). *Thinking through communication: An introduction to the study of human communication.* Allyn and Bacon.

U.S. Department of Health and Human Services-HHS. (2000). *Healthy people 2010: Understanding and improving health.* U.S. Department of Health and Human Services.

U.S. Department of Health and Human Services-HHS. (2008). *America's health literacy: Why we need accessible health information.* Available at: https://www.aaaceus.com/courses/nl0610/article2.html

Vaz de Almeida, & Belim, C. (2019). Health literacy and health professionals: Open the door of communication for better outcomes. *Archives in Biomedical Engineering & Biotechnology*, 1-16.

Vaz de Almeida, C., & Belim, C. (2021). Health professional's communication competences as a light on the patient pathway: The assertiveness, clarity, and positivity (ACP) model. *International Journal of Applied Research on Public Health Management*, *6*(1).

Wakefield, M. A., Loken, B., & Hornik, R. C. (2010). Use of mass media campaigns to change health behaviour. *Lancet*, *376*(9748), 1261–1271. doi:10.10160140-6736(10)60809-4

Watzlawick, P., Beavin, J., & Jackson, D. D. (1967). *Pragmatics of human communication: A study of interactional patterns, pathologies and paradoxes.* W. W. Norton.

World Health Organization (WHO). (2020). *The top 10 causes of death.* Available at: https://www.who.int/news-room/fact-sheets/detail/the-top-10-causes-of-death

Chapter 1
To Be, or Not to Be Healthy: A Question of Communication!

Célia Belim
ISCSP, University of Lisbon, Portugal

ABSTRACT

This chapter, as the starting point of the book, (re)constructs the substantive setting and puzzle of health communication, being a reflection and discussion based on the literature review on fundamentals and practices of health communication and the contributions and implications of informative and persuasive messages and communication practices to health. The literature review results show the essential role that communication has assumed in the context of health, having several positive effects, such as the treatment effectiveness, the improvement of the therapeutic relationship and health literacy, the penetration of certain health issues in the public agenda. It has also highlighted the need to strengthen and rethink, in the name of individual and social well-being, the relationship between health and communication. Particularly, in the therapeutic relationship, the need for the health professional to have adequate communication competences to interact with patients is emphasized. Additionally, the media prove to be a versatile tool in the achievement of health promotion aims.

DOI: 10.4018/978-1-7998-4396-2.ch001

INTRODUCTION

Communication "keep us healthy" (Floyd, 2011, p. 4) and has been described as an art and a science (Perkins, 2010), a key (Belim & Almeida, 2018), power (Sugai, Deptula, Parsa & Parsa, 2013), a solution or panacea (Samuel, 2016) for health. The literature is consensual on the contribution of health communication. It has been reported the need for communication to improve health outcomes and to promote well-being. For example, health communication, when delivered effectively in mass-mediated contexts, "has considerable potential to promote the health" (Ahmed & Bates, 2013, p. 4) and to shape general understandings (p. 3).

The role of communication is also highlighted by physicians from the earliest stages in their training in medical school (Sugai et al., 2013). There is an art behind delivering information to patients and this topic has been reported on extensively in the literature. For example, the importance of patient communication in surgery is "paramount" and is not only a means of educating the patient, but it is also a way of preserving a patient's well-being after a surgical procedure (Sugai et al., 2013). Mazor et al. (2012) discover that, of the 93 patients who experienced problems with their cancer treatment, 44 (47%) reported communication breakdowns, including fundamental problems in information sharing, emotional support, and care coordination. The authors postulate that effective communication between patients and clinicians can prevent lapses in quality and, when problems occur, can mitigate harm and restore trust.

On the other hand, although the mechanisms of media effectiveness are not entirely understood, "the media play a vital role in assuring the health of the public in the twenty-first century" (Institute of Medicine US Committee on Assuring the Health of the Public in the 21st Century, 2002). Snyder (2001), in a series of meta-analyses, observes that media messages about health can create about 8% of the behavior change. Studies have shown that media effectiveness depends, among other factors, on the health objective to be achieved. Media communication creates more change when promotes the adoption of new behavior (prevention of HIV-AIDS) than when attempts to change addictive behaviors (tobacco or alcohol use). Flynn et al. (1992, 1994) discover that media campaigns, combined with other strategies such as school smoking prevention programs, are effective in changing behavior.

Ahmed and Bates (2013) argue that these mass-mediated messages are more likely to be successful in affecting health knowledge, attitudes, behavior, practice, and policy if they include and absorb the health communication theory (p. 4). In this context, this chapter attempts to compile and discuss insights and inputs from the literature review on the contribution of health communication, considering the two main configurations of health communication and different levels of communication strategies, and to (re)construct, based on literature review, the substantive setting and puzzle and some fundamentals or principles and practices of the health communication.

"THE FIRST WEALTH IS HEALTH"

The American philosopher Ralph Waldo Emerson wrote in 1860 that "the first wealth is health", reminding that "good health is the foundation on which to build – a life, a community, an economy" (Hayden, 2014). Good health is the desire of every human, depending on his/her ability to live a positive lifestyle. But it is difficult to be attained absolutely as human needs cannot be completely satisfied at any given time.

Arthur Schopenhauer also captured perfectly a deeply felt human need when he wrote that "health is not everything, but without health everything is nothing". This assumption is following the argumentation of Stiglitz, Sen, and Fitoussi (2009) that health is probably the most fundamental aspect of quality of life since without health all other components of quality of life have little value (pp. 156-157). Discussing this causality, there is a vast literature revealing the nefarious consequences for the individual derived from negative health shocks.

Cieza et al. (2016) clarify that it is a mistake to adopt the Banks et al. (2006) understanding of health merely as the absence of disease, once health needs to be measured as a factor of functioning in a parsimonious set of domains that matches the intuitive notion of health (p. 586). Brüssow (2013) explains that the preferred view on health was the ability to adapt and to self-manage (p. 343). Regarding physical health, the term "allostasis" was introduced – the maintenance of physiological homeostasis through changing circumstances. In the field of mental health, a sense of coherence was identified as defining criterion. Social health refers to people's capacity to accomplish their potentials and obligations, the ability to manage their lives, and to participate in social activities including professional ones (Brüssow, 2013, p. 343).

WE ARE COMMUNICATION

Communication defines what we are as humans, being at the heart of the human identity (Rimal & Lapinski, 2009, p. 247). Communication is, simultaneously, a way of exchanging information and a symbolic capability (Rimal & Lapinski, 2009, p. 247). In Carey's words are, respectively, the transmission and ritual forms of communication. As Carey (2008) explains: "a fully developed understanding of communication involved both a ritual and a transmission view and that for a modern society to exist both forms of communication would be at play" (p. xviii).

Rimal and Lapinski (2009) explain that this dual view of communication conduces to three intervention considerations: (1) the realization that communication interventions do not fall into a social vacuum; (2) like Hall (1980) identified and named as "oppositional code or reading" (p. 127), it is reasonable to expect discrepancies between messages disseminated and received; (3) communication is a dynamic process in which sources and receivers of information continuously interchange their roles. Effective communication happens when the message that is sent is the same message that is received (Erozkan, 2013, p. 742).

Communication defines the human essence to a point that we can say that the Man is "a communicational animal", apprehending the evidence that "communication is all we have" and "it is what makes us human" (Macnamara, 2017). Communication is the cornerstone of the interaction with people (Erozkan, 2013, p. 739) and refers to a set of strategies and actions to enhance reciprocity, mutual understanding, and decision-making (Edelman & Mandle, 2010, p. 96).

FROM COMMUNICATION TO HEALTH COMMUNICATION

Health communication "is at the heart of health care and health promotion" (Gully, 2009, p. xxvii). Gully (2009), agreeing with Kurtz, Silverman, and Draper (2004), refers that communication can significantly improve patient's health outcomes, where effective communication makes a difference in their health (p. 26).

There is no consensus on the specific temporal genesis of health communication studies. Thompson (2003) and Harrington (2015) mention that health communication became, in 1975 at the annual conference of the International Communication Association (ICA), a sub-discipline of communication. However, Thompson (2003) argues that studies on health communication began before 1975 (p. 1). Blatt, Spinazzi, and Greenberg (2014) place, from the 60s and 70s, the greatest attention of communication to clinical care between doctor and patient (p. 295).

Health communication has been defined – and it is tending to be a consensual definition – as the study and use of communication strategies to inform, influence, and motivate individuals, institutions, and communities in making effective decisions to improve health and enhance the quality of life (e.g., U.S. Department of Health and Human Services, 2005, Wallington, 2014, p. 169). It is the study and practice of communicating health content such as in health education, public health campaigns, and in the therapeutic relationship between health professional and patient (National Communication Association, 2013).

Cline (2003) understands health communication as a theoretical-practical area that pays special attention to the relationship between communication and health, health attitudes, beliefs, and behaviors (p. 285). By optimizing the understanding of health information that circulates in various media and forms of language, whether interpersonal, verbal, auditory, or digital, the population health and disease prevention is improved (Almeida, 2014, p. 155). Harrington (2015), in this sense, emphasizes that health communication plays a key role in preventing disease and premature death, increasing longevity (p. 2).

Health communication is a subset of a much larger communication science discipline and has an interdisciplinary matrix, growing from diverse roots in sociology, psychology, anthropology, political science, electrical engineering, cybernetics, and, more recently, neuroscience (Storey et al., 2014, p. S241).

It is gaining consistency with the assumption that health communication can become far more effective in the digital world (Thorson & Duffy, 2009, p. 438), reinventing the way of communicating health. For example, two surveys confirm the role of social media platforms for transplant health care professionals: 1. in a survey with a sample of 299 American Society of Transplant Surgeons (ASTS) members, most of the respondents reported that social media is influential in increasing awareness of deceased organ donation and increasing living organ donation, despite most reported that their transplant center does not do social media outreach (Henderson et al., 2018). According to Henderson et al. (2018), social media participation is promising, due to may offer transplant surgeons and other transplant professionals the opportunity to leverage social media to deliver high-quality information to patients and potential donors (p. 15); 2. in the online survey distributed through the European Society for Organs Transplantation's social media tools, transplant professionals recognize the role of social media platforms in promoting organ donation, sharing information, and providing knowledge for trainees of for research purposes (Bellini, Parisotto, Dor & Kessaris, 2020). Additionally, Belim (2020), analyzing the potential of digital media for benefiting rare diseases, observes that "knowledge is power". This is justified due to digital media can be used in modes (e.g., rhetorically, in terms of the type of content) that can aware and offer accurate and reliable information to individuals with rare diseases and their families who can better decide.

Two Main Configurations of Health Communication

In practice, health communication can assume the interpersonal configuration, as in the therapeutic relationship, and the media configuration, with the communication campaigns. So, the research of health communication anchors on messages about health, the dissemination of health-related information through broadcast, print, and electronic media, and the role of interpersonal relationships in health communities. Health communication includes messages, which can serve several purposes, such as: to promote health and to educate for health; to avoid risks and to help to deal with health threats, to prevent diseases; to suggest and recommend behavior changes; to recommend screening examinations; to report on health and disease; to report medical examinations; to prescript medicines; to recommend preventive measures and self-care activities in individuals (Alves, 2011, Benson, 2014, Bittner, Jonietz, Beickert & Harendza, 2015, Cegala, 2011, Hargie, 2011, Teixeira, 2004, Viswanath, 2006).

Communication demands competences to fulfill objectives. Communication competence can be understood as a complex construct that has been vastly debated (Allen, 2017). McCroskey (1982) inaugurated this debate in the early 1980s when he discussed competence in terms of skills, performance, and effectiveness. This discussion, then, inspired Spitzberg (2003) to propose a precise definition, clarifying that communication competence entails three interdependent constructs: knowledge, skill, and motivation. In other words, communication competence refers to an individual's knowledge, skill, and motivation to accomplish a concrete aim. There is a pattern constituting about how skills (know how to do), knowledge (know), and, additionally, personal attributes (know how to be) lead to broader competencies (Tench & Moreno, 2015, p. 43). Gregory (2008) explains that competencies are how knowledge and skills are used in performance (p. 216). To a complete version, personal attributes should be included (Tench et al., 2013, p. 17; Tench & Moreno, 2015, p. 44).

Contributions and Implications of Communication Fundamentals and Practices for Health

Health communication has much to celebrate and contribute (Rimal & Lapinski, 2009, p. 247). Communication alone can: increase the intended audience's knowledge and awareness of a health issue, problem, or solution; influence perceptions, beliefs, and attitudes that may change social norms; prompt action; demonstrate or illustrate healthy skills; reinforce knowledge, attitudes, or behavior; show the benefit of behavior change; advocate a position on a health issue or policy; increase demand or support for health services; and refute myths and misconceptions (U.S. Department of Health and Human Services, 2005, p. 3).

However, some barriers difficult the efficiency of health communication, such as: low health literacy, poor communication links, poor research (Nkanunye & Obiechina, 2017), the wrong person sending messages, lack of receivers, unclear messages, inappropriate channel, inadequate feedback, and noise distorting the message (Achalu, 2008), anxiety, attitudes, gaps between sender and receiver, resistance, transference and countertransference, sensory barriers, failure to address concerns or needs (Edelman & Mandle, 2010, pp. 107-109)

Informative and persuasive campaigns can use a panoply of media and tools to aware the public of a healthy lifestyle and the benefits of adopting or changing behaviors that can optimize the quality of life. Designing health campaigns demands consistency simultaneously in substance and form (e.g., aesthetic appearance, linguistic style, tone) and there is no single strategic communication response to health-related challenges (Servaes & Malikhao, 2010, p. 43).

Noar, Benac, and Harris (2007) explain that, despite the large and growing literature on tailored print health behavior change interventions, there is no confirmation if or to what extent tailoring works. The authors, through a meta-analytic review of literature, including 57 studies, reveal that tailored messages within these intervention studies have outperformed comparison (e.g., generic/targeted) messages and even further outperformed no-treatment control conditions (p. 681).

To achieve long-term aims of health for people, five levels of communication strategies for health behavior can be included in health communication planning and implementation (Servaes, 2007b, 2008; Servaes & Liu, 2007) (Table 1).

Table 1. Levels of communication strategies for health behavior

Health communication strategies	Specificities
Behavior change communication (BCC)	mainly interpersonal communication
Mass communication (MC)	community media, mass media, and information and communication technologies (ICT)
Advocacy communication (AC)	interpersonal and/or mass communication
Participatory communication (PC)	interpersonal communication and community media
Communication for structural and sustainable social change (CSSC)	interpersonal communication, participatory communication, and mass communication

Source: *(Servaes, 2007b, 2008; Servaes & Liu, 2007)*

Nkanunye and Obiechina (2017) identify as health communication strategies: a) traditional and rural-based communication (e.g., town crier, age-grade meetings). A town crier is a significant village "broadcaster" who summons villagers or decision makers on discussing community problems. An "age grade meeting" consists of organizing various groups, in different days/ months, in meetings and represents an avenue for health educators; b) media (e.g., radio, television, newspapers, posters/billboards, internet/social media): Broadcast media can capture a wide audience within a defined time frame.

The search for the ingredients that define effective health communication has been a challenge for researchers and health actors. Martin and DiMatteo (2014) explain that communication is the key to achieving health behavior change, treatment adherence, and patients' motivation, but only on the condition that there is a clear understanding of patients' life circumstances, concerns, ideals, and goals (pp. 3-4).

Persuasive messages tend to use a basic expectancy-value mechanism to influence beliefs related to the subjective likelihood of various outcomes occurring. The operational formula for preventing risky behaviors is susceptibility multiplied by severity, using a loss frame to motivate the public with a high likelihood of suffering painful effects (Atkin & Rice, 2013, p. 9). Atkin and Rice (2013) explain that incentive appeals often build on the existing values of the target public, so the message tends to reinforce the predispositions (p. 9).

Nabi (2014), centered on the emotional dimension of the message (*pathos*), refers that fear, guilt, and humor are the emotional appeals that have received the most attention (p. 115). Contrary and arguing a solution focused on *logos* (logic), Haines and Rogers (2001, p. 164) and O'Keefe (2014) highlight that the strength of evidence for specific recommendations should be explicit.

In a medical context, Haines and Rogers (2001) refer that some available checklists, endowed with scientific validity, can help clinicians. There are three criteria for a good guideline (Haines & Rogers, 2001): 1) the important options and outcomes in the decision process are considered and the evidence on which the guideline is drawn is gathered in an explicit and systematic form; 2) the relative values of different outcomes are considered and the guidelines are regularly updated; 3. the guidelines should be peer-reviewed and piloted to ensure that they are pertinent and appropriate to the clinical setting and the patient group (p. 164). O'Keefe (2014) notes that decisions to adopt specific message strategies for use in persuasive health interventions should be evidence-based, just as evidence-based medicine informs health screening and treatment decisions. For example, in deciding to adopt a narrative or a statistical approach, the campaigner should look for evidence in the literature for which will be more effective in influencing attitude, intention, or behavior change.

In instituting change within practices in response to research-based information, some variables have to be under attention, such as (Haines & Rogers, 2001): the nature of the message, what processes in the practice need to be changed, the key players who can promote or retard change, the obstacles and levers for change, the concrete interventions that can promote change, and how change can be monitored (p. 163). Regarding the message and its presentation, some aspects have to be considered, such as the scope and content, the scientific (internal) validity (the message's scientific basis), generalizability and applicability (external validity), target audience, channels for dissemination, format, and presentation (e.g., the clarification of the nature of the message), mechanisms for updating.

An influential message should have some appeal, such as (Atkin & Rice, 2013, p. 9): 1. Credibility, by exposing the trustworthiness and competence of the source and convincing evidence; 2. The engaging manner of presenting style and ideas via a combination between arousing substance and attractive stylistic execution; 3. The personally involving and relevant selection of content and style, so receivers regard the behavioral recommendation as applicable to their situation and needs; 4. Understandability in the sense that the presentation of content should be simple, explicit, and detailed and consequently comprehensive and comprehensible to receivers; 5. The motivational incentives of the message, that are the gratifications the recipients can get by complying with health recommendations.

Health communicators can use a wide range of "multiple methods" of influence, such as media literacy, media advocacy, public relations, advertising, education entertainment, individual and group instruction, and partnership development (U.S. Department of Health and Human Services, 2005, p. 4).

So, the research on health communication brings implications related to the identification and provision of better and more effective communication strategies that will improve the overall health of society (Stacks & Salween, 2009, p. 489).

Interpersonal Communication

Interpersonal communication matters in a relationship because it is contributing to relational and health improvement (Floyd, 2011). The quality of interpersonal communication depends on interpersonal competence, which is the ability to deal effectively with interhuman relationships, with interlocutors, in a manner that suits their situational needs and demands (Moscovici, 1981, p. 17). Moscovici (1981) distinguishes three components of interpersonal competence (pp. 17-18):

a) the perception that has to be trained for an accurate view of the interpersonal situation, requiring a long process of personal growth, encompassing simultaneously self-perception, self-awareness, and self-acceptance;
b) competences components, such as the perceptual and behavioral flexibility ability, which means being able to see multiple angles of the same situation and act differently, the creative ability to find more original and rewarding solutions, the ability to give and receive feedback, building an I-you and not an I-this meeting;
c) the emotional-affective component, which must be balanced with the cognitive one.

Some criteria can be gathered to better perform interpersonal communication competences (Table 2).

Table 2. Criteria to better perform interpersonal communication competences

Criteria	Description
Dialogue	It is defined by characteristics, such as "coordination (or cooperation), coherence, reciprocity, and mutuality (e.g., concerning moral commitments)" (Linell, 1998, p. 14), empathy, confirmation, relaxed readiness, perspective reflection, meta-communication, congruence, humor, present orientation, genuineness, and egalitarianism (Kristiansen & Bloch-Poulson, 2000; Pearce & Pearce, 2000)
Clarity	It is one of the most intuitive or lay notions of competence
Understanding	Independent of the mode of expression, to what extent do interlocutors comprehend each others' intended meanings?
Efficiency	Refers to the notion that accomplishing a goal can involve less or more effortful and resource-intensive activities, being typified by statements such as "Well why didn't you just say so in the first place?" and "Why are you beating around the bush?"
Satisfaction	It is the accomplishment of the preferred outcomes through interaction, linked to the experience of a sense of positive affect. It is typified by statements such as: "I enjoyed talking with you" and "How do you feel about your consultation?"
Effectiveness	It is the extent to which preferred outcomes are achieved
Appropriateness	It is the extent to which behavior meets the standards of legitimacy or acceptability in a context

Source: *(Spitzberg, 2003)*

Kemp, Ball, Jason, Appel, and Fitzroy (2019)'s study of the processes surrounding Assisted Living (AL) residents' health status changes in the context of communication identifies four basic and interrelated processes that comprise a model of communicative competence: identifying change; assessing the significance of the change; responding to change; and communication, consisting of informing, consulting, and collaborating regarding the change (p. 9).

Each therapeutic encounter encompasses verbal communication and nonverbal communication (Table 3). Nonverbal communication, seeming to have a certain primacy over the verbal content (Mast & Cousin, 2014, p. 39), is commonly defined as communication behavior without linguistic content (Knapp & Hall, 2010), often interacting with verbal behavior, once it has potential to stress, complement, substitute, repeat, regulate or contradict verbal behavior (Mast & Cousin, 2014, p. 39). But research shows that 65% of interpersonal communication is nonverbal and that, when verbal messages contradict nonverbal ones, adults usually believe the nonverbal messages over the verbal ones (Burgoon, Guerrero & Floyd, 2016, p. 3).

The significance of nonverbal communication can be best captured by the axiom "actions speak louder than words" (Edelman & Mandle, p. 99). Several possible arguments justify the force of influence of nonverbal communication (Burgoon, Guerrero & Floyd, 2016, pp. 3-9): a) is omnipresent as nonverbal facets pervade virtually every communicative act; b) is multifunctional, assuming different functions, such as create a favorable first impression, persuade; c) may form a universal language system once it tends to be transnationally understood; d) can lead to misunderstanding as well as understanding; e) has phylogenetic primacy once predated language in the evaluation of human communication; f) has ontogenetic primacy once the first manifestation of language in a human being is nonverbal; g) has interaction primacy once before people even open their mouths, their nonverbal behaviors are supplying an informative wealth to onlookers; h) can express what verbal communication can't or shouldn't, and i) is trusted considering the naïve belief that nonverbal behaviors are the "windows to the soul".

Table 3. Composition of nonverbal communication

Component of nonverbal communication	Manifestation
Face	smiling, gazing, frowning, eyebrow-raising facial expressivity
Body / kinesics	posture, like arm and leg positions (crossed versus uncrossed) body orientation (toward the interaction partner or not) interpersonal distance emblematic gestures (e.g., thumb up), illustrative gestures (e.g., indicate the size of an object) regulating gestures that coordinate the verbal exchange (e.g., to slightly open one's mouth and lean forward to manifest one's intention to speak) adaptive gestures that satisfy a personal need (e.g., scratching oneself to relieve a sensation of itching) emotional gestures (e.g., to clench one's first when expressing hostility)
Voice	loudness voice pitch (low versus high) monotony (versus variations) speech rate
Physical appearance	clothes hair shoe makeup adornments
Touch/haptics	Hetero (affability, care) and self-touch (nervousness, serenity)
Timing / chronemics	Relation to time: punctuality, that can reveal a commitment to exactitude

Source: *(Burgoon, Guerrero & Floyd, 2016, p. 3, 19; Mast & Cousin, 2014, p. 39)*

Mechanic and Meyer (2000) note, through semi-structured interviews with 90 U.S. patients with serious illness from New Jersey, that interpersonal competence focused on listening carefully and providing responsive feedback, minimizing interruptions, maintaining eye contact, conveying an understanding of patients' distress and vulnerabilities are behaviors valued by patients and skills that can be teachable (p. 667).

Good and effective communication helps interactants understand each other and brings them closer to each other (Markides, 2011, p. S123). In the health field, good communication helps health professionals identify the patients' needs and the modern perspective assumes that the two actors need to work together as a team (p. S123). The quality of the relationship can be therapeutic for the patient and, in this relation, trust and listening are a key of quality. Trust is not something that can be bought but is gained, demanding that before trusting there must be respect. Listening means not interrupting neither command, warn or judge. It implies emphatically trying to understand the discourse of the patient and using open-ended questions, to learn about the experience of illness by the patient but also about the patient as an individual (p. S124). Additionally, practitioners who enhance how they express empathy and create positive expectations of benefit can improve patient outcomes (Howick et al., 2018, p. 1). Table 4 gathers communication practices that should be adopted in health interpersonal relations.

The therapeutic encounter has been changed by significant digital developments (Eckler, Worsowicz & Downey, 2009). Research has shown that the complexities related to this type of encounter have been mitigated by new media interventions, like e-mail, telemedicine, online health information, wireless handheld devices like PDAs and cell phones, blogs, and laptops (Eckler, Worsowicz & Downey, 2009).

Mass Media Communication

Much of the publics' comprehension of health and health policy is not derived from direct experience (Ahmed & Bates, 2013, p. 3). One evidence is that most of the human understanding is mediated. So, media channels affect the health care system and individuals' use of that system (Friedman, 2004) and media representations of health and illness shape our understanding of the experiences related to health issues (Seale, 2002, 2004). Media "can be a delivery mechanism for getting the right information to the right people in the right way at the right time to promote personal change" (Wallack, 2000,

p. 338) and can be a vehicle for promoting social change (p. 338), often demanded in the health field.

Table 4. Practices associated with interpersonal health communication

a) Permit people to tell their stories in their own words and chronology
b) Use a conversational interviewing style
c) Be friendly through humor and social, conversational, and nonverbal cues, such as smiling
d) Elicit patients' views, perspectives, thoughts, wishes, goals, values, and expectations
e) Inquire about the nature of the patient's life
f) Attend to the person's needs
g) Avoid overemphasis on technical aspects of care and tasks
h) Not be too busy to talk
i) Respond to cues concerning emotional issues and problems
j) Give information about self-care and participation in decision-making
k) Develop mutual understanding
l) Create collaborative health care plans
m) Show empathy and concern for the individual's well-being
n) Connect with individuals through humor, touch, and selective self-discourse
o) Turn into the individual's preferences and style
p) Attend to and advocate for individuals' needs
q) Maintain confidentiality
r) Focus on the clinical discussion on the person's story rather than a version reformulated by the provider (e.g., use open-ended questions)
s) Attend to the process that represents the clinical encounter: respect, preparation, listen first, the "story", progressive dialogue, and review and summation – inform, teach-back, support, and comfort
t) Consider the steps to functional communication: firmly state the case, clarify the message, seek feedback, and be receptive to feedback when it is received
u) Adopt the characteristics associated with therapeutic effectiveness: self-awareness and self-reflection, openness, self-confidence and strength, genuineness, concern for the individual, respect for the individual, knowledge, ability to empathize, sensitivity, acceptance, creativity, ability to focus and comfort
w) Practice a supported communication concentrated on rapport, trust, empathy, goal direction, and ethics
v) Maintain eye contact

Source: *(Edelman & Mandle, 2010, p. 98; Harner, 2011; McCabe, 2004; Moyle, 2003; Welch, 2005)*

There is ample agreement that awareness leads to knowledge, and knowledge leads to behavior modification (Rimal, 2000, p. 232). Various theories and models acknowledge the contributions of the mass media in creating awareness in society. The agenda-setting theory (McCombs & Shaw, 1972), that preconizes that the media can tell audiences what issues are major and relevant, thus setting the agenda, is one example. The media can achieve this by choosing what stories to consider newsworthy and how much prominence and space they give those stories (Folarin, 1998). In other words, this theory explains that the mass media through their presentations of event(s) and other kinds of information selected for public dissemination ascribe prominence to the stories selected. The underlying assumption is that the mass media attract attention to certain issues: they build up public images of issues, they constantly present objects, suggest what the audience should think about, know about, have feelings about, agitate about, and eventually call for legislation about (Anaeto, Onabajo & Osifeso, 2008; Folarin, 1998; McCombs & Shaw, 1972). In sum, the mass media influence pre-determine issues that people should be aware of in society.

The precaution adoption model (Weinstein & Sandman, 1992) also recognizes that the media plays a pivotal role in disseminating information and raising awareness. According to this model, awareness is an essential component that moves an individual in various stages. For example, stage one stresses when an individual becomes aware of a health issue – "aware of the issue, but not personally engaged"; stage two focuses on when an individual decides to act or not to act – "engaged and deciding what to do". In stages three and four, the individual either acts or does not (Weinstein & Sandman, 1992). The mass media not only informs individuals about health issues but its message can also be used to influence individuals to action. The diffusion of innovation theory (Rogers, 2003) advocates that the mass media can be a crucial component in influencing beliefs and attitudes that will eventually lead to a behavior. Four elements influence the spread of a new idea: the innovation itself, communication channels, time, and social system.

Similarly, one of the major constructs of the health belief model is the cue to action that helps trigger a particular behavior. A cue to action is something that helps move someone from wanting to make a healthy change to make the change. These cues to action range from bodily events to environmental factors that stimulate an individual to act. The health belief model recognizes media campaigns and promotion as one of the effective environmental cues to action (Janz, Champion & Strecher, 2002).

In fact, the mass media can prove to be a versatile tool, assuming certain contributions (Corcoran, 2013, pp. 76-77): 1. Achieve wide coverage; 2. Impact on behaviors receptive to change; 3. Convey simple information; 4. Increase knowledge; 5. Put health on the public agenda.

Mass media can operate through direct or indirect routes to change the health behavior of the population. Many media campaigns are intended to directly influence the public instigating cognitive or emotional responses, but behavioral change might be concretized by the indirect pathway (Wakefield, Loken & Hornik, 2010, p. 1262).

Snyder et al. (2004) performed a meta-analysis of studies of mediated health campaigns in the United States of America (USA), to examine the effects of the campaigns on behavior change. The authors observe that mediated health campaigns have small measurable effects in the short-term, that the type of behavior that is intended (e.g., cessation of old behavior, prevention of a new undesirable behavior) influence campaign effect sizes, and that campaigns with an enforcement component are more effective than those without.

Wakefield, Loken, and Hornik (2010) identify the benefits for the mass media option (p. 1262): a) mass media messages can define an agenda for and increase the frequency, depth, or both, of interpersonal discussion on a specific health issue within an individual's social network, which, in combination with individual exposure to messages, might reinforce (or undermine) specific behavioral changes; b) once mass media messages reach ample audiences, behavioral changes, that become norms within an individual's social network, might influence that person's decisions without them having been directly exposed to or initially persuaded by the campaign; c) mass media campaigns can prompt public discussion of health issues and lead to changes in public policy, resulting in constraints on individuals' behavior and, thereby, changes.

Interventions, using mass media campaigns, are usually aimed at influencing the secular or the normal trend in the amount of information available on a given topic in a system. The influence may take two forms: a) an attempt to increase the amount of available information on the topic of interest; b) an effort to redefine or frame the issue as a public health problem to make it salient, attract the attention of the target audience, and suggest a solution to resolve that problem (Randolph & Viswanath, 2004, p. 420).

Some conditions can influence a successful campaign (Table 5).

Table 5. Conditions influencing a successful campaign

Conditions	Description
Manipulation of the informative environment	by campaign sponsors to ensure sufficient exposure of the audience to the campaign messages and themes (e.g., attention to the amount of available information on the health issue)
Use of social marketing tools: creative marketing, messages, and message effects	to create the appropriate messages for distribution and, where possible, message theory and tailoring; careful attention to the messages; use of message effects theories to design messages and of fear appeals; consideration of effects of message framing and ethnic targeting; the combination of media campaigns and other strategies, such as community-based programs
Creation of concomitant structural conditions / Supportive environment	opportunity structure that allows the target audience to make the recommended change
Clear and complete understanding of the determinants of health behavior	this type of understanding can potentially lead to desired health outcomes (theory-based campaigns)
Process analysis and exposure assessment	can serve as useful intermediate markers, both in making the midcourse correction and in explaining final campaign outcomes

Source: *(Randolph & Viswanath, 2004)*

Effective health communication has to accomplish some criteria when constructing the contents that will be disseminated (Healthy People 2010), for example, within a campaign: a) accuracy: the content is valid and without errors of fact, interpretation, or judgment; b) availability: the content is delivered or placed where the audience can access it. Placement varies according to the audience, message complexity, and purpose; c) balance: where adequate, the content refers the benefits and risks of potential actions or recognizes different and valid perspectives on the health issue; d) consistency: the content remains internally coherent over time and also with information from other sources; e) cultural competence: the design, implementation, and evaluation process that focuses on special questions targeting special population groups has to consider the cultural dimension of these groups (e.g., ethnic, linguistic, educational, and disability traits); f) evidence-based: the content concentrates on scientific evidence and demands rigorous analysis to formulate practice guidelines; g) reach: the content is available to the amplest possible number of people in the target publics; h) reliability: the source of the content is credible, and the content itself is kept up to date; i) repetition: the delivery of/ access to the content is continued or repeated over time, both to reinforce the impact with a specific audience and to reach new generations; j) timeliness: the content is provided when the publics are more receptive to, or in need of, the concrete information; and k) understandability: the content considers the health literacy of the target publics.

Advocacy Strategies

Advocacy can be understood as the process of speaking out for something, such as a cause or a policy (WHO, 2004, p. 2), an action directed at changing the policies, positions, or programs of any type of institution or is putting a problem on the agenda, providing a solution to that problem, and building support for acting on both the problem and solution (Sharma, 1997).

As a "powerful health communication strategy", media advocacy performs a pivotal role in engaging people in dialogue about health promotion and disease prevention, facilitating community organizing to generate demand or support for health services, and potentially influencing policy-making on critical public health issues (Ahmed & Bates, 2013, p. 4). Generally, these efforts are likely to be grounded in communication theories from the realm of rhetoric, public relations, and agenda-setting (Ahmed & Bates, 2013, p. 5).

Cullerton, Donnet, Lee, and Gallegos (2018) suggest a range of strategies available that can increase the influence of advocates in the policy process: a) invest in relationships strategically; b) develop a clear, unified solution; c) employ or develop the skills of a policy entrepreneur; d) secure a policy champion; e) reframe the issue to appeal to values and beliefs; f) amplify the frame, and g) increase public will (pp. 6-9).

The choice of advocacy strategies will vary with the nature of the issue or characteristics of policy problems (interdependence, subjectivity, artificiality, dynamics of policy problems) and the expectation of the people or the stakeholders (Servaes & Malikhao, 2010, p. 43) (Table 6).

Table 6. Communication instruments adjusted to policy life-cycle phases

Policy life-cycle phase	Communication instruments
Identifying the public health problem	Regular opinion/attitude surveys (Mass) Media content analysis Analysis of communication materials (newsletters, leaflets, websites) of non-governmental organization (NGO)'s, consumer groups, etc. Systematic and continuous network (both in real and virtual spaces) with NGO's, interest groups, scientific institutions Regular briefings/interviews and meetings with interest and lobby groups
Understanding the public health problem	Knowledge/attitude/practice (KAP) surveys Integrating communication in the mix of policy instruments Design of health communication strategy Informative extension/communication (to disclose issues and policy options) to those who will get involved
Solving the public health problem	Communication as an independent instrument Communication complementary to other instruments Informing groups on the use of other instruments (e.g., new laws, subsidies) Ex-ante evaluation through qualitative research
Controlling the public health problem	Public information Informing on changes of policy design and implementation Regular opinion/attitude surveys (since age-linked target groups will be replaced slowly by younger generations)

Source: *(Servaes & Malikhao, 2010, p. 43, Winsemius, 1986)*

CONCLUSION

There is a consensus in the literature review on the importance of communication for health: communication is endowed with the power to optimize health outcomes and individual and collective well-being. Health communication has two main configurations – interpersonal and media ones –, that preconize assumptions that orient the best forms of performance.

The optimization of results depends on communication that absorbs and reflects evidences and theoretical basis and that takes advantage of the confluence of previously tested and confirmed teachings. It can be said that "the first wealth is health" and that the first wealth of health is communication, because "we are communication". Therefore, understanding the essence, functionality, and impact of communication can enhance the effect of the medication and can be the key to health promotion and disease prevention.

REFERENCES

Achalu, E. I. (2008). *Communication skills in Health Education and Public Health: Methods & Resources*. Port Harcourt: Pam unique.

Ahmed, R., & Bates, B. R. (2013). Communicating health through mass media: An overview. In R. Ahmed & B. R. Bates (Eds.), *Health communicating and mass media: An integrated approach to policy and practice* (pp. 3–18). Routledge.

Ahmed, R., & Bates, B. R. (Eds.). (2013). *Health communication and mass media: An integrated approach to policy and practice*. Gower.

Allen, M. (Ed.). (2017). *The SAGE encyclopedia of communication research methods*. Sage. doi:10.4135/9781483381411

Almeida, C. (2014). Comunicação e literacia em Saúde. In M. Cruz, T. Ventura, M. Cardim, & N. Melim (Eds.), *Cidadania na sociedade do conhecimento* (pp. 151–160). Centro de Filosofia das Ciências da Universidade de Lisboa.

Banks, J., Marmot, M., Oldfield, Z., & Smith, J. P. (2006). Disease and disadvantage in the United States and in England. *Journal of the American Medical Association*, *295*(17), 2037–2045. doi:10.1001/jama.295.17.2037 PMID:16670412

Belim, C. (2020). Digital media in rare diseases or "knowledge is power": The role of EURORDIS in creating awareness and diagnosing rare diseases. In L. V. Costa & S. Oliveira (Eds.), *Communicating rare diseases and disorders in the digital age* (pp. 154–178). IGI Global.

Belim, C., & Almeida, C. V. (2018). Communication competences are the key! A model of communication for the health professional to optimize the health literacy – Assertiveness, clear language and positivity. *Journal of Healthcare Communications*, *3*(31). Advance online publication. doi:10.4172/2472-1654.100141

Bellini, M. I., Parisotto, C., Dor, F., & Kessaris, N. (2020). Social media use among transplant professionals in Europe: A cross-sectional study from the European Society of Organ Transplantation. *Experimental and Clinical Transplantation, 18*(2), 169–176. doi:10.6002/ect.2019.0078

Blatt, B., Spinazzi, N., & Greenberg, L. (2014). Communication skills training for resident physicians: a physician-educator perspective. In H. Hamilton & W. Chou (Eds.), *The Routledge handbook of language and health communication* (pp. 294–326). Routledge.

Brüssow, H. (2013). What is health? *Microbial Biotechnology*, *6*(4), 341–348. doi:10.1111/1751-7915.12063 PMID:23647782

Burgoon, J. K., Guerrero, L. K., & Floyd, K. (2016). *Nonverbal communication*. Routledge. doi:10.4324/9781315663425

Carey, J. W. (2008). *Communication as culture: Essays on media and society*. Routledge.

Cieza, A., Oberhauser, C., Bickenbach, J., Jones, R. N., Üstün, T. B., Kostanjsek, N., Morris, J. N., & Chatterji, S. (2016). Health is not just the absence of disease.... *International Journal of Epidemiology*, *45*(2), 586–587. doi:10.1093/ije/dyw063 PMID:27174840

Cline, R. (2003). Everyday interpersonal communication and health. In T. Thompson, A. Dorsey, K. Miller, & R. Parrott (Eds.), *Handbook of health Communication* (pp. 285–313). Lawrence Erlbaum Associates.

Corcoran, N. (2013). *Communicating health: Strategies for health promotion*. Sage. doi:10.4135/9781526401588

Cullerton, K., Donnet, T., Lee, A., & Gallegos, D. (2018). Effective advocacy strategies for influencing government nutrition policy: A conceptual model. *The International Journal of Behavioral Nutrition and Physical Activity*, *15*(1), 83. Advance online publication. doi:10.118612966-018-0716-y PMID:30170610

Eckler, P., Worsowicz, G. M., & Downey, K. (2009). Improving physician-patient communication. In J. Parker & E. Thorson (Eds.), *Health communication in the new media landscape* (pp. 283–302). Springer.

Edelman, C. L., & Mandle, C. L. (Eds.). (2010). *Health promotion throughout the life span*. Mosby Elsevier.

Emerson, R. W. (1860). *The conduct of life*. Ticknor and Fields.

Erozkan, A. (2013). The effect of communication skills and interpersonal problem solving skills on social self-efficacy. *Educational Sciences: Theory and Practice*, *13*(2), 739–745.

Floyd, K. (2009). *Interpersonal communication: The whole story*. McGraw-Hill.

Flynn, B. S., Worden, J. K., Secker-Walker, R. H., Badger, G. J., Geller, B. M., & Costanza, M. C. (1992). Prevention of cigarette smoking through mass media intervention and school programs. *American Journal of Public Health*, *82*(6), 827–834. doi:10.2105/AJPH.82.6.827 PMID:1585963

Flynn, B. S., Worden, J. K., Secker-Walker, R. H., Pirie, P. L., Badger, G. J., Carpenter, J. H., & Geller, B. M. (1994). Mass media and school interventions for cigarette smoking prevention: Effects 2 years after completion. *American Journal of Public Health*, *84*(7), 1148–1150. doi:10.2105/AJPH.84.7.1148 PMID:8017542

Friedman, L. D. (Ed.). (2004). *Cultural sutures: Medicine and media*. Duke University Press. doi:10.1215/9780822385530

Gregory, A. (2008). Competencies of senior communication practitioners in the UK: An initial study. *Public Relations Review*, *34*(3), 215–223. doi:10.1016/j.pubrev.2008.04.005

Gully, P. (2009). Foreword. In J. Parker & E. Thorson (Eds.), *Health communication in the new media landscape* (pp. xxvi–xxix). Springer Publishing Company, LLC.

Haines, A., & Rogers, S. (2001). Integrating research evidence into practice. In C. Silagy & A. Haines (Eds.), *Evidence-based practice in primary care* (pp. 157–176). BMJ Books.

Hall, S. (1980). Encoding/decoding. In S. Hall, D. Hobson, A. Lowe, & P. Willis (Eds.), *Culture, media, language: Working papers in cultural studies, 1972-79* (pp. 117–128). Routledge.

Harner, R. N. (2011). Patient-provider communication. In C. F. Parvanta, D. E. Nelson, S. A. Parvanta, & R. N. Harner (Eds.), *Essentials of public health communication* (pp. 313–326). Jones & Bartlett Learning.

Harrington, N. (2015). *Health communication: Theory, method, and application*. Routledge.

Hayden, J. (2014). *Why good health is the first health*. World Economic Forum. Retrieved from https://www.weforum.org/agenda/2014/12/why-good-health-is-the-first-wealth/

Healthy People. (2010). Retrieved from https://www.healthypeople.gov/2010/document/HTML/Volume1/11HealthCom.htm

Henderson, M. L., Adler, J. T., Van Pilsum Rasmussen, S. E., Thomas, A. G., Herron, P. D., Waldram, M. M., ... Segev, D. L. (2018). How should social media be used in transplantation? A Survey of the American Society of Transplant Surgeons. *Transplantation*, *1*. Advance online publication. doi:10.1097/TP.0000000000002243 PMID:29684002

Howick, J., Moscrop, A., Mebius, A., Fanshawe, T. R., Lewith, G., Bishop, F. L., Mistiaen, P., Roberts, N. W., Dieninytė, E., Hu, X.-Y., Aveyard, P., & Onakpoya, I. J. (2018). Effects of empathic and positive communication in healthcare consultations: A systematic review and meta-analysis. *Journal of the Royal Society of Medicine*, *111*(7), 240–252. doi:10.1177/0141076818769477 PMID:29672201

Institute of Medicine (US) Committee on Assuring the Health of the Public in the 21st Century. (2002). *The future of the public's health in the 21st century*. Washington, DC: National Academies Press.

Kemp, C. L., Ball, M. M., Jason, K., Appel, J. A. D., & Fitzroy, A. F. (2019). Communicative Competence: Responding to Residents' Health Changes in Assisted Living. *The Gerontologist*, gnz119. Advance online publication. doi:10.1093/geront/gnz119 PMID:31504482

Kurtz, S., Silverman, J., & Draper, J. (2004). *Teaching and learning communication skills in medicine*. CRC Press.

Markides, M. (2011). The importance of good communication between patient and health professionals. *Journal of Pediatric Hematology/Oncology, 33*(Supplement 2), S123–S125. doi:10.1097/MPH.0b013e318230e1e5 PMID:21952568

Martin, L. R., & DiMatteo, M. R. (2014). 2. Barriers and keys to treatment adherence and health behavior change. In L. R. Martin & M. R. DiMatteo (Eds.), *The Oxford handbook of health communication, behavior change, and treatment adherence* (pp. 9–22). Oxford University Press.

Mast, M. S., & Cousin, G. (2014). 4. The role of nonverbal communication in medical interactions: Empirical results, theoretical bases, and methodological issues. In L. R. Martin & M. R. DiMatteo (Eds.), *The Oxford handbook of health communication, behavior change, and treatment adherence* (pp. 38–53). Oxford University Press.

Mazor, K. M., Roblin, D. W., Greene, S. M., Lemay, C. A., Firneno, C. L., Calvi, J., Prouty, C. D., Horner, K., & Gallagher, T. H. (2012). Toward patient-centered cancer care: Patient perceptions of problematic events, impact, and response. *Journal of Clinical Oncology, 30*(15), 1784–1790. doi:10.1200/JCO.2011.38.1384 PMID:22508828

McCabe, C. (2004). Nurse-patient communication: An exploration of patients' experiences. *Journal of Clinical Nursing, 13*(1), 41–49. doi:10.1111/j.1365-2702.2004.00817.x PMID:14687292

McCroskey, J. C. (1982). Communication competence and performance: A research and pedagogical perspective. *Communication Education, 31*(1), 1–7. doi:10.1080/03634528209384654

Mechanic, D., & Meyer, S. (2000). Concepts of trust among patients with serious illness. *Social Science & Medicine, 51*(5), 657–668. doi:10.1016/S0277-9536(00)00014-9 PMID:10975226

Moscovici, F. (1981). Competência interpessoal no desenvolvimento de gerentes. *Revista de Administração de Empresas, 21*(2), 17–25. doi:10.1590/S0034-75901981000200002

Moyle, W. (2003). Nurse-patient relationship: A dichotomy of expectations. *International Journal of Mental Health Nursing, 12*(2), 103–109. doi:10.1046/j.1440-0979.2003.00276.x PMID:12956021

National Communication Association. (2013). *What is communication?* Retrieved from https://www.natcom.org/about-nca/what-communication?id=236&terms=health%20communication

Nkanunye, C. C., & Obiechina, G. O. (2017). Health communication strategies as gateway to effective health promotion and well-being. *J Med Res Health Educ.*, *1*(3), 13.

Noar, S. M., Benac, C. N., & Harris, M. S. (2007). Does tailoring matter? Meta-analytic review of tailored print health behavior change interventions. *Psychological Bulletin*, *133*(4), 673–693. doi:10.1037/0033-2909.133.4.673 PMID:17592961

Perkins, P. S. (2010). *The art and science of communication: Tools for effective communication in the workplace*. John Wiley & Sons.

Randolph, W., & Viswanath, K. (2004). Lessons Learned from Public Health Mass Media Campaigns: Marketing Health in a Crowded Media World. *Annual Review of Public Health*, *25*(1), 419–437. doi:10.1146/annurev.publhealth.25.101802.123046 PMID:15015928

Rimal, R. N. (2000). Closing the knowledge-behavior gap in health promotion: The mediating roles of self-efficacy. *Health Communication*, *12*(3), 219–237. doi:10.1207/S15327027HC1203_01 PMID:10938914

Rimal, R. N., & Lapinski, M. K. (2009). Why health communication is important in public health. *Bulletin of the World Health Organization*, *87*(4), 247–248. doi:10.2471/BLT.08.056713 PMID:19551226

Rogers, E. (2003). *Diffusion of innovations*. Free Press.

Samuel. (2016). Effective xommunication as a panacea for gaining acceptance of hospital services by clients. *Texila International Journal of Public Health, 4*(4).

Seale, C. (Ed.). (2002). *Media and health*. Sage Publications.

Seale, C. (Ed.). (2004). *Health and the media*. Wiley-Blackwell.

Servaes, J., & Malikhao, P. (2010). Advocacy strategies for health communication. *Public Relations Review*, *36*(1), 42–49. doi:10.1016/j.pubrev.2009.08.017

Sharma, R. (1997). An introduction to advocacy: training guide. Washington, DC: Support for Analysis and Research in Africa (SARA).

Snyder, L. (2001). How effective are mediated health campaigns? In R. Rice & C. Atkin (Eds.), *Public communication campaigns* (pp. 181–190). Sage. doi:10.4135/9781452233260.n10

Snyder, L. B., Hamilton, M. A., Mitchell, E. W., Kiwanuka-Tondo, J., Fleming-Milici, F., & Proctor, D. (2004). A meta-analysis of the effect of mediated health communication campaigns on behavior change in the United States. *Journal of Health Communication, 9*(sup1), 71-96. doi:10.1080/10810730490271548

Spitzberg, B. H. (2003). Methods of interpersonal skill assessment. In J. O. Greene & B. R. Burleson (Eds.), *Handbook of communication and social interaction skills* (pp. 93–134). Lawrence Erlbaum Associates, Publishers.

Stacks, D. W., & Salwen, M. B. (Eds.). (2009). *An integrated approach to communication theory and research.* Routledge.

Stiglitz, J. E., Sen, A., & Fitoussi, J.-P. (2009). *Report by the Commission on the Measurement of Economic Performance and Social Progress.* Technical report.

Storey, D., Seifert-Ahanda, K., Andaluz, A., Tsoi, B., Matsuki, J. M., & Cutler, B. (2014). What Is Health Communication and How Does It Affect the HIV/AIDS Continuum of Care? A Brief Primer and Case Study From New York City. *JAIDS Journal of Acquired Immune Deficiency Syndromes, 66*(Supplement 3), S241–S249. doi:10.1097/QAI.0000000000000243 PMID:25007193

Sugai, D. Y., Deptula, P. L., Parsa, A. A., & Parsa, F. D. (2013). The importance of communication in the management of postoperative pain. *Hawai'i Journal of Medicine & Public Health: a Journal of Asia Pacific Medicine & Public Health, 72*(6), 180–184. PMID:23795326

Tench, R., & Moreno, A. (2015). Mapping communication management competencies for European practitioners. *Journal of Communication Management (London), 19*(1), 39–61. doi:10.1108/JCOM-11-2013-0078

Tench, R., Zerfass, A., Verhoeven, P., Moreno, A., Okay, A., & Verčič, D. (2013a). *ECOPSI Benchmarking Report.* Leeds Metropolitan University.

Thompson, T. (2003). Introduction. In T. Thompson, A. Dorsey, K. Miller, & R. Parrott (Eds.), *Handbook of health communication* (pp. 1–5). Lawrence Erlbaum Associates.

Thorson, E., & Duffy, M. E. (2009). Health communication in the new media landscape: A summary. In J. Parker & E. Thorson (Eds.), *Health communication in the new media landscape* (pp. 437–446). Springer.

U.S. Department of Health and Human Services. (2005). *Making health communication programs works.* Retrieved from https://www.cancer.gov/publications/health-communication/pink-book.pdf

Wakefield, M. A., Loken, B., & Hornik, R. C. (2010). Use of mass media campaigns to change health behaviour. *Lancet, 376*(9748), 1261–1271. doi:10.1016/S0140-6736(10)60809-4 PMID:20933263

Wallack, L. (2000). The role of mass media in creating social capital: A new direction for public health. In B. D. Smedley & S. L. Syme (Eds.), *Promoting health: Intervention strategies from social and behavioral research* (pp. 337–365). National Academy Press.

Wallington, S. (2014). Health disparities research and practice: The role of language and health communication. In H. Hamilton & W. Chou (Eds.), *The Routledge handbook of language and health communication* (pp. 168–183). Routledge.

Weinstein, N. D., & Sandman, P. M. (1992). A model of the precaution adoption process: Evidence from home radon testing. *Health Psychology, 11*(3), 170–180. doi:10.1037/0278-6133.11.3.170 PMID:1618171

Welch, M. (2005). Pivotal moments in the therapeutic relationship. *International Journal of Mental Nursing, 14*, 161–165. PMID:16181152

WHO. (2004). *Health research for policy, action and practice.* Alliance for Health Policy and Systems Research, Council on Health Research for Development, Global Forum for Health Research, INCLEN Trust. Retrieved from http://www9.who.int/alliance-hpsr/resources/ModuleIII_U3_AdvocacyV2.pdf

Chapter 2
In Principio Erat Verbum:
The Origins of the Communication Models in Health

Cristina Vaz de Almeida
ISCSP, University of Lisbon, Portugal

ABSTRACT

This chapter discusses the origins of the various models used as a basis for health communication through a literature review. Models seek to represent reality and are dynamic constructs that evolve as the world's own needs and discoveries are made. Particularly in health, a territory for a long time dominated by the biomedical model and a passive view of its recipients, the models have brought a breath of fresh air to the true human dimension. Among the various models that have been defended based on a biopsychosocial perspective, the cognitive, behavioral, emotional components of the human being are reflected, as well as their context and environment in which they move, namely the social, economic, cultural, political, and other dimensions. It is also the determinants of health that influence the whole and that make the interpersonal relationship in health richer and representative of the complex human dimension seen in a holistic way.

DOI: 10.4018/978-1-7998-4396-2.ch002

INTRODUCTION

Models are simplified images of parts of the real world according to Cobley and Shulz (2013). One model represents part of the characteristics of the world and moves towards becoming a theory, which is in fact a symbolic construction of concepts (Kaplan, 1964, p. 296) that present a systematic vision and explain and predict phenomena (Kerlinger & Lee, 2000).

The communication models allied to health (from biomedical to biopsychosocial) have evolved and integrated elements related to the person and his/her essence. The person and his/her essence cannot be left out of this chess of solutions.

Communication cannot be performed in a *vacuum*, and must be integrated in each context, itself affected by attitudes, social norms, behaviors, beliefs, stress, and goals to be achieved on a permanent basis. And it is in this framework that models are built.

First, communication models emerged, associated with theories related to personal interaction and media efforts, originally explained by social scientists, like Lazarfeld, with works related to the analysis of campaigns associated with the voting process in the United States of America (1944), or Lasswell (1948) through the model that proposes basic elements of communication: "who?", "says what?", "through which channel?", "to whom?", and "to what effect?" that proposes a structure and function of communication in society.

Katz (1955) contributes with the two-step flow communication theory and the studies on personal influence elaborated with Lazarsfeld (1955). Schramm's works (1954; 1955) are also important. Hall (1980), in Schramm line, structures and grounds the encoding/decoding approach and deepens cultural studies.

These models were gradually associated with models of health communication and drinking from them the complex dimension of health, whether at the individual, group or mass level.

Health communication is a complex problem of solving tasks, in a continuous process of detecting objectives and forming responses. Communication, as Dance (1970) explained, is a process through which we understand other, and we are understood. It is a dynamic, constantly changing and transformative process.

It is important, therefore, that the actors in the health process, health professionals, decision-makers, can identify the theories and models that are suitable to promote the management of behavior change aimed at improving the health of individuals and communities (Pearson et al., 2005).

MODELS: ITS CONSTRUCTS

In order to focus on the concept of health communication models, we must start from the definition of each of its constructs, and the evolution of the concept "model".

Starting from Deutsch (1952) who considers the model as a structure of symbols and operational rules that aggregates relevant points in an existing structure or process (p. 357), Engel (1981), highlights the importance of the models' usefulness (p. 122) and Littlejohn (1999) again reinforces the need for "symbolic representation of an underlying thing, process or idea" (1999, p. 19). According to this author, all theories and all models contain concepts, but the conceptual type varies significantly (Littlejohn, 1999, p. 22).

Each model implies judgments of relevance and a theory that combines the structural correspondence between the model and certain aspects of the thing it is supposed to model (Deutsch, 1952, p. 358) (Figure 1)

Figure 1. Models conceptualization
Source: (Author based on Deutsch, 1952; Littlejohn, 1999)

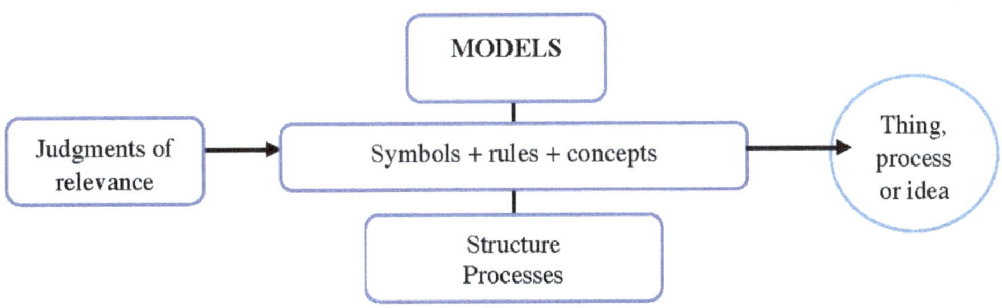

According to Deutsch (1952), the role of each models can be: 1) Organizational; 2) Predictive; 3) Heuristics; 4) Measurement (pp. 360- 361).

Models have an organizational function because they can order and relate data that are separate and are able to present similarities or connections (p. 360). This organization facilitates memory storage and recall when necessary.

Prediction presupposes verification by physical operations, ranging from a simple "yes-no" to high degrees of qualitative prediction of similarity or correspondence, to the other extreme of quantitative predictions, which give us time series and answer questions about when and how much (Deutsch, 1952, p. 361).

The heuristic function is independent of the degree of order, organization, prediction or measurement.

The operational function (measurement) allows teaching or training to facilitate the transfer of habits from a familiar environment to an unfamiliar one, that is, it transfers a familiar behavior to a "new" problem, the explanation of which is satisfactory.

Deutsch reinforces that models are evaluated for their simplicity or economy of means (1952, p. 362) and communication is what makes the organization coherent, and control is what regulates the behaviors (p. 367).

In turn, Engel (1981) states that the value of a scientific model is measured, not because it is right or wrong, but because of its usefulness (p. 122). Later, Littlejohn (1999) states that we can consider a model as a short form of a theory (p. 5).

BIOMEDICAL PERSPECTIVE

The biomedical perspective assumes patients as passive receivers of doctors' instructions (Munro et al., 2007, p. 3; Ross & Deverell, 2004).

Health or illness goes back to biomedical causes, such as bacteria or viruses, and the treatment focuses on the patient's body (Ross & Deverell, 2004). It is understood that non-adherence is motivated by patient's traits, such as sex and age.

The biomedical model in medicine represents medicine's application of the classical factor analysis approach, characterized in Western science for many centuries. The biomedical model considered reductionist, because it intends to find it as quickly as possible through simple explanations, looking at the "unique" disease and seeing the rest as "complications" (Engel, 1981, p. 108) (Figure 2).

The patient's need is to relieve the tension correctly or incorrectly attributed to the disease (Engel, 1981, p.102), and his/her expectation is that the other party has the professional competence and the motivation to provide this relief (p. 102).

The biomedical model is an adequate scientific model, but it does not include the patient and his/her attributes as a person and a human being (Engel, 1981, p. 103) and therefore, more than looking at the body and the disease, he/she must not neglect the patient as a "person" (p. 107).

Figure 2. The biomedical model
Source: (The author)

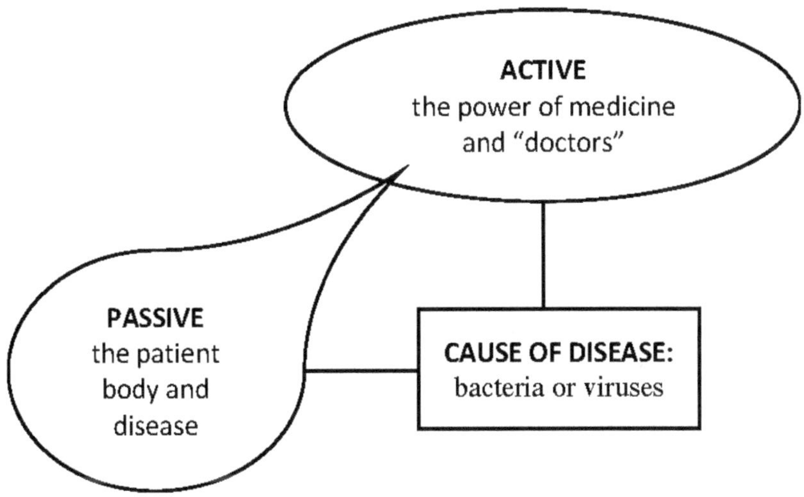

In this dual tension relationship, patients must be given a voice. Patients must be able to develop the health behaviors they aspire to have (Martin & DiMatteo, 2014, p. 16). The doctor's first source is the patient (Engel, 1981, p. 107) and it is necessary to ensure that, at least, the most credible source historically (Hovland, 1953; Lawrence, 2008) that is, the health professional, fulfill his/her mission.

Biomedicine, like medicine from other cultures, is influenced by conditions and beliefs in the culture and, therefore, reflects the value and norms of its creators (Weber, 2016, p. 2)

Medical hegemony dominates the biomedical model with the active suppression of alternatives, as well as a corporatism of personal and clinical medicine and hospital-centered pharmaceutical treatment (Weber, 2016).

Within the scope of the biomedical model, health professionals (especially doctors and nurses) are probably among the most careful professionals in our society (Leape, 1994, p. 1851).

It is not supposed to make mistakes, to have unforeseen events, to indulge in the task or to be exhausted and worried, with a strong emphasis on perfection, whether in diagnosis or treatment (Leape, 1994, p. 1851). In this demand for perfection, centrality operates through the health professional's power over his/her patient in a relationship between the expert and the layman.

Engel (1981) reinforces that the judgments and decisions of the health professional with a "biomedical" stance on decisions related to the patient's interpersonal or social aspects are taken with the least amount of information about people, their relationships and circumstances and even with less knowledge and understanding basic principles in the context of interpersonal and social transactions (Engel, 1981, p. 120).

According to Munro et al. (2007, p. 3), a fundamental limitation of this theory is that it ignores other factors besides the patient's characteristics, which may have an impact on health behaviors such as 1) the patient's perspective on his/her illness; 2) psychosocial influences; 3) the impact of the socio-economic environment.).

Although with diverse criticisms (Engel, 1977, 1981; Kurtz, Silverman & Draper, 2005; Munro et al., 2007, Sasz & Hollender, 1956), biomedical theory has recently been integrated into a broader theory incorporating the context of the social environment (Munro et al., 2007, p. 3).

THE BEHAVIORAL PERSPECTIVE

The behavioral perspective incorporates the theory of behavioral learning, which focuses on the environment and teaching skills to manage adherence (Munro et al., 2007, p. 3; WHO, 2003).

Learning theories aim to explain how experience changes what we do or feel and focus on how we react to stimuli or events, rather than focusing on the individual's actions

It is characterized using the principles of antecedents, consequences and their influence on behavior (WHO, 2003).

The antecedents are internal (thoughts) or external (environmental suggestions), while the consequences can be punishments or rewards for a behavior (WHO, 2003).

Antecendents can be achieved through patient education and good health care worker communication skills, that places emphasis on the timing of treatment, instruction and comprehension (Munro et al., 2007, p. 4).

However, there are studies, (Blackwell, 1992) that show that external rewards have no effects, sometimes even having negative effects (e.g., with electronic recall systems).

Munro et al. (2007) argue that behavioral perspective ignores attitudinal, motivational and interpersonal factors that may interfere with the reception of the message and the translation of knowledge into behaviour change (Munro et al., 2007, p. 4).

The Behavioral Learning Theory is criticized for its focus on influences external to behavior and for lacking an individualized approach, and for not considering less conscious influences of behavior that are not linked to immediate rewards, such as past behavior, habits or lack of encouragement diagnosis (Blackwell, 1992; Munro, et al., 2007, p. 4). In this sense, it is necessary to consider the individual perceptions of appropriate rewards in order to have better results (Munro et al., 2007, p. 4).

COMMUNICATION PERSPECTIVE

From a communicational perspective, the improvement in professional-patient communication will increase patient compliance, assuming that adherence depends on the patient's literacy and the professional's communication skills (Leonard, Graham & Bonacum, 2004, p. 187; Ross & Deverell, 2004; Sawyer & Aroni, 2003, p. 2).

Communication must be clear and understandable to be effective, which adds to the treatment time, the patient's instruction and his/her understanding (Munro, et. al. 2007, p. 4).

In the field of public health, communication is considered "scientific in the strategic dissemination and critical and relevant, accurate, accessible and understandable evaluation of health information for specific audiences for the advancement of public health (Bernhardt, 2004; Parvanta & Bass, 2020, p. 28; *US Dep. of Health and Human Services,* 2000).

Interpersonal communication is a process of continuous development and not just a discreet set of interactions. The exchanges of messages that took place in the past end up influencing future exchanges (Kreps, 2001, p. 599). There is a transactional process here, which, according to Kreps (2001) define and redefine interpersonal relationships (Figure 2).

There is a hierarchical structure (Argyle et al., 1994) in interpersonal skills as the larger and higher-level units are sequences that integrate the lower level units (p. 20). Starting at the lowest level are the primary components that consist of verbal and non-verbal behavior, that is, what we say and what we do (Wright & Taylor, 1994).

If people have interpersonal skills at the verbal level, they ask questions, make statements, can select the verbal component most appropriate to the situation in question, are able to act and use non-verbal suggestions adapted to that situation.

Moving to a second level, involves the structure or the way in which the primary components of behavior are sequenced. Competent people in this level organize and use verbal and non-verbal components in specific sequences to achieve a certain objective, such as solving problems by using open-ended questions to start the conversation and then start to funnel and ask closed questions (from answer yes or no) (Wright & Taylor, 1994). In the upper floor of the competencies, other arguments are used, such as congruence and the expectation of the results and reactions of others (anticipation). For example, managers who want to help their team members become more effective may decide to adopt a help style that involves empowering them, so that they can experiment and learn from their own mistakes and not substitute for tasks and functions (Hayes, 2005).

Also, in the Theory of Communicative Competence (Spitzberg, 2013, p. 126) there is an integration of individual and institutional concerns, and there may be a conceptual framework where these concerns can be elaborated and compared through programs. According to Spitzberg (2013, p. 126), communicative competence is defined as an impression of adequacy, effectiveness and efficiency, which is functionally related to individual motivation, knowledge, skills, contextual facilitators and constraints, thus questioning the ideas of Munro and others (2007).

Interpersonal relationships also guide individual communication responses. A relational orientation in the study of communication between healthcare providers and healthcare consumers (Kreps, 2001) should examine how message exchanges influence what it is established (p. 599).

The study of communication must consider the development and maintenance of interpersonal relationships in healthcare (Kreps, 2001, p. 599).

It is therefore necessary to investigate the perspectives of both stakeholders: healthcare professional and patient. According to Thompson (1998) in the relational communication, the expression and development of empathy, therapeutic communication, social support and psychosocial adjustment is quite important.

Lewin, Skea, Entwistle, Zwarenstein and Dick (2001) say that the elements of communication in the relationship in health effectively allow: 1) improving communication in consultations, 2) increasing patient satisfaction, 3) increase health outcomes.

Criticisms to Communication Perspective

Criticisms made to the perspective of the communication approach emphasize that this approach cannot be seen in isolation (Munro et al., 2007, p. 4) because there is an influence of external factors, such as access costs as well as, for example, ignoring attitudinal, motivational and interpersonal factors that can interfere with the reception of messages and changes, both in knowledge and behavior (Munro et al., 2007, p. 4).

COGNITIVE AND EMOTIONAL PERSPECTIVE

According to Ogden (2004, p. 39), cognitive models analyze the predictive factors and precursors of health behaviors and have their origin in Edwards (1954) in the Theory of Subjective Expected Utility.

These theories focus on the cognitive variables of change behavior, such as self-efficacy, attitudes, and beliefs (Bandura, 1977; Rosenstock, Strecher & Beckr, 1988; Stroebe, 2000), expectations of events and future results (Gebhardt & Maes, 2001), as determinants of behavioral change (Munro, Lewin, Swart, Volmink, 2007, p. 4). Faced with a set of alternatives, individuals choose the action that leads to positive results (Munro et al. 2007, p. 4). Non-voluntary factors can affect behaviors (Gebhardt & Maes, 2001).

People today live in a multifaceted consumer society and need to navigate complex health systems, and have all the time to make decisions, and their choices have an impact on their health (Kickbusch, 2019). Kickbusch (2019) defines health literacy through two strands on the one hand, the set of knowledge, skills, motivation, and correct information, which allows people to make decisions in their lives, on the other the environment that influences these decisions and that it can make it easy or difficult to make healthy choices correctly or use the health system properly (Table 1).

At an individual level of behavioral intentions, studies suggest that the likelihood that the target audience will adopt a desired behavior can be predicted by assessing the attitudes and perceptions of benefits, as well as assessing the opinion that their peers will have regarding this behavior (Fishbein & Ajzen, 1975). These authors (Fishbein & Ajzen, 1975) argue that the perceived attitudes of individuals and society are predictors of future actions, so an important step in influencing behavior is to make a preliminary assessment of the attitudes of the target audience, and it is necessary to follow-up to identify any change in attitude (U.S. Department of Health and Human Services, 2004, p. 220).

Table 1. Theories from the cognitive perspective

• The Locus of Control Model (Wallston & Wallston, 1982; Rotter, 1966) based on specific beliefs that a person may have about the way he or she controls significant events in his/her life; • The Social-Cognitive Theory (Bandura, 1977) based on modeling and behaviors and self-efficacy; • The Health Belief Model (Rosenstock, 1974) based on susceptibility, severity of occurrence, benefits and barriers to behavior change; • The Rational Action Theory and Planned Behavior Theory (Fishbein & Azjen, 1975; Armitage & Connor, 2001; Azjen, 1991) in which behaviors depend on subjective intentions and norms and behavioral control; • The Theory of Self Determination (Decy & Ryan, 1985, 2002) based on the psychological needs for autonomy, relationship and competence as a key to understanding human motivation; • The Theory of Motivation for Protection (Rogers, 1975, 1983), and similar ones like the Health Action Process (HAPA) – Health Action Process, based on the role of expectations the adoption and maintenance of health-promoting behaviors (Schwarzer, 1992, 2008).

Source: (The author)

Cognitive models describe behavior as a process of rational information, highlighting individual cognitions but not the social context where these cognitions occur (Ogden, 2004, p. 29).

According to Cobley and Shulz (2013), the domain of "cognitive theories of communication" is tremendously broad and encompasses a variety of only-partially-overlapping approaches to theorizing (p. 182).

THE LOCUS OF CONTROL MODEL (ROTER, 1966)

The Locus of Control Model (Wallston & Wallston, 1982; Rotter, 1966) refers to the specific beliefs that a person may have about the way he or she controls significant events in his/her life. The locus of control has to do with the individual's internal and external attributions.

Individuals may consider that the events that occur in their lives are controlled by themselves (locus of internal control), or on the other hand, they cannot be controlled or are controlled by others (for example by their doctors).

According to Ogden (2004), it was demonstrated that this locus of health control is related to the fact that individuals change their behaviors or not and to the communication style they expect from their health professionals (p. 35).

The locus of control model theory states that people are more likely to engage in behavior when they perform that the previous reinforcements they had, came directly because of their own behavior (locus of internal control).

The potential for behavior change is less when people perceive that these reinforcements occurred due to other behaviors or due to external factors (external locus of control).

According to Ogden (2004) there are questions that should be asked regarding this theory, namely: 1) is the locus of health control a state or a (personality) trait, that is, the person will always make internal assignments?; 2) can it be both internal and external? For example, going to the doctor is something external, because the person thinks that the doctor is the other powerful person who can do him/her good, or else the person assumes that he/she is influencing his/her health status by looking for the health professional in an appropriate way.

SOCIAL-COGNITIVE THEORY (BANDURA, 1977, 1986)

Social-Cognitive Theory-SCT (Bandura, 1977, 1986), originated from the Theory of Social Learning (Bandura, 1977), maintains that behavior is determined by expectations, incentives and social cognitions. This theory, evolved from the theory of social learning, may be the most comprehensive theory for behavior change.

The determinants that interact with each other are: 1) behavior, 2) cognitive and other interpersonal factors, 3) and environmental events.

The social cognition model includes measures of individual representations of the respective social world, trying to place the individual in the context of other people in the wider social world (Ogden, 2004, p. 48).

SCT advocates that behaviors are determined dynamically: they are influenced by personal factors and the environment. Changes in any of these three factors (behavior, cognition, and environment) can cause changes in the others.

One of the key concepts of this theory (SCT) is the environmental variable: which is reflected in what is observational learning.

In contrast to previous behavioral theories, this theory considers the environment as a variable that is preponderant in reinforcing or punishing behaviors. However, it also allows, by comparison, that the individual can observe the actions of others and thus be able, through modeling, to learn the consequences of adopting these behaviors.

The social learning process goes through the following steps presented in the table 2.

Table 2. Social learning process

Observational learning processes
• Attention - gaining and maintaining attention • Retention - to be remembered / remembered • Reproduction - reproduce the observed behavior • Motivation - the stimulation that aims to produce the behavior

Source: (Based on Bandura, 1977)

In the SCT there is a multifaceted causal structure (Munro et al., 2007, p. 6) in the regulation of human motivation, action and well-being.

There is a reciprocal determinism that is based on a continuous and dynamic interaction between the individual, the environment and the behavior (Redding, Rossi, Rossi, Velicer, & Prochaska, 2000).

This theory sugests that the prerequisites for change are: 1) knowledge of health risks; 2) the benefits; 3) the selfinfluences associated with the beliefs about personal effectiveness (could yourself doing this?) and 4) the expected results, which may include social approval or disapproval or the subject's positive or negative self-evaluation.

The change in behavior may be due to the reduction or elimination of barriers: the person realizes that he/she has control over the results and that there are few external barriers, and the person thus has confidence in his/her competence to execute the respective behavior. According to Keller, Fleury, Gregor-Holt & Thompson (1999), self-efficacy can explain 4% to 26% of the variation in behavior.

Social cognitions are a central component of social cognition models, which attempt to place the individual in the context of other people in the wider social world, and therefore include measures of individual representations of the social world (Ogden, 2004, p. 48).

Expectations can be divided, according to Rosenstock (1988) in: a) expectations about environmental clues, that is, beliefs about how events are interconnected; b) expectations about the consequences of each person's action, that is, opinions about how the behavior of individuals influences results, and c) expectations about their own competence to perform the behavior necessary to influence results, that is, self-efficacy.

In turn, incentives (or reinforcements) can be defined as the value of a particular object or result. This result can be health status, physical appearance, approval from others, economic gain or other consequences (Rosenstock, 1988, p. 176).

Social cognitive theories are concerned with how people make sense of their environment (including their message environment), others, and themselves (Cobley & Shulz, 2013, p. 187).

THE HEALTH BELIEF MODEL (1966, 1974)

The Health Belief Model (Rosenstock, 1966, 1974) is an cognitive model and was developed to explain preventive health behaviors, thus aiming at prevention by the person who does not "have" the disease (Rosenstock, 1974, p. 328), as well as the answer from behaviors to the treatment of acute and chronic patients (Ogden, 2004, p. 40).

Rosenstock (1974) says that the researchers who were at the origin of this model of health beliefs were influenced by a phenomenological orientation and by the theories of Kurt Lewin represented by the individual existence in a living space composed of "regions" in which some are positively valued and others negatively valued (p. 329). In this sense, the "disease" is in the "negative region" so one can expect the person to leave that region (p. 330).

The author of the health belief model (Rosenstock, 1974), states that the person to avoid the disease has to believe in susceptibility, that is, in the subjective risk of contracting the disease, in the severity of it, in a greater benefit and being able to overcome barriers (p. 330). It also stresses that researchers were concerned with building a theory and not just solving practical problems, with a strong component of motivation and perception on the part of those who exhibit behaviors (Rosenstock, 1974, p. 329). If the perception of severity is high and susceptibility is low, it is assumed that the probability of the action will be high. Intuitively it can be assumed that the probability in this case of occurring will be low when both variables are high.

In this model, behavior results from a set of central beliefs, which are the individual perceptions about (Rosenstock, 1974, Ogden, 2004, p. 40): susceptibility to the disease; severity of the disease; the costs involved; the benefits involved; the clues for action (internal and external).

Risk learning models have been utilized in a wide variety of contexts (Pechmann, 2001, p. 191).

According to Ogden (2004, p. 41), several studies confirm the hypotheses raised by the health belief model, namely that you want to follow a dietary regime, practice safe sex, be vaccinated, make regular visits to the dentist or have regular exercise, it will relate to the factors involved in the model: the person's perception of the susceptibility of having a problem, the belief in the severity / severity of the problem, the perception that the benefits will outweigh the costs (Becker, 1974, Rosenstock, 1974).

Criticisms to the Health Belief Model

Some of the criticisms pointed out that the health belief model does not produce results in Africa, Asia or Latin America because it is an individual, rational and linear model (Airhihenbuwa, 1995, p. 8).

According to Airhihenbuwa (1995), theories based on individuals and their individual decisions do not work in these societies where the family and the community are central to the construction of the concepts of health and well-being (p. 9). According to this author (Airhihenbuwa, 1995), the locus of control is outside the "self", in the community and in the family. Using the proper opinion of "agree or not to agree" within these cultural contexts is considered disrespectful (p. 9).

For Blackwell (1992, p. 165), Munro et al. (2007, p. 5), Stroebe (2000) and Stroebe and de Witt (1996), the weaknesses of the model are as follows (Table 3).

Table 3. Weaknesses of health belief model

• Perceived threats (especially severity) have a weak correlation with health action and may result in avoiding protection. The perception of severity may not be as important as the perception of susceptibility. Recently, self-efficacy has been integrated into this theory of health beliefs, incorporating the need for a person to feel competent before long-term change (Munro et al., 2007, p. 5; Strecher & Rosenstock, 1997); • There is no clear explicit relationship between the variables; • No definitions were made for the individual components or clear rules of combination; • It is assumed that the variables are not moderated by each other or that they have additional effects; • The theory does not include the important determinants of health behavior as positive effects of negative behaviors, as well as social influences (Munro et al. 2007, p.5; Stroebe, 2000; Stroebe & de Witt, 1996); • While the health belief model theory can predict adherence in certain situations, it does not provide for the reduction of risky behaviors that are more linked to social or unconscious motivations (Blackwell, 1992, p. 165).

Source: (The Author based on literature).

Differences Between Helth Belief Model and Social Cognitive Theory

The difference between the health belief model and SCT is that it has at least two contributions to the explanation of health-related behavior that do not exist in the health belief model (HBM), namely the emphasis on the various sources of information such as the informative and motivational role of reinforcement and the role of learning by observation (modeling / imitation), as well as the introduction of the concept of effectiveness (expectation of effectiveness) different from the expectations of the results, which is the assessment made by the person who a certain behavior will lead to a certain result, which is similar in HBM to the "perceived benefits" (Rosenstock, 1988, p. 178).

For example: For a person to quit smoking (behavior) for health reasons (results), she/he must believe that cessation will benefit their health (expectation of results) and that she/he is able to stop (expectation of effectiveness) (adapted from Rosenstock (1988, p. 178). This theory advocates the promotion of self-efficacy, a necessary requirement for the health professional to close the cycle of the therapeutic relationship successfully.

Associated with this self-efficacy is the confidence established in the therapeutic relationship, which leads the patient to know how to perform the task or action that results from health instructions and, therefore, from adherence. In addition, the motivation generated, which in turn, is also the result of demonstrated self-efficacy (Figure 3).

Figure 3. Expectation, behavior, and outcomes
Source: (Based on Bandura, 1977)

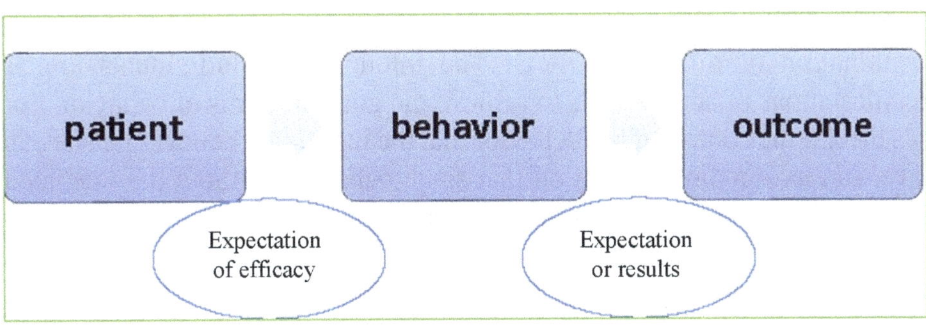

REASONED ACTION THEORY AND PLANNED BEHAVIOR THEORY (AZJEN & FISHBEIN, 1970; FISHBEIN & AZJEN, 1975)

Reasoned Action Theory (Azjen & Fishbein, 1980; Fishbein & Azjen, 1975) highlights the role of social cognitions in the form of subjective norms (individual beliefs), including both the beliefs and the assessments that are made these same beliefs (Ogden, 2004, p. 49).

The importance of this theory is revealed by the fact that it integrates the individual in his/her social context, assigning a role to values and thus contrasting with the traditional and rational approach to behaviors (Ogden, 2004, p. 49).

The Theory of Reasoned Action (TRA) was the first cognitive model that included measures of individuals' cognitions about their social world, that is, the importance of the social context, through subjective norms (Ogden, 2004, p. 237). The TRA explains about 25% of variance in behavior from intention alone and explains slightly less than 50% of variance in intentions (Munro et al., 2007, p. 3).

The TRA was subsequently extended in Ajzen's (1991) Theory of Planned Behavior (TPB).

The TPB is an extension of the theory of reasoned action (Ajzen & Fishbein, 1970; Fishbein & Ajzen, 1975) made necessary by the original models' limitations in dealing with behaviors over which people have incomplete volitional control (Azjen, 1991, p. 181)

The TPB posits that, in addition to attitudes toward the behavior and subjective social norms, there is a third factor, perceived behavioral control (Cobley & Shulz, 2013, p. 189).

Also, TPB highlights the behavioral intentions that result from the combination of different beliefs. The intentions of individuals are as manifestations of action plans to achieve the goals in terms of behavior. For this theory, the control of the behavior that the individual believes he/she can have, can have a direct effect on that same behavior, without the mediated effect of the behavioral intentions (Ogden, 2004, p. 50).

The theory of planned behavior states that the intentions to have a certain behavior result from the following beliefs: 1) attitudes towards behaviors, which are the positive and negative evaluations made about that behavior, the subjective norms that integrate the perception of norms and existing social pressures (for example, criticism from family or friends) and behavioral control, which consists in the individual perceiving that he/she can master his/her behavior through internal control factors (for example, not smoking) (Ogden, 2004, p. 50).

Schwarzer (1992) criticizes the theory of planned behavior because it states that the temporal element is not considered and that the order of the different beliefs and the direction of causality are not described. However, according to Ogden (2004), this model includes a level of irrationality, that is, evaluations, as well as considering social and environmental factors (normative beliefs) and attending to past behavior (p. 51).

PROTECTION MOTIVATION THEORY (ROGERS, 1975, 1983)

The Protection Motivation Theory developed by Rogers (1975, 1983) is a cognitive model and includes additional factors to the health belief model (Ogden, 2004, p. 43).

In this theory, the person estimates the severity of the disease (perceived severity) and estimates the chance of contracting the disease (perceived vulnerability).

This theory postulates that the one generated by this estimate influences attitudes and behaviors when the person assesses the severity of the danger.

The person tends to execute the recommendations in order to remove the threat (effectiveness of the response) and has a belief in his/her ability to successfully carry out the recommended action (self-effectiveness).

The model includes four components: 1) severity (e.g., smoking causes cancer); 2) vulnerability (e.g., the chances of having cancer for those who smoke are high); 3) effectiveness of the response (e.g., if I quit smoking would improve my health), 4) self-efficacy (e.g., I believe I can quit smoking). With these components it would be possible to predict the intentions of behavior (e.g., I intend to change my behavior).

According to Rogers (1975), there are three elements, namely, 1) the severity, 2) the vulnerability and 3) the fear that involve the threat assessment, while the 4) effectiveness of the response and 5) self-efficacy are associated with the coping assessment, this with the ability to cope with the disease (Ogden, 2004, p. 44).

There may be a change in behavior when appealing to individuals' fears. There are thus threw components of fear: 1) the magnitude of the evil in each event; 2) the probability of events to occur and 3) the effectiveness of the protective response. Thus, there may be a change in behavior when individuals' fears are appealed, with a multiple combination for the intensity of protection resulting in an activity that results from a desire for self-protection (Munro et al. 2007, p. 6). According to a meta-analysis carried out by Munro and other researchers (2007), this is the only theory with a broad cognitive perspective that explicitly uses the costs and benefits of a behavior (p. 6).

The most recent version of the motivation protection theory, assumes that motivation to protect a person from a certain danger is a positive linear function of beliefs in which 1) the threat is severe; 2) the person is personally vulnerable, 3) the person may have a coping response (self-efficacy), 4) the coping response is effective (response effectiveness).

People do not consider themselves able of performing the action without having the means to do so (Bandura, 1997; Munro et al., 2007, p. 6).

Criticisms to the Protection Motivation Theory

The criticisms to the Protection Motivation Theory are:

1. It does not consider usual behaviors, nor does it include a role for social and environmental factors (Ogden, 2004, p. 45).
2. Not all environmental and cognitive variables that can have an impact on changing attitudes are identified (such as pressure to conform to social norms).
3. A meta-analysis found moderate effects on behaviors (Floyd, Prentice-Dunn & Rogers, 2000).
4. It is necessary to consider the influence of social, psychological and environmental factors on motivation.

Pechmann says (2001) when efficacy (coping) is perceived to be very poor, increasing risk perceptions may inadvertently lower intentions because people feel they have no recourse and react defensively (p. 190).

Floyd, Prentice-Dunn and Rogers (2000) report that the increased severity of the threat, the vulnerability of the threat, the effectiveness of the response and self-efficacy facilitated adaptive intentions or behavior. On the other hand, decreases in rewards for non-adaptive responses and the costs of an adapted response have increased adaptive intentions or behavior (Table 4).

Table 4. Criticism to the cognitive theories

Some of the criticism to the cognitive theories (Ingham et al., 1991; Munro et al., 2007; Ogden, 2012; Weinstein, 1983) are based on the follow ideas: 1- They do not consider the behavioral skills necessary to ensure adherence (Munro et al., 2007, p. 4); 2- These theories pay little attention to the origin of beliefs and how these beliefs can influence other behaviors (Weinstein, 1983); 3- These theories ignore other impacting factors such as the power of relationships and social reputation (Ingham, Woodcock & Stennerk, 1991); 4- The possibility of risk may involve more than one person; 5- They criticize because they focus on a single threat or preventive behavior instead of including competing threats (Weinstein, 1983).

Source: (The authors based on Ingham et al., 1991; Munro et al., 2007; Ogden, 2012; Weinstein, 1988)

THE SELF-REGULATORY PERSPECTIVE

The self-regulatory perspective assumes that subjects are motivated to avoid and treat disease threats, and that they are active and self-regulating problem solvers (Bandura, 1969; Leventhal, Meyer & Nerenz, 1980; Rosenstock, Stercher & Beckr, 1988; Rotter, 1954).

From the perspective of self-regulation (Leventhal, Leventhal & Schaefer, 1992) it is necessary to examine the patient's subjective experience in the face of health threats, in order to understand his/her way of adapting to these threats (Munro et al., 2007, p. 8).

Individuals form cognitive representations of health and threats (and related emotional responses) and combine new information. It is these representations (in a complex interaction with environmental perceptions, symptoms and beliefs about the cause of the disease) that "guide" (Munro et al., 2007, p. 8) the patient in choosing strategies to deal with health threats and influence results (Munro et al., 2007, p. 8).

LEVEL PERSPECTIVE

The Transteoric Model (Prochaska & DiClemente, 1983; Sutton, 2000) is the most relevant model among those who take the perspective of "levels".

The model presents a different qualitative number of discrete levels and their processes of change, as well as the reasons why people move between these levels, going back and revisiting the previous levels (Munro et al. 2007, pp. 58-59).

Thus, the model raises the hypothesis of several qualitatively different stages and processes of change, where subjects go through these stages, typically falling back and revisiting previous stages before success (Prochaska & DiClemente, 1983; Sutton, 2000).

In this perspective of the existence of several levels, Prochaska and DiClemente (1982) refer that, before making changes, people evolve on a series of levels, from pre-contemplation to maintenance of action. The theory offers an "integrated perspective on the structure of intentional change where perceptions about the advantages and disadvantages of behavior are crucial to behavior change.

Criticism to The Transtheoretical Model

Criticism to the transtheoretical model is made at its levels, its coverage, definitions and descriptions of the change (Munro et al., p. 9).

Analyzing Bandura's critical perspective on this model, Munro et al. (2007, p. 9) state that the theory violates the three basic assumptions of stage theories, namely: a) qualitative transformations across discrete stages; b) invariant sequence of change and c) non-reversibility.

Munro et al. (2007) suggest, following Bandura's (1997) perspective, that the human function is too multifaceted to fit into these separate and discrete levels, and argue that thinking by levels constrains the objective of interventions promoters of change (Munro et al., 2007, p. 9)

Sutton (1997) also states that the definitions of levels in the model are "false" and that the time periods assigned by each level are arbitrary. For Munro et al. (2007, p. 10) the strength of this theory is that it allows to make interventions tailored to individual needs.

CONCLUSION

Health communication models and theories are used to understand, explain and predict the beliefs, attitudes, intentions and behaviors of individuals, groups and mass audiences (Cameron, 2009, p. 309), allowing professionals to better understand their interactions with patients and their behavior (Cameron, 2009, p. 309).

The perspective of individual cognition, the assessment of risks by the individual of their beliefs, barriers, knowledge are evaluated in parallel with all the influences of the environmental context in which the individual is inserted or reflected in his/her conduct.

Theories seek to resolve issues associated with the attitudes and behaviors of individuals, with a strong communicative component in all of them.

Communication becomes the permanent factor in all solutions for improving the behavior and health of the individual, even if this component is not listed in the various models and theories developed. Without communication, it is impossible to pass any message and for the patient to understand both verbal and non-verbal language are critical factors in the assimilation, understanding and use of health information and the correct navigability in the system.

REFERENCES

Airhihenbuwa, C. O. (1995). *Health and culture: Beyond the Western paradigm*. Sage Publications.

Ajzen, I., & Fishbein. (1970). The prediction of behaviour from attitudinal and normative beliefs. *Journal of Personality and Social Psychology*, *6*, 466–487.

Ajzen, I. (1991). The theory of planned behavior. *Organizational Behavior and Human Decision Processes*, *50*(2), 179–211. doi:10.1016/0749-5978(91)90020-T

Argyle, M. (Ed.). (1981). *Social skills and health*. Methuen.

Argyle, M. (1994). *The psychology of interpersonal behaviour*. Penguin.

Armitage, C. J., & Conner, M. (2000). Social cognition models and health behaviour: A structured review. *Psychology & Health*, *15*(2), 173–189. doi:10.1080/08870440008400299

Bandura, A. (1977). *Social learning theory*. Prentice Hall.

Bandura, A. (1977). Self-efficacy: Toward a unifying theory of behavioral change. *Psychological Review*, *84*(2), 191–215. doi:10.1037/0033-295X.84.2.191 PMID:847061

Bandura, A. (1986). *Social foundations of thought and action: A social cognitive theory*. Prentice-Hall.

Bandura, A. (1997). *Self-Efficacy: The exercice of control*. W.H. Freeman and Company.

Becker, M. H. (1974). The health belief model and personal health behavior. *Health Education Monographs*, *2*(4), 324–508. doi:10.1177/109019817400200407

Becker, M. H., & Rosenstock, I. M. (1984). Compliance with medical advice. In A. Steptoe & A. Mathews (Eds.), *Health care and Human Behavior*. Academic Press.

Bernhardt, J. M. (2004). Communication at the core of effective public health. *American Journal of Public Health*, *84*(12), 2051–2053. doi:10.2105/AJPH.94.12.2051 PMID:15569948

Blackwell, B. (1992). Compliance. *Psychotherapy and Psychosomatics*, *58*(3-4), 161–169. doi:10.1159/000288624 PMID:1488500

Cameron, K. A. (2009). A practitioner's guide to persuasion: An overview of 15 selected persuasion theories, models and frameworks. *Patient Education and Counseling*, *74*(3), 309–317. doi:10.1016/j.pec.2008.12.003 PMID:19136229

Chaffee, S. H., & Rogers, E. V. (Eds.). (1997). *The beginings of communication study in America. A personal memoir*. Sage Publications.

Cobley, P., & Schulz, P. J. (2013). *Theories and models of communication. Handbook of Communication Science* (Vol. 1). De Gruyer Mouton. doi:10.1515/9783110240450

Dance, F. E. X. (1970). The "concept" of Communication. *Journal of Communication*, *20*(2), 201–210. doi:10.1111/j.1460-2466.1970.tb00877.x

Engel, G. L. (1977). The need for a new medical model: A challenge for biomedicine. *Science*, *196*(4286), 129–136. doi:10.1126cience.847460 PMID:847460

Engel, G. L. (1981). The clinical application of the biopshychosocial model. *The Journal of Medicine and Philosophy*, *6*(2), 101–123. doi:10.1093/jmp/6.2.101 PMID:7264472

Fishbein, M., & Ajzen, I. (1975). *Belief, Attitude, Intention, and Behavior: An Introduction to Theory and Research*. Addison-Wesley.

Floyd, D. L., Prentice-Dunn, S., & Rogers, R. W. (2000). A Meta-Analysis of Research on Protection Motivation Theory. *Journal of Applied Social Psychology*, *30*(2), 407–429. doi:10.1111/j.1559-1816.2000.tb02323.x

Gebhardt, W. A., & Maes, S. (2001). Integrating social-psychological frameworks for health behaviour research. *American Journal of Health Behavior*, *25*(6), 528–536. doi:10.5993/AJHB.25.6.2 PMID:11720300

Hall, S. (1980). Encoding/decoding. In S. Hall, D. Hobson, A. Lowe, & P. Willis (Eds.), *Culture, media, language: Working papers in cultural studies* (pp. 128–138). Hutchinson.

Hayes, J. (2005). *Interpersonal skills at work*. New York: Taylor & Francis e-library.

Hovland, C., Janis, I., & Kelley, H. (1953). *Communication and persuasion*. Yale University Press.

Ingham, R., Woodcock, A., & Stenner, K. (1991). Getting to know you… Young people's knowledge of their partners at first intercourse. *Journal of Community & Applied Social Psychology*, *1*(2), 117–132. doi:10.1002/casp.2450010206

Ishikawa, H., & Kiuchi, T. (2010). Health literacy and health communication. *BioPsychoSocial Medicine*, *4*(18), 1–5. PMID:21054840

Kaplan, A. (1964). *The conduct of inquiry. Methodology for behavioral science*. Transaction.

Katz, E. (1957). The Two-Step Flow of Communication: An Up-To-Date Report on an Hypothesis. *Public Opinion Quarterly*, *21*(1), 61. doi:10.1086/266687

Katz, E., & Lazarsfeld, P. (1955). *Personal influence: the part played by people in the flow of mass communication*. Free Press.

Keller, C., Fleury, J., Gregor-Holt, N., & Thompson, T. (1999). Predictive ability of social cognitive theory in exercise research: An integrated literature review. *The Online Journal of Knowledge Synthesis for Nursing*, *5*(6), 2. doi:10.1111/j.1524-475X.1999.00019.x PMID:12870090

Keller, D. B., Sarkar, U., & Schillinger, D. (2014). Health literacy and information exchange in medical settings. In L. R. Martin & M. R. DiMatteo (Eds.), *The Oxford handbook of health communication, behavior change, and treatment adherence* (pp. 23–37). Oxford University Press.

Kerlinger, F. N. & Lee, H. B. (2000). *Foundations of behavioral research*. Wadsworth: Thomson Learning.

Kickbusch, I. (2019). Health promotion 4.0. *Health Promotion International*, *34*(2), 179–181. doi:10.1093/heapro/daz022 PMID:30939200

Kreps, G. L. (2001). History of health communication. In T. L. Thompson (Ed.), *Encyclopedia of Health Communication*. Sage Publications. doi:10.4135/9781483346427.n219

Kreps, G. L. (2009). Applying Weick's Model of organizing to health care and health promotion: Highlighting the central role of health Communication. *Patient Education and Counseling, 74*(3), 347–355. doi:10.1016/j.pec.2008.12.002 PMID:19150591

Kurtz, S., Silverman, J., & Draper, J. (2005). *Teaching and learning communication skills in medicine*. Radcliff Publishing.

Lasswell, H. (1948). Structure and Function of Communication in Society. In L. Bryson (Ed.), *The communication of ideas*. Institute for Religious and Social Studies.

Lawrence, W. (2008). Advancing health literacy: Building health communication from the patient side. *Journal of Communication in Healthcare, 1*(2), 182–193. doi:10.1179/cih.2008.1.2.182

Lazarsfeld, P. E., Berelson, B., & Gaudet, G. (1944). *The people's choice: How the voter makes up his mind in a presidential campaign*. Duell, Sloan and Pearce.

Leape, L. L. (1994). Error in medicine. *Journal of the American Medical Association, 272*(23), 1851–1857. doi:10.1001/jama.1994.03520230061039 PMID:7503827

Leonard, M., Graham, S., & Bonacum, D. (2004). The human factor: the critical importance of effective teamwork and communication in providing safe care. *Quality Safe Health, 13*(1), i85-i90. Doi: doi:10.1136/qshc.2004.0110033

Lewin, S. A., Skea, Z. C., Entwistle, V., Zwarenstein, M., & Dick J. (2001). Interventions for providers to promote a patient-centred approach in clinical consultations. *Cochrane Database Syst ver, 4*, CD003267.

Littlejohn, S. W. (1999). *Fundamentos teóricos da comunicação humana*. Zahar Editores.

Munro, S., Lewin, S., Swart, T., & Volmink, J. (2017). Review of health behavior theories: How useful are these for developing interventions to promote long-term medication adherence for TB and HIV/AIDS. *BMC Public Health, 7*(1), 104. doi:10.1186/1471-2458-7-104 PMID:17561997

Ogden, J. (2004). *Psicologia da saúde*. Climepsi Editores.

Pearson, A., Vaughan, B., & Fitzgerald, M. (2005). *Nursing models for practice*. Butterworth-Heinemann.

Pechmann, C. (2001). A Comparison of Health Communication Models: Risk Learning Versus Stereotype Priming. *Media Psychology*, *3*(2), 189–210. doi:10.1207/S1532785XMEP0302_04

Prochaska, J. O., & DiClemente, C. C. (1983). Stages and processes of a self-change of smoking: Toward an integrative model of change. *Journal of Consulting and Clinical Psychology*, *51*(3), 390–395. doi:10.1037/0022-006X.51.3.390 PMID:6863699

Redding, C. A., Rossi, J. S., Rossi, S. R., Velicer, W. F., & Prochaska, J. O. (2000). Health behaviour models. *Int Electr J Health Education, 3,* 180-193. Retrieved from https://www.oiiq.org/SanteCoeur/docs/redding_iejhe_vol3_nospecial_2000.pdf

Rogers, R. M., & Kinkaid, D. L. (1981). *Communication Networks: Toward new paradigms for research.* Free Press.

Rogers, R. W. (1975). A protection motivation theory of fear appeals and attitude change. *The Journal of Psychology*, *91*(1), 93–114. doi:10.1080/00223980.1975.9915803 PMID:28136248

Rosenstock, I. M. (1974). Historical origins of the health belief model. *Health Education Monographs*, *2*(4), 328–335. doi:10.1177/109019817400200403

Rosenstock, I. M. (1990). The health belief model: Explaining health behavior through expectancies. In *Health behaviour and health education*. In K. Glanz, F. M. Lewis, & B. K. Rimer (Eds.), *Health behavior and health education: theory, research, and practice* (pp. 39–62). Josey-Bass.

Rosenstock, I. M., Strcher, V. J., & Becker, M. H. (1988). Social learning theory and health belief model. *Health Education Quartely*, 175-183.

Ross, E., & Deverell, A. (2004). *Psychosocial approaches to health, illness and disability: A reader for health care professionals.* Van Schaik.

Rotter, J. B. (1966). Generalized expectancies for internal versus external control of reinforcement. *Psychological Monographs*, *80*(1), 1–28. doi:10.1037/h0092976 PMID:5340840

Sawyer, S. M., & Aroni, R. A. (2003). Sticky issue of adherence. *Journal of Paediatrics and Child Health, 39*(1), 2–5. doi:10.1046/j.1440-1754.2003.00081.x PMID:12542804

Schramm, W. (1954). *Process and effects of mass communication*. University of Illinois Press.

Schramm, W. (1955). How communication works. In W. Schramm (Ed.), *The process and effects of mass communication*. University of Illinois Press.

Schwarzer, R. (1992). Self-efficacy in the adoption and maintenance of health beahaviors: Theoretical approaches and a new model. In R. Schwarzer (Ed.), *Self-efficacy: Thought control of action* (pp. 217–243). Herisphere.

Spitzberg, B. H. (2013). (Re) Introducing communication competence to the health professions. *Journal of Public Health Research, 2*(3, e23), 126–135. doi:10.4081/jphr.2013.e23 PMID:25170494

Strecher, V., & Rosenstock, I. (1997). The health belief model. In *A. Baum, S. Newman, J. Weinman, R. West & C. McManus (Eds.), Cambridge Handbook of psychology, health and medicine* (pp. 113–116). Cambridge University Press.

Stroebe, W. (2000). *Social psychology and health*. Open University Press.

Stroebe, W., & de Wit, J. (1996). Health impairing behaviours. In G. R. Semin & K. Fiedler (Eds.), *Applied Social Psychology* (pp. 113–143). Sage. doi:10.4135/9781446250556.n5

Sutton, S. (1997). Theory of Planned Behavior. In *A. Baum, S. Newman, J. Weinman, R. West & C. McManus (Eds.), Cambridge Handbook of psychology, health and medicine* (pp. 180–182). Cambridge University Press.

Szasz, T., & Hollender, M. (1956). A contribution to the philosophy of medicine: The basic models of doctor-patient relationship. *Archives of Internal Medicine, 97*, 585–592. PMID:13312700

Szasz, T. S., & Hollender, M. H. (1956). A contribution to the philosophy of medicine: The basic models of the doctor-patient relationship. *A.M.A. Archives of Internal Medicine, 97*(5), 585–592. doi:10.1001/archinte.1956.00250230079008 PMID:13312700

U.S. Department of Health and Human Services. (2004). Making Health Communication Programs Work. Washington, DC: National Cancer Institute.

Wallston, K. A., & Wallston, B. S. (1982). Who is responsible for your health? The construct os health locus of control. In G. S. Sanders & J. Suls (Eds.), *Social pshychology of health and Ilness* (pp. 65–95). Lawrencer Erlbaum.

Weber, D. (2016). Medical hegemony. *International Journal of Complementary & Alternative Medicine*, *3*(2), 00065. doi:10.15406/ijcam.2016.03.00065

Weinstein, N. (1983). Reducing unrealistic optimism about illness susceptibility. *Health Psychology*, *2*(1), 11–20. doi:10.1037/0278-6133.2.1.11

WHO. (2004). *What are the advantages and disadvantages of restructuring a health care system to be more focused on primary care*. WHO.

WHO. (2009). *Background Note: regional preparatory meeting on promoting health literacy*. UN ECOSOC.

WHO. (2019). Improving health through health literacy. *Journal of The Who Regional Office for Europe Public Health - Panorama, 5*(2-3), 123-329.

Wiemann, J. W. (1977). Explication and test of a Model of Comunicative Competence. *Spring, 3*(3), 195-213.

Wright, K. B., Rosenberg, J., Egbert, N., Ploeger, N. A., Bernard, D. R., & King, S. (2013). Communication Competence, social support and depression among college students: A model of facebook and face-to-face support network influence. *Journal of Health Communication*, *18*(1), 41–57. doi:10.1080/10810730.2012.688250 PMID:23030518

Chapter 3
Communication on All Sides:
Models of Health Communication

Cristina Vaz de Almeida
ISCSP, University of Lisbon, Portugal

ABSTRACT

People seek to solve problems, either through cognitive or emotional means or both, including behavioral ones. Health professionals have a specific mission to care and heal and they do so through their skills, behaviors, knowledge, and beliefs. To fulfill this mission of promoting satisfactory results in health relationships, the therapeutic relationship can be approached in several ways and based on different models. If there are trends of great centralization of consultation in the health profession, an effort has been made for patient-centered decision. The path of this relationship in health allows for a mutually beneficial interaction with commitment and better health results. Without wishing to be exhaustive and knowing that many models are left out, the authors explore the evolution of models applied to health throughout history.

INTRODUCTION

In the consultation, the patient is in a state of tension and wants a relief response to this feeling, even if it is not directly related to the disease (Engel, 1981, p. 102).

Adults with low health literacy pose significantly less health care questions (four on average compared to six with high literacy) (Katz et al., 2007, p. 782), which can affect their ability to learn conditions and medical treatments

DOI: 10.4018/978-1-7998-4396-2.ch003

(Katz et al., 2007, p. 782). Moreover, many times, the patient's expectation is that the other party, the health professional, has the professional competence and the motivation to provide this relief.

There is also tension in the therapeutic relationship, often brought by this patient-system, who brings with him, for consultation or therapeutic interaction, not only himself, but his family, the influences of his neighborhood and community, his psychosocial, family, economic status influence this relational process that converges in the consultation (Pendleton et al., 2003).

For example, managing life on a low income is very stressful, has a huge impact on the body and the regulatory system, and is associated with unhealthy behaviors (Buck, Baylis, Dougall, & Robertson, 2018, p. 21). In this context, Teixeira (2006, p. 410) reflects on the consequences of the increase of social inequalities and situations of social fragility, oppression and violence that "facilitated the appearance of victimization behaviors, which often correspond to an experience of lack personal power characterized by a reduced critical conscience, a fatalistic attitude and a posture of social conformism, which causes an inability to construct meanings and develop projects (p. 410).

On the other hand, patient brings to the therapeutic relationship needs, beliefs, and senses that he wants to be satisfied. In this sense, the entire communication process implies a good identification of relevant objectives, in which the intervention models allow to sustain the interventions and the strategic alignments of the consultation with a view to immediate and future results.

Based on the therapeutic relation and on the path traced by the biopsychosocial model (Engel, 1981), there are central tasks for the health professional. (Table 1)

Table 1. Three central tasks of the health professional

Step 1: Learning how and what the patient felt and experienced. **Step 2:** Involve the patient's participation. **Step 3:** Request the patient's cooperation for tension relief activities and correct actions because the patient's responsibilities and tasks are complementary to those of the health professional.

Source: (Based on Engel, 1981)

Patients, with some frequency, even if they are activated to make shared decisions, voluntarily delegate their health decisions to professionals, such as knowledge about subjects (Levinson, Kao & Thisted, 2005, p. 531).

If a mechanism does not exist that stimulates the situational motivation to solve a problem, the patient's passive attitude in the acquisition, selection and transmission of information will be maintained, considered as dependent variables in the problem solving theory (Kim & Grunig, 2011).

Thus, even if the patient wants to delegate this responsibility for the decision to the professional, it is necessary to move towards appropriate and conscious decision making. Communication is a bridge to problems resolution on consultation.

BEYOND THE BIOMEDICAL MODEL

The ability to actively involve the patient in their health care, allowing them to decide, presupposes the adoption of models that go beyond the biomedical model.

Biopsychosocial and cognitive models that consider motivation, social norms, beliefs and self-efficacy value the human model and its complexity, showing what neurosciences have been warning about the complexity of changing behaviors.

Decision making by the patient also activates parts of his brain and encourages active behaviors, which remain even after the consultation. In this multi-level environment, the patient moves between environments - consultation - family - other healthcare providers - community - system. For example, in the United Kingdom, there has been greater investment in the knowledge of patients and the public in recent years, with a clear commitment to greater patient involvement, demonstrated in 2001 with the publication of the "Specialist Patient" (Department of Health, 2001). The knowledge and experience of patients, especially with chronic diseases, implies them as active participants. Thus, in addition to these patients with chronic diseases being the recipients of care, they can also be the main decision makers in the treatment process (U.S. Department of Health, 2001). In this sense, the empowerment of patients to assume some responsibility in the management of their conditions also allows for a strengthening of doctor-patient relations, particularly in the field of shared decision. (Table 2)

A research on patient participation and duration of consultations, was conducted by Greenfield, Kaplan and Ware (1985), with an experimental group (n = 23) and a control group (n = 22), carried out at the Center for Ulcer Research and Education. The meetings between health professional and patient were audio recorded, with the patients self-completing two questionnaires (one at home and one after the consultation), measuring health status, involvement in medical decision and knowledge and satisfaction with care. (p. 521).

Table 2. Shared Decision

The main characteristics of the shared decision are:
Step 1: The involvement of at least two parties (the patient and the professional) in decision making
Step 2: Sharing information between the parties
Step 3: Making a treatment decision based on a mutual agreement

Source: (Based on Charles, Gafni and Whelan,1997)

The study by Greenfield, Kaplan and Ware (1985) took place in an outpatient clinic of a Hospital in Los Angeles, California, with 8 doctors, and 200 patients with peptic ulcer, of which 45 people under 75 years old were selected, who did at least one appointment in the last six months. The results on the duration of the consultation in the experimental group and in the control group did not change significantly (16 minutes), however the two groups differed in the way they used their time. In the experimental group, patients were more significantly involved in interactions and were more assertive in the direct flow of communication and in the professional's behaviors (p. 523).

Patient-centered communication is a highly recommended model and a key element in interpersonal behavior between doctors and patients. Lewin et al. (2001) said that training in patient-centredness for healthcare providers may improve communication with patients, enable clarification of patients' concerns in consultations and improve satisfaction with care (p. 2).

Cegala, McNeilis, Mcgeee and Jonas (1995), in an experiment that was supported by video and a post-consultation questionnaire, studied how 16 doctors and 32 North American patients process information through interactions. The results indicate that the concerns of both stakeholders in the medical consultation are identical, with patients significantly distancing themselves from doctors in two categories: negative focus on interaction and negative provision of information (p. 195).

Patients assumed that they were unhappy with their information and that of the doctor (Cegala et al., 1995, p. 196), suggesting that it is a matter to improve in medical consultations.

The relationship between the health professional and the patient must be balanced and the patients, motivated, must recognize that the professional is genuinely interested in them and in their care, and both reach a common platform in the care process (Kaplan et al., 1997, p . S49). However, there are many cases of professional hegemony, in which there is an implicit position of the professional as the first influence to shape the patient's sense of decision (Nimmon & Regehr, 2018, p. 2).

As a result of this reflection and literature review, we can show that, through the development of interpersonal relationships, based on solid structures of communicative and clinical skills, health professionals are able to offer health care that meets the needs and the essence of what patient seeks in the health relationship.

COMMUNICATION IN HEALTH

Communication allows a positive domino effect of the results of the consultation.

Communication transforms the way people see health as a "fountain of hope or a font of despair" (Williams & Calnan, 1996, p. 1609).

Communication between professional and patient is an interpersonal, communicational, critical, care-giving process (Kreps, 2001, p. 598), which takes place within a specific cultural framework (Cline & Mcenzie, 1998).

Health communication is a strong promoter of public health in conjunction with other health promoting factors when it is assertive, clear, positive, appropriate, permanent or always reinforced in positive behaviors (Vaz de Almeida, 2018, 2019) that motivate and help in perception and then in memorization and with themes that interest the individual and the community.

The National Cancer Institute and the Centers for Disease Control and Prevention use the following definition for health communication: The study and use of communication strategies to inform and influence individual and community decisions that enhance health (U.S. Department of Health and Human Services, 2004).

A patient which is informed and aware of the attitudes, behaviors and actions should adopt, the information out of the consultation, and share it with family, friends, spreading knowledge and reinforcing behaviors.

In this dynamic process of interpersonal therapeutic relationship, the languages used, verbal and non-verbal, shape the development of that person's health history.

With a wide scope and in a circular view, Watzlawick et al. (1967) claim that "all communication affects behavior" (p. 19) and that all behavior in an interactional situation is communication (Watzlawick et al., 1967, p. 46), even when it is not successful (Watzlawick et al., 1967, p. 45).

As much as the individual tries, "it is impossible for him not to communicate" (Watzlawick et al., 1967, p. 45). As Ruesh and Bateson (1951) refer, we can never refrain from communicating, as human beings and members of a society, with our organs and senses constantly on the alert and never resting, so "we are biologically obliged to communicate" (Ruesh & Bateson, 1951, p. 7).

In this great diversity of reflections on its characteristics, functions and effects, several authors describe communication as discourse, understanding, interaction, relationship, social process, reduction of uncertainty (Salter, 1949; Wolpe, 1968), connection, acquisition, transfer and information retention (Ruesch & Bateson, 1951, p. 7), response, stimulus, intention, power (Dance, 1970, pp. 204-208).

Kim and Grunig (2011) reinforce the importance of the dimension of organized communication for problem solving, in which feedback or feedback means that there is control of the action through the incorporation of information about the effects (Ruesch, 1956, p. 161). It appears, therefore, that there is an ethical imperative in communication, in order to avoid conflict and its consequences.

In addition, Dance (1970) had already mentioned that "there is a common theme that cuts across all definitions (of communication) which is the notion of "process" (p. 208) and of system (Engel, 1981; Littlejohn, 1982; Pendleton, Schofield, Tate & Havelock, 2003; Ruesch & Bateson, 1951). Berlo (1977), for example, describes, operationally (p. 13), that "communication is a process", of "organization of relationships" (p. 14), including the "complex organization of an individual or groups of individuals" (p. 13), which implies a "change over time" (p. 18) and "activities that take root in natural events, that is, symbols that constitute the sensory messages we exchange" (p. 19).

Frey, Botan and Kreps (2000) also adopt a procedural version of communication: they refer to it as the process of managing messages and media, with the aim of creating meaning, being itself considered as a sequence of objectives, responses and effects (Hulsman, 2009, p. 303). In this procedural line, Littlejohn (1982), when listing the theories of communication, states that they can be of two types: those that explain nature and essence, as a whole, and those that explain the parts of the process (p. 41).

It is in the specific *medium* of social and cultural interaction of reciprocal creation of meaning (Sherko, Sotiri & Lika, 2013, p. 457) that this unique framework (consultation) of someone who has the (professional) expertise in face of biological need is structured, psychological and emotional manifestation of the other (the patient) and where there needs to be a result (prevention, promotion or health care).

The generated moment wich combines rational and emotional factors, allows effects that propagate outside the consultation in a structure of multiple influences (social, economic and cultural framework). There must be a concerted effort between the sender and the receiver so that the codes are perceptible, with a view to understanding by the part of the patient, health instructions, and on the part of the professional the understanding that the other party actually understood what was said.

One of the key elements of the understanding and adherence process is the attitudes and behaviors of health professional and the communication established with the patient (Bittner, Jonietz, Bittner, Beickert & Harendza, 2014).

Interpretative theories are phenomenological and pragmatic regarding people's intention for action (LitlleJohn, 1999, p. 561). The interpretivists share the characteristics of common pragmatism, phenomenology and hermeneutical heritage for whom the social world is constituted through actions and experiences.

In human interaction there is a shared, meaningful and real understanding, where people's ideas are respected and human diversity is emphasized (LittleJohn, 1999, p. 561). Hermeneutics is based on a philosophy of interpretation and understanding, which aims to examine how language and dialogue contribute to the process of interpretation. (LittleJohn, 1999, p. 558).

It is in this urgent need for balance and respect for human beings that the meeting in health takes place (consultation) motivated by those looking for answers and support (patient), even if in a minimal degree of suffering (as occurs, for example, in regular family planning consultations), through the expertise of the other (professional) that reinforces the dialogue between two interactants.

In a dynamic and transactional process of encoding and decoding (Hall, 1980) of messages (of healing and care), relationships in health that produce results beyond the space and time of the consultation grow and mature.

Social reality is built in the minds of social actors, and it is, in part, sociological studies that allow recognizing, expanding, and validating the ways in which individuals interpret and create the social world. (LittleJohn, 1999, p. 557).

In this line of analysis LitlleJohn (1999) enunciates the common characteristics of interpretive theories (p. 561):

1 - Empathic identification: to understand the meaning of communication and social action, the person must assume the role of the one who seeks to understand. The role of the health professional in this dimension of understanding is highlighted, until reaching the subjective awareness of the other. You enter the actor's mind and perspective to discover the reasons, ideas, objectives and circumstances surrounding that person who uses services to find an answer

2 - Intentionality: the capacity for action is the direct manifestation of this intentionality. It is the deepest human desire people share experiences, meanings, interpersonal communication and collective actions.

3 - Reflexivity - the vision of humanity that is based on the reflective power of human beings. Reflexivity is the individual's human capacity to imagine himself through other people's point of view (to imagine himself from the perspective of the other). The person imagines himself using the perspectives of others.

This act of seeing people as their reflexes encourages interpretivists to focus on the construction and reproduction of their social reality, which is subject to a continuous reassessment and reinterpretation.

4 - Nominality / nominative - human beings make their lives meaningful by creating symbols, names, categories, rules for social objects (LitlleJohn, 1999, p. 561).

ENCODING-DECODING: A COMMON BASIS TO BE EFFECTIVE - SCHRAMM (1955) and HALL (1980)

Among the new ways of thinking about communication, some prominent authors such as Schramm (1955) and Hall (1980) stand out in the evaluation of the key elements of the content and effects of the communication process, namely the coding and decoding process (Schramm, 1955; Hall, 1980)

Schramm (1954) highlights the role of the "founding fathers" in the investigation of communication in the United States such as Katz, Berelson, Lazarsfeld, Hovland and Hall (Buttle, 1995, p. 298).

For Schramm (1954), communication is an act of sharing and involves knowledge, experience and culture. More than "something someone does for someone else" (p. 8) is the true fundamental social process (Schramm,

1955, 1960), with an emphasis on the study of culture as a component of the communication effects (Schramm, 1997, p. 115).

In the book on the process and effects of mass communication (Schramm, 1954), the author reinforces that when we communicate, we try to establish a "similarity / commonality" with someone '(1954, p. 3). According to this author, communication involves at least three elements: the source, the message and the recipient.

The source encodes the message and transmits it while the receiver decodes it. The encoding and decoding depend on the individual experience of the sender and the receiver, so there may be distortion of the message at any point in the process, so there is no link between encoding and decoding. If the encoding directly reflects the meaning of the decoding, it is because there was a good result of this "commonality" or similarity.

Schramm (1954) says it is "misleading to think of the communication process as starting somewhere and ending somewhere else" (p. 8) because we are constantly receiving signals and decoding them from the surrounding environment, interpreting those signals and then immediately coding something like Schramm also adds a final element to his model: Feedback, which allows us to reveal how our messages are interpreted.

For Schramm (1954) in an effective communication, coding and decoding are the two essential processes and communication is complete only when the sender receives a feedback from receiver in a constant feedback.

When in 1973 Stuart Hall launched his work «Encoding / Decoding», he again used Schramm's guidelines regarding the symmetrical process existing in each of the participants as encoders / decoders, offering a theoretical basis on how messages are produced and disseminated. It considers four stages: production, circulation, use (distribution and consumption) and reproduction. Each stadium has its limits and possibilities. The process of decoding the message depends, according to Hall on the cultural past, on the economic aspects and personal experiences of the individual. Communication or language is done through codes within the discourse chain.

Hall (1980) associates the encoding of the message with its production, resulting in a system of encoded meanings intended to be understood by the audience. In this process the encoder uses verbal and non-verbal language that can be understood by its recipient, its decoder, that is, its audience.

Decoding is a process of interpreting and translating information by its "audience" who processes the message, "decodes it" and interprets it. t is in this discursive environment that the product moves, as well as being distributed to different audiences/publics.

There is only effective communication when the message is understood as it was proposed by the encoder (hegemonic readind).

When the message is interpreted differently, there are distortions or lack of understanding that there is a "lack of equivalence" between what the encoder intended to transmit and what the decoder understood, and there may be an oppositional reading.

Thus, every moment according to Hall (1980) is necessary to make the whole circuit, but none of the moments guarantees the next moment with which it is articulated. The discursive form of the message has a privileged position in the exchange of communication (from the point of view of circulation) and the moments of encoding and decoding are relatively autonomous in the communication process.

The steps of symmetry or asymmetry (understanding or misunderstanding) depend on the symmetry / asymmetry (equivalence relations) established between the personifications of the product / encoder and the receiver / decoder.

In the Schramm model (1955) and, later, Hall (1980), which focus on encoding /decoding (sender) and encoding/decoding (receiver), it is assumed that communication is a system of constant feedback, in which each participant is simultaneously a communicator that encodes and decodes the message (Ho, 2008, p. 8). In this process, the messages from each individual are changed or affected by feedback from the other participant. The general implication of this binomial is that encoding, and decoding may not be "perfectly symmetrical" (Hall, 1980, p. 54).

What Hall (1980) considered to be "distortions" or "misunderstandings" happens and is augmented by the "lack of equivalence" between the two parties involved in the exchange of communication (Hall, 1980, p. 54). It means that the decoded meaning does not necessarily correspond to the encoded meaning, even despite the use of shared language systems. Decoding can follow a different path than intended (Hall, 1980, p. 67). Therefore, it assumes that the receivers can read between the lines and even reverse the intended direction of the message (oppositional reading), which will compromise the communicational result. This model incorporates fundamental principles to be considered for communicational success (preferential reading): the multiplicity of meanings of the content; the existence of various "interpretive" communities; and the primacy of the recipient in determining meaning (Hall, 1980, p. 67).

According to Hall (1980) and in the perspective of evaluating a "hegemonic position" (p. 59), in which there is a coincidence between the sender's message and its interpretation by the recipient (encoding-decoding), full understanding is promoted. Also, the therapeutic relationship aims to achieve balance, reciprocity, symmetry and equality (Ledingham & Bruning, 1998). In this hegemonic position, health professionals establish a relational basis with the patient, with ambitions of symmetry and equality (centered on the person), in which the dimensions of trust, openness, commitment, involvement and investment are present (Ledingham & Bruning, 1998; Ledingham, 2003).

It was Schramm (1955) who started the process of evaluating communication models, which range from the simplest to the most complex and which represent the steps of coding and decoding between the subjects in a communicative relationship. We then evaluate the four models proposed by this author, from the simplest to the most complex.

Starting from Model 1 (Schramm, 1955, p. 4) the source is a simple "encoder" that emits a signal to its receiver, which represents the "decoder". This model is like the Lasswell Model (1948), which considers the communicative process in a sequence of: Who? Say what? Which channel? To whom? To what effect?

Figure 1. Model 1 - adapted from Schramm, 1955
Source: (Adapted from Ho, 2008; Schramm, 1955)

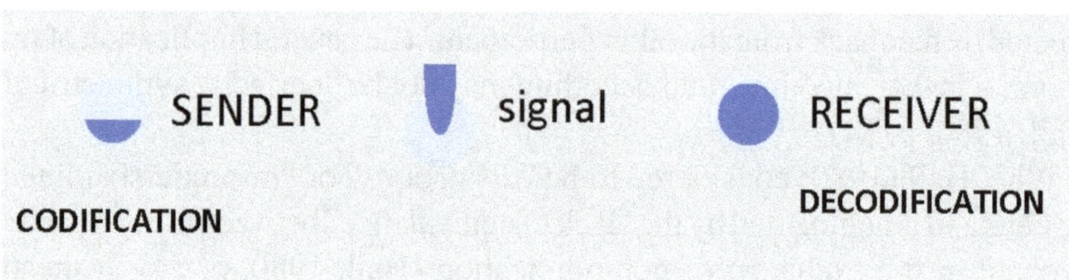

Schramm's model 2 (1955, p. 6) highlights the accumulated experiences (Ho, 2008, p. 7) of the sender and the receiver, as important elements in communication. (Figure 2)

In Schramm's model 3 (1955, p. 7) each participant becomes a sender and receiver, who interprets the received signal and responds based on their experience. (Figure 3)

The Scharmm model has evolved and latest model, communication appears as a system in permanent feedback and each participant is simultaneously a communicator, who encodes and decodes the message, which is dynamic, according to the feedback of the other participant. (Figure 4)

Figure 2. Model 2 of Schramm, 1955
Source: (Adapted from Ho, 2008; Schramm, 1955)

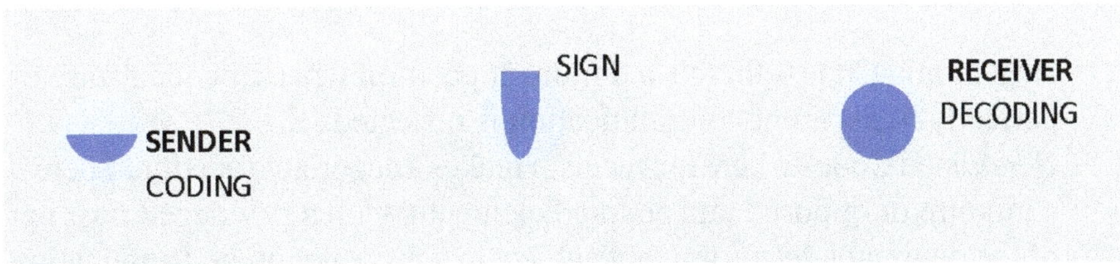

Figure 3. Model 3 of Schramm, 1955
Source: (Adapted from Ho, 2008; Schramm, 1955).

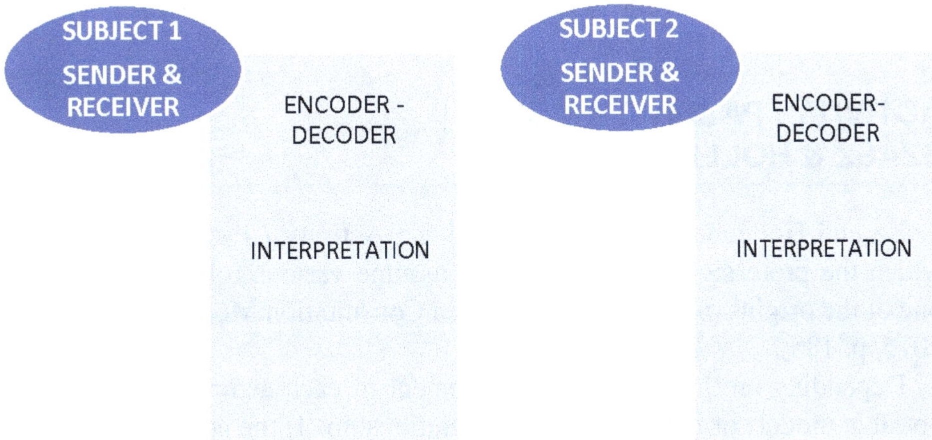

Figure 4. Model 4 of Schramm, 1955
Source: (Adapted from Ho, 2008; Schramm, 1955).

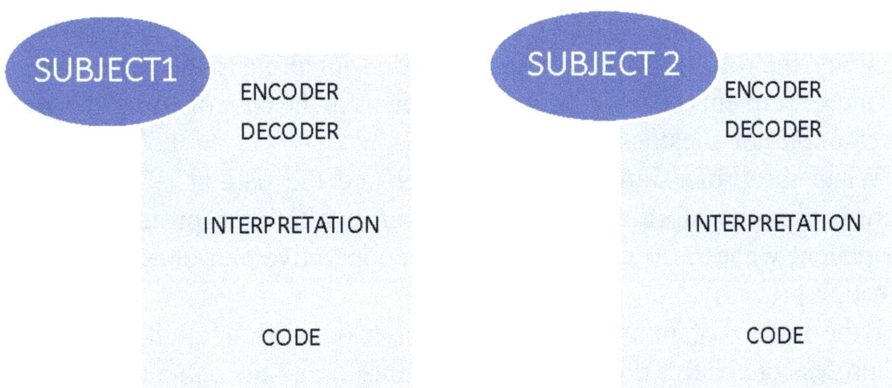

After Schramm (1955), Hall comes later (1980) to present the three hypothetical positions of communication:

1. Hegemonic Code – there's a dominant position where the ideal case of perfectly transparent communication is reflected.
2. Negotiated Code - where the receiver makes a negotiated version. There's a mixture of opposed and adapted elements, with a privileged position of the dominant definition, but subject to a more negotiated application under local conditions.
3. Oppositional Code – This position determines that it is possible for the receiver understand the literal and connotative inflection given by a speech, but to decode in a globally contrary way (opposite).

ACTIVITY / PASSIVITY MODEL | SZASZ & HOLLENDER, 1956

Szasz and Hollender (1956) developed the Activity / Passivity Model in which the professional and the patient assume various roles, having been one of the origins of the Patient-Centered Consultation Model (Cheng et al. 2015, p. 185).

Depending on the degree of involvement of each actor, there are three possible models of the doctor-patient relationship: 1. the activity-passivity, in which the physician is active and the patient is passive, 2. the guidance-co-operation, in which the physician is active, and the patient follows the doctor's advice, and 3. the mutual participation, in which the doctor guides the patient, helping him/her (Szasz & Hollender, 1956).

When the model is based on a "Father - Baby" relationship, of activity / passivity, the role of the professional is to do something to the patient and he is a mere recipient (because he can't answer, as in the case of coma, delirium, for example) or anesthesia).

When the professional is like a father and the patient is like a child, there is a model of guidance / cooperation in which the professional tells the patient what to do and the patient is cooperative and obeys (e.g. in an infection process).

If the model is of mutual participation, based on an adult / adult relationship, the professional helps the patient to help himself and the patient participates in a partnership, using the professional's competence.

Table 3. Szasz and Hollender Model (1956)

Atittudes	Model	Professional role	Paciente behavior
Father - Baby	Activity/ Passivity	Do something to patient	Acts as a receiver and is unable or unwilling to respond
Father - Child	Guide and Cooperation	Tells the patient what to do	Is cooperative and obedient
Adult - Adult	Mutual participation	Helps the patient to help himself	Participates, cooperates in the professional-patient partnership

Source: (Szasz and Hollender, 1956)

BALINT MODEL | 1957

Balint (1957) stands out in the innovative approach in the practice of medicine, introducing the biopsychosocial perspective, through the work developed with other doctors in primary health care.

Balint (1957) defends a genuine doctor-patient relationship. It refers to the doctor as "drug doctor", characterizing the therapeutic relationship and its therapeutic potential with a view to the best results for the patient. The beginning of the therapeutic relationship, seen from a biopsychosocial perspective, Balint (1957) highlights the importance of active listening and the existence of a hidden agenda.

In this sense, the health professional must start to discover the real problem that motivated the patient to seek his health care. This correct assessment of the "hidden agenda" is what will allow the diagnosis with greater certainty and the most effective strategy to solve the problem that has been identified.

The search for this "hidden agenda" defended by Balint (1957) reveals the concern of the health professional, the sender to decode the meaning of the other, that is, of the patient who receives the message (the receiver).

There is a need on the part of the health professional, to open the "relationship map" and present solutions to the other (receiver): this process underlines the importance, at least for one of the parties (health professional) in coding - sending the message and, at the same time, obtaining its decoding, but controlling the health relationship.

A criticism made of Balint's model is that, despite exploring the doctor-patient relationship, it remains very centered on the professional (Pawlikowska, Leach, Lavallee, Charlton & Piercy, 2007, p. 186).

WESTLEY AND MACLEAN COMMUNICATION MODEL | 1957

The communication model of Westley and MacLean (1957) was developed to substantiate that, unlike Dance, Westley and MacLean, the communication process in human beings starts, not in the first moment, when the person starts communication (Dance, 1970; Watzlawick, Beavin, & Jackson, 1967) but only when the individual receives signals or messages from his or her external environment.

It means that the communicative process is triggered by external factors, with a dense relationship between the signs of the environment and the beginning of the communication process. This entire communicative flow begins through the reception of messages, instead of sending them.

The signals emitted by the environment can be intentional or accidental (like a sudden storm for example).

This model does not integrate the fact that the whole process in which the individual moves, being communication by itself (Watzlawick et al. 1967).

According Bajracharya (2018) the advantages of Westley and MacLean's Model of Communication are: 1) the model has the advantage of integrating feed back; 2) as the message comes from the environment, sensory field improves the message formation; 3) social and other factors are included in objects of orientation; 4) the model can be applied to interpersonal, group communication as well as mass communication; 5) the model is very descriptive.

Being a two-dimensional model, the model does not apply when there are communication events that may involve a broader context as well as a wider range of communication messages.

TRANSCULTURAL THEORY OF CARE OR THEORY OF THE DIVERSITY OF CARE AND CULTURE | 1968

Leininger (1968, 1997) proposes the Transcultural Theory of Care or Theory of Diversity in Care and Culture (Leininger, 1997, p. 34) based on the assumption that cultures and subcultures differ in terms of care behaviors and beliefs of health, both in the roles of the caregiver and the person being cared for.

This theory focuses on the discovery of the universal and cross-cultural phenomenon of care (Leininger, 1997, p. 33) and highlights the importance of nurses moving from a unilateral thought and perspective to a comparative, multicultural and holistic perspective (Leininger, 1997, p. 34).

Within this approach, there is no cure without care, and the more the technological elements of care were present, the greater the interpersonal distance between "nurse" and the patient, and the less the patient's satisfaction (Raingruber, 2013, p 76).

TRANSACTIONAL COMMUNICATION – BARNLUND | 1970

Barnlund's (1970) transactional model of communication emphasizes the transaction that exists when individuals exchange meaningful information that intends to follow a path towards their goals. This production of meaning results from encoding and decoding:

The sender encodes, that is, transmits his thoughts by words, symbols or gestures through a channel (oral, gestures, signals) to the receiver, who decodes them.

This encoding and decoding process occurs at the same time (Parvanta & Bass, 2020), and there may be "noises" (p. 22) such as there is noise in the space where the communication takes place, thinking with another issue besides the one that is be debated at the moment, the person has another language, the gesture made (finger in the air, for example) has different connotations in the culture of one of the actors (Parvanta & Bass, 2020).

For this reason, communication is the transfer of symbolic information within a common symbol system (Bass & Parvanta, 2020, p. 21). It therefore assumes that the symbol must be understood in the same way between both parties, which can be difficult if the symbols change or are used differently, as is the case when we use only capital letters in the email text and the recipient can to think that we are angry or irritated (Parvanta & Bass, 2020, p. 21)

INTERPERSONAL CONTENT: THE IMPORTANCE OF RECIPROCITY - WEBB MODEL | 1975

For Webb (1975), interpersonal communication is based on human relationships and systematization of four aspects:

1. Interpersonal communication relationships develop over time.

2. The focal point is the relationship between people.
3. Interpersonal communication is a dynamic relationship and that both communicators send and receive signals simultaneously.
4. Interpersonal communication is a transactional relationship, that is, a relationship with the other and with their environment, in each context. (Figure 5)

Figure 5. The Webb Model (1975)
Source: (Adapted from Fisher and Adams, 1997; Webb's Model, 1975, p. 24)

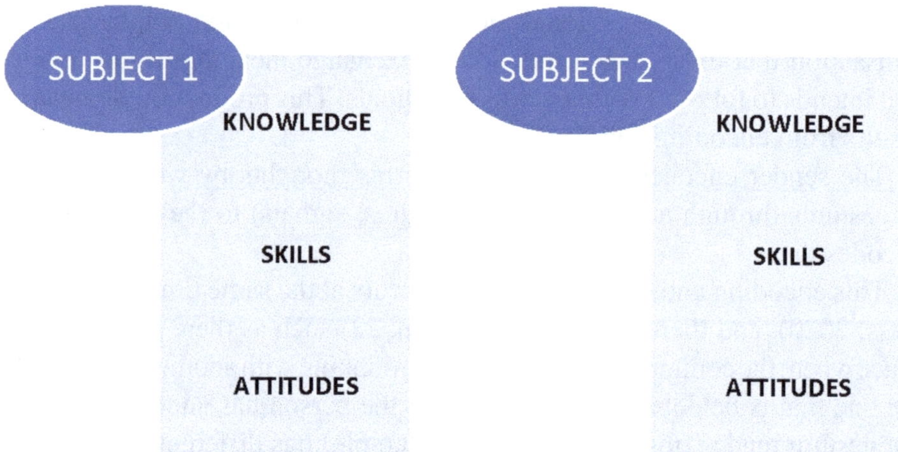

Fisher and Adams in 1994 innovate by including interpersonal relationships in the communication model. The interpersonal relationship is the prerequisite for the optimization of health care (Ong et al., 1995, p. 904). An important aspect of interpersonal communication is the establishment of relationships, and a relationship is a pattern of interaction between two people based on their reciprocal perceptions (Littlejohn, 1999, p. 206). In this interaction and according to Parsons (2012), there are three elements that affect a situation at the interpersonal level: 1) the relationship with the other person; 2) the aspects of the two communications (the receiver is also the transmitter (encoder / decoder) and 3) the Dialogue (p. 34).

According to Vaz de Almeida and Sebastião (2018) health professionals are the main sources / coders of information that allow the pursuit of health and health education. In other words, they are the information-sender element in a therapeutic relationship. This is a communicative and collaborative interpersonal relationship between professional and patient (or caregiver), in a given space and time, which aims at valuing and training the person, so that he / she can understand and adhere, in an autonomous way, to health instructions (message), with a view to better health outcomes (2018, p. 27).

Wiemann (1977), in turn, states that a competent communicator is oriented towards the other, while maintaining his interpersonal goals: he is empathetic, has and supports his interlocutor, he is calm while interacting (p. 211). It can be assumed that this concept of communicative competence is analogous to that of assertiveness in the therapeutic relationship. There is the idea, in Wiemann's theory (1977, p. 197), of mutual satisfaction with the situation, leaving openness so that one of the actors may be able to persuade the other to accept the situation. Persuasion makes sense within the margins of competent communication, if the result is functional for maintaining the long-term relationship (Wiemann, 1977, p. 197).

McGuire (1961, 1964, 1968, 1989) described the steps by which an individual to be persuaded must undergo assimilate desired behavior. And the steps to provoque influence are as follows:

Step 1: Exposure to the message;
Step 2: Attention to the message, the personal interest or relevance of the message;
Step 3: Understanding the message;
Step 4: Accept this change;
Step 5: Remember the message and continue to agree with it, be able to think about it;
Step 6: Make decisions based on that message that is remembered; behave as decided;
Step 7: Receive positive reinforcement for this adopted behaviour;
Step 8: **A**ccept behavior in someone's life.

Reinforcing Wiemann and Backlund (1980, p. 185) emphasize that the component of communicative competence is based on empathy, flexibility of behavior and management of interaction. In a "process" perspective, Kreps, (2001, p. 598) focuses on interpersonal communication between the professional and the patient, describing it as:

1. A critical process necessary to provide patients with informed consent when they select treatment strategies.
2. As a primary social process used to describe patient care strategies and encourage them to follow treatment regimens.

3. As a process that consumers and service providers use to gather information needed to monitor responses to treatment and make decisions to redefine long-term strategies.

There are several benefits as shown in the following table (4):

Table 4. Consultation satisfaction and benefits

- Measure the quality of care
- Predict health outcomes
- Predict commitment to treatment
- Economic implications
- Treatment continuity
- Effectiveness of therapeutic interventions
- Effectiveness of preventive interventions
- Increased health "status"

Source: (Based on Meakin e Weiman, 2002, p. 258)

The sense of reciprocity and the search for balance between the parts of the therapeutic relationship contributes to increased participation and the development of the patient-centered relationship. In this context, the increase in interpersonal communication skills of health professionals, allows a constructive dynamic of the therapeutic relationship.

According to Vaz de Almeida and Sebastião (2018, p. 39), the professional and the patient tend to make nonverbal behaviors reciprocal, such as sounds, response latency, body orientation and gestures (Street & Buller, 1987, p. 234). These health professionals also tend to estimate the amount of information given to their patients taking into account their education, income, sex and age (Street, 1991, p. 541).

INFORMATION-PERSUASION MODEL (IPM) | MCGUIRE (1976, 2001)

Mcguire (1968) developed an Information-Persuasion Model (IPM) that can be used as a Communication-Persuasion Model.

The Mcguire's model is based on communication "inputs" (which make up the message side of the communication) and in "outputs" (which make up the receiver's side of the communication).

Mcguire's communication model has an information and persuasion matrix that consists of the following elements:

Input: the source, the message, the channel, the receiver and the destination (Corcoran, 2007, p. 23)

Output: it is based on persuasion techniques such as:1) exposure to the message; 2) attention to the message; 3) like the message and be interested; 4) understand the message; 5) related cognition; 6) skills acquisition; 7) keep in memory/, memorisation; 9) recover the memory message when received; 10) attitudes, action and performance of action; 12) integration of action into behaviour; 13) behaviour change/appropriate behavior.

The basis of Maguire's IPM (1968, 2001) is mainly rooted in advertising. It has been used in the mass media (Corcoran, 2007, p. 22).

The Model assesses consumer behavior in response to different messages. For example, Kaphingst et al (2004) used the Mcguire Model matrix to analyze television advertising about prescription drugs.

Corcoran (2007, p. 23) states that Mcguire's model (1976, 2001) examines consumers' behavior in relation to advertising messages.

The advantage of the model is that it presents a clear planning of phases that can be followed to obtain a result.

THEORY OF HUMANISTIC NURSING | 1976

Theory of Communication in Humanistic Nursing | 1983

Paterson and Zderad (1976/1988) proposed the theory of humanistic nursing, which describes the total experience between patient and "nurse" as a living (McCamant, 2006, p. 335) and humanized dialogue. Humanistic nursing emerges from interactions between the nurse and the patient. Nursing presence is a concept experienced in the interaction between the nurse and the patient (Yesilot & Oz, 2016, p. 95).

In this interaction, patients and nurses test their limits, and share experiences and this effort illustrates the concept of Kleiman (2010). Thus, the nurse must have an open, receptive and prepared attitude so that she can offer her true "presence" (Paterson & Zerad, 1976).

The theory was developed since the beginning of the sixties and continuously refined in the following 20 years with the support of students, they describe nursing not as a profession or a calling but as a human response from one person to another in need (Decker-Brown, 2003). As nursing expresses in all contexts, it can be considered a meta nursing theory. (McCamant, 2006, p. 334).

Yeşilot and Oz (2016) point out that the theory of humanistic nursing is based on a dialogue, in a human-to-human relationship between the patient and the nurse (p. 95). Nursing is conducted through the call, the response and the dialogue experienced in these moments, where the nurse, increases her awareness of her role and evaluates the calls and understands what the patient really needs.

Duldt, Giffin and Patton (1983) later developed the Humanistic Nursing Communication Theory (1983) based on the Humanistic Nursing Theory, focusing exclusively on interpersonal communication between the "nurse", patient, peers and colleagues, highlighting the three characteristics of the human being: 1) living: being able to function biologically and physiologically as a viable animal entity; 2) communicate: be able to label things and talk about them when they are not present. 3) negative: being able to talk about the symbolic negative (-1, no, none), creating rules (laws about "you will not do it") and being concerned about what may not happen, as well as considering your own non -existence (p. 4).

The person will tend to feel recognized and accepted as a human being, depending on the degree to which he receives a humanizing communication from others (p. 4).

Duldt, Giffin and Patton (1983) suggest a variant of the approach of Paterson and Zderad (1976), differing from this in that: a) it defines the human being poured into nursing practice; b) Provides expressions of relationship; c) Provides a structured body of knowledge that can be implemented in nursing education programs.

The authors (Duldt et al., 1983) reflect that when humanized communication is used in the face of a critical life situation for a client / patient, the client's health tends to move in a positive direction.

WEICK'S COMMUNICATION MODEL | 1979

Weick's model (1969, 1979) is based on three phases of the theory of socio-cultural evolution that shape the communication process: regulation, selection and retention (Kreps, 2009, p. 348).

The regulation phase focuses on health-related challenges, and at this stage, professionals and patients must develop good communication strategies to deal with health issues.

In the selection phase, decisions are focused on increasing the patient's understanding of communication.

In the retention phase, the processes serve to preserve what has already been learned, creating a repository of experiences about what has worked and what has not worked (Raingruber, 2014, p. 71).

In each phase, the participant strives to transform equivocal messages into predictable and understandable messages (p. 71), by emphasizing that it is a process in permanent feedback and that all phases are mutually dependent (Kreps, 2009, p. 349).

The socio-cultural evolutionary theory explains that people adapt to changes, often due to social pressures, in their social and cultural relationships in order to survive (Kreps, 2009, p. 348).

Weick (1979) introduces a concept of "uncertainty" in his model: the actors of the organization (health professionals) reduce uncertainty through the use of organization and communication rules in order to improve their patient's understanding. As Kreps says: Weick's model explains the uncertain situations (2009, p. 347).

Uncertainty is compared to "mistakes". It is through the health professional, who adapts the existing rules to the profile of his patient, especially the one with limited health literacy. The model shows the important roles that communication performs in enabling health care consumers and providers to make sense of the complexities of modern health care and health promotion (Kreps, 2009. p. 377).

According to Kreps (2009), the Weick Model (1979) is a contemporary social-scientific theory that allows to resolve mistakes and uncertain situations, and to promote problem solving. The model explains the uncertain situations that organizational actors (patients and health professionals) face. Problem solving (Kim & Grunig, 2011) covers the set of equivocal information inherent in the many complex situations and the problems and issues that exist in this system (Kreps, 2009, p. 347)

Weick's organization model is an excellent framework for understanding the complexities inherent in many health care and health promotion situations, as well as a model for guiding effective health communication interventions (Kreps, 2009, p. 347).

BIOPSYCHOSOCIAL MODEL | 1977

Engel (1981) was the exponent of the biopsychosocial model and a fierce critic of the biomedical model.

The way health professionals approach patients and the problems they present is influenced by the conceptual model in which they organize their knowledge and experience (Engel, 1981, p. 101). According to Engel (1981), this tension between science and humanism could be attenuated or eliminated if the physician were to approach clinical problems from the more inclusive perspective (p. 107).

Connecting professional perspectives, communication tasks and the principles of the biopsychosocial model, Engel (1977) assumes that the patient is a "systemic creature" with permeable boundaries made up of mind and body, organism and environment, more than one complex set of isolated symptoms (Engel, 1977, p. 131).

In view of the patient's need to discharge his anxiety, the professional has the competence and motivation to give relief and involve the patient. The expectation of the patient is that the physician, has the professional competence and motivation to provide such relief (Engel, 1981, p. 102).

In this process, the patient's tasks and responsibilities are complementary to the professional.

According to Engel (1981, p. 121), the biopsychosocial model offers a conceptual framework that allows the professional to act rationally in areas where this type of approach is excluded. It motivates the professional to become more informed in the psychosocial areas, disciplines seen as "aliens and remote" (Engel, 1981, p. 121). For the author of the model, it is expected that the biopsychosocial professional has a job of knowing the principles, language and basic facts of each relevant discipline, not being expected to be an expert in everything.

RELATIONAL MODEL IN HEALTH | 1988

Kreps (1988) highlights in his Relational Model of Health skills that, in addition to the interrelationships between communication skills and social support, respond to the results of increased communication skills and health outcomes.

Communication skills lead to greater therapeutic communication, social support, satisfaction, exchange of information and cooperation (Query & Kreps, 1996, p. 336). Kreps (1988) stipulates that it is, at the interpersonal level of health communication, that meaningful relationships are established between those who seek and those who provide health care services (p. 344).

This model, created based on the "wheel of the health care delivery system" (Query & Kreps, 1996, p. 336), assumes that the competence of health communication includes: knowing how to listen empathically; verbal and non-verbal sensitivity; the ability to encode, decode, and manage the interaction (Query & Kreps, 1996, p. 337).

Also, for Rungapadiachy, (1999, p.193), the communicational skills are those that each one needs to communicate effectively with another person or group of people. Query and Kreps (1996) partially test the model (p. 335), examining the relationship between communication skills, social support and depression of caregivers of people with Alzheimer's, demonstrating that the communication skills of caregivers are related, in a positive way, with psychological health results, reducing depression (p. 335).

Wright, Rosenberg, Egbert, Ploeger, Bernard and King (2013) rely on this model to assess the effect of face-to-face and Facebook support on 361 students at a university in the southeastern United States (p. 48) who participated in a survey (p. 47), noting that the increase in communication skills through face-to-face support has a greater effect in reducing depression than support through Facebook (p. 52).

MODEL OF THE THREE FUNCTIONS OF THE MEDICAL INTERVIEW | 1990

Bird and Cohen-Cole (1990, p. 65), anticipate some problems with the Model of the Three Functions of the medical interview (1990): communication skills of health professionals are inadequate, that professionals interrupt patients after 18 seconds (Beckman & Frankel, 1984; Nørgaard, 2011; West, 1984), and that only 23% completed their statements without interruption by the doctor (Nørgaard, 2011, p. 1).

Considerering that interruptions lead to an incomplete and inaccurate data collection, as well, health professionals forget their patients' psychosocial problems, Bird and Cohen-Cole (1990) proposed a new educational support: the Model of three functions of the medical interview (1990).

The Model explains that the medical interview has three main functions based on skills and emotions, and they are:

1. The emotions that through communication promote positive relationships between the professional and the patient
2. The behavior that motivates and educates patients to better understand their problem and what they need to do to promote their health. Among the skills, we highlight the way in which the patient is approached, clear and immediate counseling, the rational approach, the verification of understanding and the strengthening of the partnership and a common base
3. The collection of data that must be accurate and appropriate for the approach to the patient. This process requires attentive listening, open and closed questions, use of understandable words, evaluation of other problems, clarification and summary of the consultation (Cohen & Bird, 2000).

This tool was developed to improve and teach communication skills to medical students and doctors. It incorporates validated educational empirical principles that aim to facilitate the acceptability and attractiveness of the biopsychosocial interview, as well as helping the participants to understand and remember the facts and principles of communication with patients. This model of the three functions of the medical interview aims to "raise the emotional, educational and behavioral aspects" of the doctor-patient relationship to a level of equal importance in the information gathering process.

THE PRECEDE – PROCEDE MODEL (PPM) |1991

The Precede – Procede Model (PPM) (Green & Kreuter, 1991) is a planning model that comes from John Hopkins University and was designed to teach students about health promotion, created within a framework of planning, intervention and evaluation.

Green first developed Precede in 1974 and Green and Kreuter added Proceed in 1991 (Porter, 2015).

It assumes that interventions are effective if they come from the community, are planned through it, are based on data, include feasible interventions with multiple strategies and are based on feedback and the progress of assessments (Table 5).

Table 5. Phases of Precede & Procede

The Precede phases are:	The Proceed phase integrates:
1) Predisposing 2) Reinforcing and Enabling Constructs in Educational Diagnosis 3) Evaluation) (map educational 'diagnosis' and planning)	1)Policy 2) Regulatory and Organisational Constructs in Educational 3) Environmental Development) (guides socio-ecological assessment and planning

Source: (Based on Porter, 2015, p. 2).

The purpose of the PPM Model is to identify the most effective way to promote change through local needs assessment and program assessments. The model is based on cognitive social psychology, education and management of principles (Green, Kreuter, Deeds & Partridge, 1980).

The Model is divided into two steps:

- The 1st step to conduct a social assessment where community participants identify their own needs:
- In a 2nd step, an epidemiological assessment is made using vital statistics and national questionnaires to identify the health problems that have the greatest impact on a given community.

In parallel with the ACP Model (2014), in which it is necessary for the professional to be equipped with clinical and communication skills to correctly assess the patient. Above all, the previous perception of the needs of the patient that the Precede - Procede model confers, allows a final better and sound decision.

COAST MODEL - COMMUNICATION, OPTIONS, ALTERNATIVES, STANDARDS, TRUST | 1994

Based on a dyadic encounter with intensive communication acts (Ratzan, 1994, p. 230), the health communication model COAST - Communication, Options, Alternatives, Standards, Trust (Ratzan, 1994, p. 226) evokes a process of ethical and effective communication between the professional and the patient.

Through intensive communication, an honest and open exchange takes place, from which a strong and confident relationship emerges (p. 230).

COAST advocates a dialectical approach, with the opportunity to replace an existing unidirectional flow and transform, through empowerment, the therapeutic relationship between the professional and the patient (Ratzan, 1994, p. 229).

ARGYLE'S SOCIAL SKILL MODEL | 1994

One of the most cited models of social interaction is the Argyle Social Skill Model (1994) which determines that in any social encounter, individuals have plans or goals that they try to accomplish through the continuous correction of their social performance, in the face of the reactions of others.

The behavioral sequences that are generated in this social interaction are a certain type of motor skill, and social performance is presented as a set of motor responses. Just as a car driver can correct the maneuvers of his car, so the health professional can take corrective measures through Communication to control patients (eg, who get excited).

The reciprocal nature of the interactions and objectives of both participants is highlighted. The feedback comes from each one, as well as the responses of the other person. There is an influence of emotions and cognitions on the perception, interpretation and planning of responses (Figure 6).

Figure 6: Behavioral interaction (feedback)
Source: (Adaptation of the Argyle, 1994).

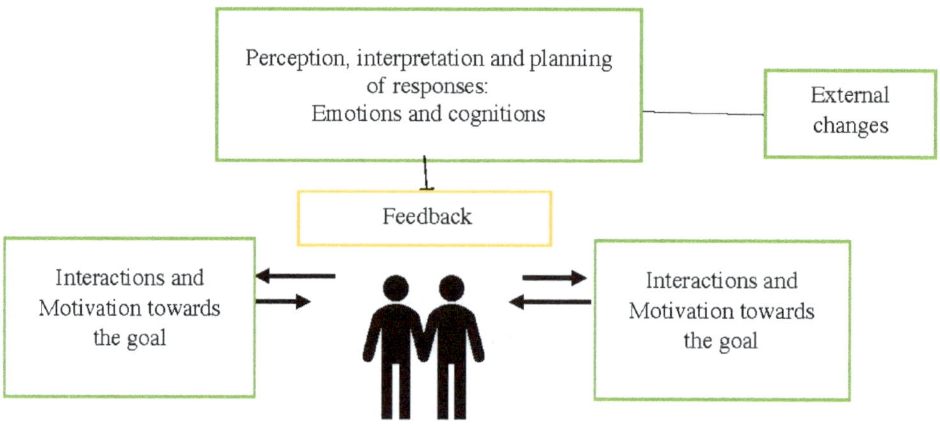

E4 MODEL | 1994

Keller and Carroll (1994) propose the E4 model for communication between the professional and the patient, where, in order to have a successful meeting, there must be human involvement (p. 134).

According to the authors (1994), there are four communication tasks in the medical meeting: to involve; empathize; to educate; and add / list (E4).

These authors consider that the communication between the professional and the patient is based on three perspectives of the professional: roles, philosophy and behavior (p. 132). More than just “healing”, there are psychological, sociological and behavioral forces present in the medical interview (Keller & Carroll, 1994, p. 134). Between 1989 and 1994, the authors proved to be a useful tool in more than 500 workshops with more than 8000 doctors (p. 134).

The exchange of meaning / meaning and understanding only exists if the professional and the patient are involved and committed to the communication process.

The professional has a unique vocabulary and knowledge and is able to solve problems (pp. 134-135), while the patient has the experience of the disease and can tell his story as a narrative. The professional must understand and encourage him to tell this story and must not interrupt it for two or three minutes (Keller & Carroll, 1994, p. 135).

Empathy can be learned by the professional (p. 136) and demonstrated through awareness of the patient’s values and feelings, accepting him and being “present” and with “the patient” (p. 136).

CALGARY CAMBRIDGE GUIDE - CCG |1997

The Calgary Cambridge Guide-CCG (1997) is a guide to medical interview related to the communication process, based on a guiding checklist and used as a guideline for students in the fields of health (Silverman, Draper, & Kurtz, 1997).

The Calgary Cambridge Guide contains six key steps and integrate a set of 71 items during the consultation (Table 6).

The guide’s own authors (CCG) imply that it is too extensive: The first issue was how to enable learners to perceive the value and helpfulness of the guide without being discouraged initially by the guide’s 70 individual communication process skills (Silverman, Kurtz & Draper, 2013, p. 6).

Table 6. Main Steps of Calgary Cambridge Guide

1) Start the session 2) Gather information 3) Build the relationship 4) Provide structure 5) Explain and plan 6) Close the session

Source: (The Calgary Cambridge Guide, Silverman et al. 2013)

The authors (Silvermal et al, 2013) refer that these 71 items may seem "scary at first" (p. 16) but warn that care must be taken not to over-simplify clinical communication, and being a complex and challenging field and "we would not do justice if we reduced the guide to just a few skills (2013, p. 16).

The CCG (1996) is mainly a tool that was designed to be used during medical learning, being considered by the authors themselves as an "educational tool" within the observation guides (Kurtz & Silverman, 1996). In 2003 Silverman, Kurtz and Draper (Silverman et al., 2013, p. 17) introduced improvements to the GCC to make it easier for students and doctors who teach them to conceptualize what happens in a health interview and how communication skills and physical examination work together in an integrated manner (p. 17).

According to Kurtz (2002) better physician communication skills improve patient satisfaction and clinical outcomes (p. S23)

Good communication skills can be taught and learned, and it is important that physicians learn physician-patient communication and apply them in clinical practice. With this view, medical education programs at all levels should include teaching of physician-patient communication (Kurtz, 2002, p. s23)

FOUR HABITS MODEL | 1999

Developed by Frankel and Stein (1999), the Models of the Four Habits aims to: a) establish relationships and create trust quickly, b) facilitate an effective exchange of information, c) demonstrate care and concern and d) increase the likelihood of adherence and positive results to health.

The term "Habit" corresponds to an organized way of thinking and acting during the clinical encounter. The four habits are:

1. Invest in the beginning;
2. To elicit the patient's perspective;

3. Demonstrate empathy;
4. Invest in the end.

In the Four Habits Model, the communication tasks that make up each Habit are organized into families of skills, techniques and rewards.

Habits are interrelated and are worked together to create mutual satisfaction and effective encounters.

It is important to 1) obtain the full spectrum of concerns at the beginning of the meeting and 2) assess the importance from the patient's point of view; 3) prioritize the patient's concerns, exploring his perspective, showing empathy and 4) preparing the ground for successfully involving the patient in joint decision-making and education.

Habit 1: Invest in the Beginning

There are three tasks that must be performed at the beginning of the interview: create rapport quickly, understand the patient's concerns and plan the meeting

To create rapport quickly, it is important for the health professional to use the first few seconds to establish a welcoming atmosphere and give the patient a sense of security (Frankel & Stein, 1999, p. 80)

Habit 2: A second habit is to ask the patient for his perspective and ideas and can even "provoke specific requests" and to verify the impact on the patient's life.

Habit 3: The 3rd habit is to show empathy and be open to the patient's emotions, and the professional must use non-verbal language as to assess changes in body language and tone of voice; use brief comments or empathetic gestures; refer to a likely emotion such as: "This looks really disturbing"; praise the patient for his efforts to solve the problem; pause, touch or facial expression; use your own emotional response as a clue as to what the patient may be feeling and take a short break if necessary.

Habit 4: And the 4th habit means investing in the end, delivering the diagnosis, doing health education, involving the patient in decision-making and closing the visit.

KALAMAZOO CONSENSUS STATMENT | 2001

In 1999 a group of 21 managers from medical and professional organizations met at the Jon Health Care Communication Bayer Institute and with the Fetzer Institute drew up guidelines on communication between the professional and health and the patient to: 1) facilitate the development, implementation and evaluation of communication in the medical curriculum; 2) inform about the development of standard rules / guidelines.

From this joint reflection in the early 2000s, this group identified seven essential communication tasks in the health field (Table 7).

Table 7. Tasks in Kalamazoo Consensus Guide

1) Build the doctor-patient relationship
2) Open the speech
3) Gather the information
4) Understand the patient's perspective
5) Share information
6) Reach an agreement
7) Closing consultation

Source: (Based on Kalamazoo Consensus Statement, 2001)

The essential communication elements defined by the Kalamazoo Consensus Statement (Egener & Cole-Kelly, 2004, p. 509) are:

1. Understand the patient's agenda
2. Achieve agreement on problems
3. Get treatment plans.

Focusing on the health professional's share of responsibility for therapeutic adherence, Baumann, Baumann, Le Bihan and Chau (2008) specifically explore the relationship between the patient's perception of clinicians' communication skills - with the "TCom- skill GP"- and therapeutic adherence, applying a self-administered questionnaire to 393 people from the same geographical area.

These researchers confirm the relationship between the TCom-skill GP scale and therapeutic adherence, which includes 15 items - among them: "allocate time to listen to the patient", "do everything so that the patient trusts the professional", "explain the purpose of the treatment", "giving the impression of respecting the patient ","emphasizing", "explaining in simple words ","discussing all the patient's difficulties in complying with the treatment".

In a qualitative and cross-sectional study, using a grounded theory approach, observing, and interviewing doctors from San Francisco (USA) and Copenhagen, the authors Barfod, Hecht, Rubow and Gerstoft (2006) refined a communication model on HIV medication centered on the doctor and with influence on adherence, which includes four steps and three factors.

The four steps are:

1. Decide whether to ask about membership or not;
2. Pre-question preparations;
3. Ask the question;
4. Answer the patient's question.

The three factors are the doctors' perceptions of

1. Adherence
2. Disability
3. Credibility

When therapeutic adherence fails, negative effects prevail and quality in health decreases (Lawrence, 2008), with costs of various kinds (Haun et al., 2015). In 2005, more than 240 million health meetings (consultations) were missed, considering the patient's non-adherence (Martin & DiMatteo, 2014, p. 2).

Like CGG (1996), KCS analyzed and predicted communicative health behaviors in seven phases of professional-patient interaction (Makoul, 2001). The mandatory phases are: 1) build the relationship; 2) open the discussion; 3) gather the information; 4) understand the patient's perspective; 5) share information; 6) seek agreement on the problems and plans and 7) close the consultation. The initial intentions of the CCG (1996) were to create an educational health communication tool for medical students to understand the importance of communication, applied to the various phases of the consultation, while KCS (2001) is more reduced in the short term. in its extension, foreseeing to be a more practical tool, for example: "encourage partnership", "actively listen", encourage issues", "encourage decisions", among others.

Egener and Cole-Kelly (2004) criticize the KCS Model because, according to the authors, there is a need for an "effective way of measuring the task of understanding the essence of the visit (p. 509) from the patient's perspective and not only from the professional. They also state that "although the Kalamazoo Consensus Statment identifies the main tasks and the subset of competencies for communication, it becomes necessary to identify and measure competence, which consists of understanding the true essence or meaning of the visit, and that competence must be added to the list of core competencies" (p. 509). The skills of collecting information, according to the authors (Egener & Cole-Kelly, 2004, p. 509) is developed through good observation and non-verbal skills, which are critical to help and facilitate this "essence" that is more difficult to measure at the meeting (p. 509).

CERC MODEL - CRISES AND EMERGENCY RISK COMMUNICATION | 2002

The CERC - Crises and Emergency Risk Communication (Reynolds, 2002) was developed by the Centers for Disease Control and Prevention, which recognized that health communication must be strategic, in an era of bioterrorism and the emergence of other potential risks (Reynolds & Seeger, 2005, p. 49).

This model integrates traditional notions of health and risk and risk communication with studies in disaster and crises communication.

The model aims to help manage the complex and often uncertain events that characterize crises (Reynolds & Seeger, 2005, p. 43). Covello (1992) considers risk communication to be one in which there is an exchange of information between stakeholders about the nature, magnitude, significance and control of risk (p. 359).

It is a five-level model that assumes that the crisis develops in a predictable and systematic way: the model assumes that crises will develop in largely predictable and systematic ways, 1) from risk; 2) to eruption; 3) to clean-up ; 4) to recovery and 5) evaluation (Reynolds & Seeger, 2005, p. 51). The systematic approach reduces uncertainty and allows for the anticipation of communication.

According to Reynolds and Seeger (2005, p. 51), the model intends to offer a comprehensive approach where each risk and warning messages and crisis communication activities can be linked in a more coordinated way with the forms of communication. Considering the pandemic situation of COVID-19, in 2005, Reynolds and Seeger stated: "this approach also acknowledges that effective communication regarding crises and emergencies must begin long before an event erupts and continue after the immediate threat has subsided (2005, p. 53). So, communication matters.

PENDLETON MODEL | 2003

Inspired by the previous tools, of using communication in the various stages of the consultation, and two years after Kalamazoo Consensus Statement (2001) Pendleton et al. (2003), structured a consultation model whose tasks also go through the various stages of the consultation.

According to Pendleton (2003), "consultation is part of a 'cycle of care' in which patients' understanding and ability to manage their own health" (p. 1).

The author (Pendleton, 2003) explains better compliance: "patient satisfaction and memory of the doctor's communication affected compliance" (p. 29). From the opening to closing health professionals seeks to assess the reasons that led the patient to the consultation, as well as the risks, to support a decision shared with the patient where understanding is an important element, within a time frame that must also be taken into account (Pendleton et al., 2003).

The steps of the Pendleton Model (2003) consist of:

1. Defining the reasons for the patient's presence, including the nature and history of the problem, patients' ideas, concerns and expectations and the effects of the problems;
2. Consider other problems and risks;
3. Choose with the patient an appropriate action for each problem;
4. Achieve a shared understanding of the problem;
5. Involve the patient in management and encourage him to accept this responsibility;
6. Use the time and resources appropriately and
7. Establish or maintain a relationship with the patient that helps him / her to perform other tasks (p. 3).

CONSULTATION MODEL AS A VALUE CHAIN | 2008

This model is based on management and its benefits obtained trough analyzing the value chain (Finset & Mjaaland, 2009). This is because patients meet with health professionals for a certain reason (Finset & Mjaaland, 2009, p. 324) and this reason is very important to be understood so that the professional can choose the most appropriate actions.

The concept of value chain was presented by Michael Porter to describe how entities can organize production management to be more competitive. The value chain is a consecutive and specific order of operations and activities where the final product is created step by step in each singular operation (Porter, 1985).

The authors (Finset & Mjaaland, 2009) present a consultation model as a value chain and apply a neurobiological perspective to analyze each element in the chain, with relevance to the regulation of emotion.

Among the tasks of the health professional is the identification and promotion of positive affects, allowing patients to show negative emotions during the consultation, such as anger or sadness (Finset & Mjaaland, 2009, p. 324). The four elements of medical consultation are presented in Table 8.

Table 8. Elements of medical consultation

The four elements of medical consultation that involve communication behaviors are:
1 - Establish the relationship
2- Collect data and emotional aspects of patients
3 - Health professional expresses empathy
4- The professional makes the review, giving a positive feed back on the patient's concerns.

Source:(Finset & Mjaaland, 2008)

Positive review involves a cognitive frame of an event to reduce its negative impact.

The authors use the metaphor of the "value chain" in an analysis of the regulation of affect in medical consultation, focusing on communicative behaviors that can be learned or trained and that can be included in the curricula (Finset & Mjaaland, 2008, p. 323) .

The communication of professionals in the consultation has an impact on the regulation of affection and becomes an activity that creates added value (Finset & Mjaaland, 2008, p. 323).

The greater the variety of communication tools that healthcare professionals have, the greater the communicative effects they can create.

And, greater the control over communication tools, greater the opportunity to create an effect, according to the intention of the interaction (Finset & Mjaaland, 2008, p. 323).

The regulation of the patient's emotions is considered a product of the consultation.

There are three qualities of the value chain (Finset & Mjaaland, 2008, p. 324): 1) consultation can be designed as a series of discrete activity sequences that professionals can train for their best performance; 2) there is an emphasis on the effects of each activity; 3) the design of the value chain is oriented towards the objectives and purpose of the consultation.

INTEGRATED COMMUNICATION MODEL, HO | 2008

This Integrated Communication Model developed by Ho (2008) integrates several factors: two communicators (in which each participant is at the same time a sending and receiving communicator); context; the channels; the message message; the relationship; the time. It also involves motivation, self-concept, needs and values, worldview, beliefs, sociocultural past, knowledge, experiences, communication skills, social norms, regulation, roles, expectations, stereotypes, the perception of others. Auditory and visual perceptions involve the process of attention, sensation, understanding and memory (Ho, 2008, p. 13).

Input- Each of the human being is individually, socially and psychologically dependent on sensory stimulation that helps maintain their normal, intelligent functioning and coordinating and adaptive behavior (Ho, 2008, p. 14).

We also have selective attention that goes through certain filters (Ho, 2008, p. 14) A filter is a limit on a person's ability to feel or perceive a stimulus. The preceptive filters are built on biological limitations.

Culture, e.g. it is a component of the relationship, being a form of selection, expectation or predisposition to respond.

Communicative messages are subdivided into verbal and non-verbal, and intentional and unintentional (Ho, 2008, p. 14)

Verbal stimuli are forms of spoken communication that use words and there may be verbal intention (conscious way of wanting to communicate with others) or unintentional (what we say meaningless).

Non-verbal stimuli do not use words, or are above words, such as facial expressions, posture, tones of you, hand movements or form of dress and can be intentional / (we want to transmit) or unintentional (we transmit without our control) .

The channels allow you to hear, see and touch cultural experiences (Ho, 2008, p. 15).

The context is the situation in which human communication takes place in environments, and the interferences may or may not distort the communication.

The interference can be technical (noise) or semantics in which the receiver does not attribute the same meaning (Ho, 2008, p. 15)

Time affects the intensity of communication relationships, the mode of communication and the style of communication (eg a mother communicates differently with her child over time)

REDE - RELATIONSHIP: ESTABLISHMENT, DEVELOPMENT, ENGAGEMENT | 2014

Windover, Boissy, Rice, Gillian, Velez and Merlino, (2014) structured the REDE model (Relationship: Establishment, Development, Engagement) in a conceptual framework organized through a database that is designed to teach and evaluate relationships centered on communication (p. 8) and communication skills that will be used in the three primary phases of the relationship: 1) preparation, 2) development and 3) commitment (p. 9).

The REDE model integrates evidence-based communication practices with experienced physicians, within a large hospital system (p. 12).

The REDE model is informative and transformative and explores their beliefs about the patient and their role with professionals (Windover et al., 2014, p. 9).

The authors consider that at the center of effective communication is the ability to develop meaningful relationships with patients (p. 12) and propose a systematization of communication skills, as if it were a "toolbox" (p. 9).

It is based on the premise that people form impressions of each other very quickly (p. 9) and, when they establish a relationship (initial phase), there is a "bank of emotions" that corresponds to a mental system that has a certain frequency of connection emotional to the other (p. 9). Each time a connection is established, it is equivalent to a "deposit" in that person's emotion account (p. 9), and in this way an "emotion account" is built with the patient and family (p. 9).

This model encourages the use of empathy, and there must also be genuine interest and curiosity, which are the necessary step in building the relationship (pp. 9-10).

The REDE model (2014) proposes that the patient be humanized, that he be involved in an effective dialogue, that his symptoms are understood to bewithin a biopsychosocial context (p. 10), motivating, in turn, the professional to be curious and open to know the person, his illness and the social response to the illness (p. 11).

This model is based on significant research, which includes the placebo effect, the therapeutic alliance, communication skills and patient centering, recognizing the healing potential of health relationships not only for patients, but also for professionals (p. 12).

VEHLS - VERBAL EXCHANGE HEALTH LITERACY | 2014

We consider it useful to leave a note of this model. Through the VEHL Model (Verbal Exchange Health Literacy), Harrington and Valerio (2014) focus on verbal exchange, which consider the key to the understanding and use of health information by the patient (p. 404).

The authors emphasize the need for the ability to speak and listen - which facilitates the exchange, understanding and interpretation of health information for decision making, disease management and navigation in the health system (p. 403).

MODELO INPUT – PROCESS – OUTCOME | 2015

The Input - Process - Outcome Model (Cheng, Bridges, Yiu & Mcgrath, 2015) is a health communication model that describes the routine of consultations in a health context (Cheng et al., 2015, p. 190) between professionals and patients having been developed by several authors (Cheng, Bridges, Yiu & Mcgrath, 2015; Donabedian, 2005; Parsons, 1951; Pendleton, 1983; Sondel & Soderfeldt, 1997; Szasz & Hollender, 1956) with origins in structural functionalism (Cheng et al. 2015, p. 185; Parsons, 1951).

In this model, "complex and rich" (Cheng et al. 2015, p. 190), personal communication is at the heart of the relationship between the professional and the patient, influenced by the content of the meeting and the style of the parties in this interaction (Cheng et al. 2015, p. 185), each of the phases influences and interacts with the others, in a sequence of effects.

The "Input" phase concerns psychosocial factors, such as age, gender, expectations, environmental factors, costs and the influence of the interaction between the professional and the patient (Pendleton, 1983; Sondel & Soderfeldt, 1997).

The "Process" phase is the phase of clinical communication, in which everyone contributes to this phase, from doctors, receptionists, nurses in an interaction with the patient. For Pendleton (1983) the communication process is a cycle of interaction repeated in the consultation.

Finally, the "Outcome" phase (results) provides the results of clinical treatment, compliance and patient satisfaction with treatment.

CARE TRANSITION MODEL - 2017

The Care Transition Model was developed to avoid health complications and readmissions for elderly patients with chronic and hospitalized diseases (Laura & John Arnold Foundation, 2017). The goal is to provide them with comprehensive hospital discharge planning and home care, coordinated by a "Transitional Care Nurse", trained in caring for people with chronic conditions.

At the time of hospitalization, the nurse: (i) performs a comprehensive assessment of the patient's health status, health behaviors, level of social support and objectives; (ii) develops an individualized care plan, consistent with evidence-based guidelines, in collaboration with the patient and her doctors; and (iii) makes daily visits to the patient, with a focus on optimizing the patient's health at discharge. (Laura & John Arnold Foundation, 2017, p. 1). According to Laura & John Arnold Foundation (2017), some of the effects of the Transitional Care Model one year after patients' hospital discharge (versus the control group) included: 22% reduction in the likelihood of re hospitalization or death; 34% reduction in the average number of re hospitalizations per patient.

ACP MODEL: ASSERTIVENESS, CLARITY, POSITIVITY | 2014 - 2019

The ACP Model (2014 - 2021) its use since 2014 for a large numbers of health professionals and was validated on 2019 (through 17 focus groups of health professionals and a questionnaire involving 389 health professionals). The model integrates in an aggregated and interdependent way three communication skills that should be used during the therapeutic relationship: assertiveness, clarity and positivity (Almeida, 2018, 2019, 2021).

These skills are used from the beginning of the relation to its closure, adapting to the circumstances and above all to the patient's profile.

The ACP model is composed of three competences that are considered useful for the quality of the therapeutic relationship when applied in an integrated manner (Vaz de Almeida & Belim, 2021, p. 205).

The patient deals with a very complex health system, and often without having the ability to understand the language used by the health professional, the guidance in the health system, feeling lost and without support to make the most correct decisions for his health.

This process can generate varying degrees of tension and anxiety (even in routine consultations). In this complex process of health, the professional is the stronger part of health relationship (Almeida, 2018, p. 36) We see this "system-patient" as a member of an intimate system that includes family members, friends, and co-workers (Vaughn & Carrol, 1994, p. 132).

Although there are unconscious competences or innate and intuitive skills of health professionals, it is necessary to know how to choose the right competence for the specific moment (e.g. when it is necessary to give instructions to the patient about his health behavior or about some treatment).

On the other hand, there are many roles between professional and patient (Vaughn & Carrol, 1994, p. 132). In addition, there are many roles on the part of the health professional (Wonca, 2002) because the professional can be a clinician, confessor, paternalistic, communicator, who must always aim to obtain a relationship of mutual partnership (Vaughn & Carrol, 1994, p. 132).

Communication means to use (skills) and to have (attributes) a clear language, which is understandable by the patient "decoder" (Schramm, 1955; Hall, 1980). Communication must be clear and accessible, considering the level and patient health literacy.

However, even those who have high health literacy also prefer simple language and texts (Doak & Doak, 1986).

It is important to establish a good connection between the health professional and the patient (Lorig, & Homan, 2003) through the construction of an articulated partnership between the professional and the patient. This dynamic also requires overcoming the biomedical and professional-centered model for a shared approach in which the patient is active in researching information and has the confidence to be actively involved in the decision-making process.

Basic communication skills in isolation are insufficient to create and sustain a successful therapeutic doctor-patient relationship (Ha, Anat & Longnecker, 2010. p. 38). The profissional must be prepared and above all master the communication skills necessary to produce health results.

There is a true subjective experience of the consultation. Communication is a powerful instrument of changing behaviors. Communication is, in fact, in all sides of our lives. The health professional goes through a complex process of understanding his patient that we can summarize in the following table 9.

Table 9: Steps in consultation: the subjective experience of the consultation

1. Evaluate and measure query essence
2. Observation skills (develop and apply)
3. Understand the patient's schedule
4. Get agreement on problems and treatment plans
5. Support in identifying conscious and unconscious needs
6. Work and apply verbal and nonverbal language (prosody, proxemia, silences, kinesthesia)
7. Work and apply verbal language - clarity and positivity
8. Use clear and accessible language for better understanding
9. Work empathy and assertiveness to perfectly elucidate the patient directly and respectfully
10. Promote meeting and satifying patient needs
11. Facilitate healing
12. Replace patient decision if this solution is evident (specially with patient very low health literacy)
13. Evaluate and anticipate patient reactions
14. Flexibility in face of the diversity of emotions that the patient presents
15. Using repetition - primacy and recession effect (more fixed at beginning and end)
16. Tailor the supports (oral, written, digital) according to the patient's health literacy - printouts, drawings, graphics, models, words / letters, numbers, etc.
17. Tailor open and closed questions according to the moment, the theme, the context in which the patient finds himself
18. Evaluate the patient's cultural context
19. Assess beliefs that drive you and beliefs that limit you
20. Recognize that health professionals also have beliefs and limitations
21. Know how to distinguish content (health and disease theme) from context (relationship, culture, beliefs, fears, etc.).
22. Assess and guide patient self-efficacy (best predictor of change behavior intent
23. Evaluate what kind of visual, auditory, audiovisual memory the patient has to be able to transmit more by voice or written health instructions
24. Give correct and enough information about the nature, development, prognosis of the disease.

Source: (Almeida, 2019; Belim & Vaz de Almeida, 2018; Chakrawarty, 2015; Harrington & Valerio, 2014, Ley, 1989; Ogden, 2004; Ranjan, Kumari & Scwarzer, 1992)

With the participation of the health professional, through the effective development of previous and adequate communication skills, in the development of trusting relationships with active listening, and adequate verbal and non-verbal language (Epstein & Street, 2007) the relationship becomes more effective. In this sense, the ACP model allows intervention in all phases of the therapeutic relationship, of communication skills that enable results: assertiveness, clarity and positivity.

ACP Model is a structured communication tool, who acts as a guideline (Hulsman, 2009) and who provides a framework for sharing mental models (Clochesy, Dolansky, Hickman, & Gittner, 2015, p. 249) that ensure that the conversation between the professional and the patient includes an important content that facilitates the establishment of the therapeutic relationship and promotes better understanding of the patient.

FUTURE RESEARCH DIRECTIONS

Models associated with health communication are stable in the literature and reinforce the conduction and management of the consultation process (Makoul, 2001; Kurtz, Silverman & Draper, 1998).

The challenge seems to be the continuous development of specific communication skills that the health professional can and must have knowledge and use during the interaction established with the patient.

Improve the understanding and use of communication skills, as in the ACP communication model, where assertiveness, clarity and positivity of the language are used specifically (Model ACP, 2014) in an already structured consultation, as proposed by the Calgary Cambridge Guide (Kurtz & Silverman, 1996) or the Kalamazoo Consensus Statement (Makoul, 2001) allows you to combine a consultation model with specific communication skills.

Hulsman (2009) highlights in this domain the importance of prior preparation of health professionals, through "previous guidelines" that allow greater control of the stages and results of the consultation and the management and coordination of the brief minutes in which the health relationship takes place.

In this limited space and time, communication skills are crucial for the patient to understand the information and reuse it in his self-care, as soon as he leaves the consultation and returns to his family, community and where decision levels are necessary.

Hulsman (2009) reinforces that the previous learning of health professionals, through support scripts, reduces the cognitive effort in performing complex tasks (p. 305). With this, it is understood that the health professional, if he / she has prior knowledge and elaboration of health communication models, available in a transversal way at all times of the consultation and in different phases, can find better answers and solutions to deal with the issues raised by the patient and also make him participate in his health in a more effective and motivated way.

CONCLUSION

We find models, in the literature, centered on the communication skills of health professionals and approaches that emphasize the humanization of the relationship and the need to contemplate cultural factors and psychosocial assumptions so that communication, in the context of health, is more effective.

We find in the literature authors who focus on communication skills and on the structure of the therapeutic relationship, which is strengthened through communication (Engel, 1977; Keller & Carroll, 1994; Harrington & Valerio, 2014; Ratzan, 1994; Wiemann, 1977; Windover, Boissy, Rice, Gillian, Velez & Merlino, 2014).

Other authors such as Kreps (1988) go further in the consequences of communication skills, which have the effect of reducing the levels of depression of caregivers of people with dementia (Kreps, 1988; Query & Kreps, 1996), or the ability to decrease levels of "uncertainty" in the relationship (Weick, 1979) or by the cross-cultural vision that the relationship must have (Leininger, 1968, 1997)

Harrington and Valerio (2014) and Windover, Boissy, Rice, Gillian, Velez and Merlino (2014, p. 8) focus on communication skills in the therapeutic relationship.

The goal of health communication models is to allow them to serve as guidance for more effective practices that establish a lasting and positive relationship between the health professional and the patient.

REFERENCES

Almeida, C. V. (2011). Communication and Literacy in e-Health. In *V SEMiME Exclusão Digital na Sociedade da Informação*. FMH-Universidade Técnica de Lisboa.

Almeida, C. V. (2018). Literacia em saúde – Capacitação dos profissionais de saúde: O lado mais forte da balança. In *Literacia em saúde: Modelos, estratégias e intervenção* (pp. 33–42). Edições ISPA.

Almeida, C. V. (2019). Modelo de comunicação em saúde ACP: As competências de comunicação no cerne de uma literacia em saúde transversal, holística e prática. In C. Lopes & C. V. Almeida (Coords.), Literacia em saúde na prática (pp. 43-52). Lisboa: Edições ISPA.

Argyle, M. (1994). *The Psychology of Interpersonal Behaviour* (5th ed.). Penguin.

Balint, M. (1957). *The doctor, his patient and the illness*. International Universities Press. doi:10.1097/00000441-195711000-00018

Barfod, T. S., Hecht, F. M., Rubow, C., & Gerstoft, J. (2006). Physicians' communication with patients about adherence to HIV medication in San Francisco and Copenhagen: A qualitative study using grounded theory. *BMC Health Services Research*, *6*(1), 154. doi:10.1186/1472-6963-6-154 PMID:17144910

Barnlund, D. C. (1970). A transactional model of communication. In J. Akin, A. Goldberg, G. Myers, & J. Stewart (Eds.), *Language behavior: A book of readings in communication* (pp. 47–57). Mouton. doi:10.1515/9783110878752.43

Baumann, M., Baumann, C., Le Bihan, E., & Chau, N. (2008). How patients perceive the therapeutic communications skills of their general practitioners, and how that perception affects adherence: Use of the TCom-skill GP scale in a specific geographical area. *BMC Health Services Research*, *8*(1), 244–253. doi:10.1186/1472-6963-8-244 PMID:19046433

Beckman, H. B., & Frankel, R. M. (1984). The effect of physician behavior on collection of date. *Annals of Internal Medicine*, *101*(5), 692–696. doi:10.7326/0003-4819-101-5-692 PMID:6486600

Belim, C., & Vaz de Almeida, C. (2017). Healthy thanks to communication: A model of communication competences to optimize health literacy: Assertiveness, clear language, and positivity. In V. E. Papalois & M. Theodospoulous (Eds.), *Optimizing health literacy for improved clinical practices* (pp. 124–152). IGI Global.

Berlo, D. K. (1977). Communication as Process: Review and Commentary. *Annals of the International Communication Association*, *1*(1), 11–27. doi:10.1080/23808985.1977.11923667

Berlo, D. K. (1985). *O processo de comunicação: Introdução à teoria e à prática*. Martins Fontes.

Bird, J., & Cohen-Cole, S. A. (1990). The three-function model of the medical interview. An educational device. In Method in Teaching Consultation Liaison Psychiatry. Basel: Karger. doi:10.1159/000418260

Bittner, A., Jonietz, A., Bittner, J., & Beickert, L. H. (2014). Translating medical documents into plain language enhaces communication skills in medical students – a pilot study. In Patient Education and Counseling. Elsevier.

Buck, D., Baylis, A., Dougall, D., & Robertson, R. (2018). *A vision for population health. Towards a healthier future. Cavendish Square London*. King's Fund.

Buttle, F. A. (1995). Marketing Communication Theories. What do the texts teach our students? *International Journal of Advertising*, *14*(4), 297–313. doi:10.1080/02650487.1995.11104621

Cegala, D. J., McNeilis, K. S., & McGee, D. S. (1995). A study of doctors and patients' perceptions of information processing and communication competence during the medical interview. *Health Communication*, *7*(3), 179–203. doi:10.120715327027hc0703_1

Charles, C., Gafni, A., & Whelan, T. (1997). Shared decision-making in the medical encounter: What does it mean? (or it takes at least two to tango*). Social Science & Medicine*, *44*(5), 681–692. doi:10.1016/S0277-9536(96)00221-3 PMID:9032835

Cheng, B. S. S., Bridges, S. M., You, C. K. I., & Mcgrath, C. P. (2015). A review of communication models and framework in a healthcare context. *Dental Update*, *42*(2), 185–193. doi:10.12968/denu.2015.42.2.185 PMID:26058232

Cline, R. J., & Mckenzie, N. J. (1998). The many cultures of healthcare: Difference, dominance and distance in physician-patient communication. In L.D. Jackson & B.K. Duffy (Eds.), Health Communication Research A guide to developments and directions (pp. 57-74). Westport, CT: Greenwood Press.

Clochesy, J.M., Dolansky, M.A., Hickman, Jr R.I., & Gittner, L.S. (2015). Enhancing communication between patients and healthcare providers: Sbar3. JHHSA FALL, 237-253.

Cohen-Cole, S. A., & Bird, J. (2000). *The medical interview: The three-function approach.* Mosby.

Corcoran, N. (Ed.). (2007). *Communicating Health: Strategies for Health Promotion.* Sage.

Dance, F. E. X. (1970). The "concept" of Communication. *Journal of Communication, 20*(2), 201–210. doi:10.1111/j.1460-2466.1970.tb00877.x

Donabedian, A. (2005). Evaluating the quality of medical care. *The Milbank Quarterly, 83*, 691–729.

Duldt, B. W., Giffin, K., & Patton, R. (1983). Interpersonal communication in nursing: A humanistic approach. F.A. Davis.

Egener, B., & Cole-Kelly, K. (2004). Satisfying the Patient, But Failing the Test. *Academic Medicine, 79*(6), 508–510. doi:10.1097/00001888-200406000-00003 PMID:15165968

Engel, G. L. (1977). The need for a new medical model: A challenge for biomedicine. *Science, 196*(4286), 129–136. doi:10.1126cience.847460 PMID:847460

Engel, G. L. (1981). The clinical application of the biopsychosocial model. *The Journal of Medicine and Philosophy, 6*(2), 101–123. doi:10.1093/jmp/6.2.101 PMID:7264472

Epstein, R. M., & Street, R. L. Jr. (2007). *Patient-centered communication in cancer care: Promoting healing and reducing suffering.* National Cancer Institute.

Finset, A., & Mjaaland, T. A. (2009). The medical consultation viewed as a value chain: A neurobehavioral approach to emotion in doctor-patient interaction. *Patient Education and Counseling, 74*, 323–330.

Fisher, B. A., & Adams, K. L. (1994). *Interpersonnal Communication: Pragmatics of human relationships*. Mcgraw-Hill.

Frankel, R. M., & Stein, T. (1999). Getting the Most out of the Clinical Encounter: The Four Habits Model. *The Permanente Journal, 3*(3), 79–88. doi:10.7812/TPP/99-020

Frey, L. R., Botan, C. H., & Kreps, G. L. (2000). *Investigating Communication: An Introduction to Research Methods* (2nd ed.). Pearson.

Green, L. W., & Kreuter, M. W. (1991). *Health Promotion Planning: An Educational and Environmental Approach*. Mayfield Publishing.

Green, L. W., Kreuter, M. W., Deeds, S., & Partridge, K. (1980). *Health Education Planning: A Diagnostic Approach*. Mayfield.

Greenfield, S., Kaplan, S. H., Ware, J. E. J. Jr, Yano, E. M., & Frank, H. J. (1988). Patients' participation in medical care: Effects on blood sugar control and quality of life in diabetes. *Journal of General Internal Medicine, 3*(5), 448–457. doi:10.1007/BF02595921 PMID:3049968

Ha, J. F., Anat, D. S., & Longnecker, N. (2010). Doctor-patient communication: A review. *The Ochsner Journal, 10*, 38–43.

Hall, S. (1980). Encoding/decoding. In S. Hall, D. Hobson, A. Lowe, & P. Willis (Eds.), *Culture, media, language: Working papers in cultural studies* (pp. 128–138). Hutchinson.

Harrington, K. F., & Valerio, M. A. (2014). A conceptual model of verbal exchange health literacy. *Patient Education and Counseling, 94*(3), 403–410. doi:10.1016/j.pec.2013.10.024 PMID:24291145

Haun, J. N., Patel, N. R., French, D. D., Campbell, R. R., Bradham, D. D., & Lapcevic, W. A. (2015). Association between health literacy and medical care costs in an integrated healthcare system: A regional populationbased study. *BMC Health Services Research, 15*(1), 249. doi:10.118612913-015-0887-z PMID:26113118

Ho, H.-K. (2008). Development of the integrated communication model. Unpublished. College of Humanities. Taiwan: Nahhua University.

Hulsman, R. L. (2009). Shifting goals in medical communication. Determinants of goal detection and response formation. *Patient Education and Counseling, 74*(3), 302–308. doi:10.1016/j.pec.2008.12.001 PMID:19135823

Kaplan, C. B., Siegel, B., Madill, J. M., & Epstein, R. (1997). Communication and the medical interview. *Journal of General Internal Medicine, 12*(S2), S49–S55. doi:10.1046/j.1525-1497.12.s2.7.x PMID:9127244

Katz, M. G., Jacobson, T. A., Veledar, E., & Kripalani, S. (2007). Asking questions in the medical encounter. *General Internal Medicine, 22*, 782–786. doi:10.100711606-007-0184-6

Keller, V. F., & Carroll, J. G. (1994). A new model for physician-patient communication. *Patient Education and Counseling, 23*(2), 131–140. doi:10.1016/0738-3991(94)90051-5 PMID:21207912

Kim, J.-N., & Grunig, J. E. (2011). Problem solving and communicative action: A situational theory of problem solving. *Journal of Communication, 61*(1), 120–149. doi:10.1111/j.1460-2466.2010.01529.x

Kleiman, S. (2010). Josephine Paterson and Loretta Zderad's humanistic nursing theory. In M. E. Parker & M. C. Smith (Eds.), *Nursing theories and nursing practice* (3rd ed., pp. 337–350). F. A. Davis Co.

Kreps, G. L. (2001). History of Health Communication. In T. L. Thompson (Ed.), *Encyclopedia of Health Communication.*, doi:10.4135/9781483346427.n219

Kreps, G. L. (2009). Applying Weick's Model of organizing to health care and health promotion: Highlighting the central role of health Communication. *Patient Education and Counseling, 74*(3), 347–355. doi:10.1016/j.pec.2008.12.002 PMID:19150591

Kurtz, S., Silverman, J., & Draper, J. (2004). *Teaching and learning communication skills in medicine*. CRC Press.

Lasswell, H. (1948). Structure and Function of Communication in Society. In Revista de comunicação e teoria da comunicação (pp. 215-228). Academic Press.

Laura & John Arnold Foundation. (2017). *Social Programs That Work Review*. Evidence Summary for the Transitional Care Model.

Lawrence, W. (2008). Advancing health literacy: Building health communication from the patient side. *Journal of Communication in Healthcare, 1*(2), 182–193. doi:10.1179/cih.2008.1.2.182

Ledingham, J. A. (2003). Explicating relationship management as a general theory of public relations. *Journal of Public Relations Research, 15*(2), 181–198. doi:10.1207/S1532754XJPRR1502_4

Ledingham, J. A. (2016). Political public relations and relationship management. In J. Stromback & S. Kiousis (Eds.), *Political public relations: Principles and applications* (pp. 235–253). Routledge.

Ledingham, J. A., & Bruning, S. D. (1998). Relationship Management in Public Relations: Dimensions of an Organization-Public Relationship. *Public Relations Review, 24*(1), 55–65. doi:10.1016/S0363-8111(98)80020-9

Leininger, M. (1968). Cultural differences among staff members and the impact on patient care. *Minnesota League of Nursing Bulletin, 16*(5), 5–9. PMID:5189191

Leininger, M. (1997). Overview of the Theory of Culture Care with the ethnonursing research method. *Journal of Transcultural Nursing, 8*(2), 32–52. doi:10.1177/104365969700800205 PMID:9369663

Levinson, W., Kao, A., Kuby, A., & Thisted, R. A. (2005). Not all patients want to participate in decision making. A national study of public preferences. *Journal of General Internal Medicine, 20*(6), 531–535. doi:10.1111/j.1525-1497.2005.04101.x PMID:15987329

Lewin, S., Skea, Z., Entwistle, V. A., Zwarenstein, M., & Dick, J. (2001). Interventions for providers to promote a patient-centred approach in clinical consultations. *Cochrane Database of Systematic Reviews, 4*, CD003267. Advance online publication. doi:10.1002/14651858.CD003267 PMID:11687181

Littlejohn, S. W. (1982). *Fundamentos teóricos da comunicação humana.* Zahar Editores.

Makoul, G. (2001). Essential Elements of Communication in Medical Encounters: The Kalamazoo Consensus Statement. Participants in the Bayer–Fetzer Conference on Physician–Patient Communication in Medical Education. *Academic Medicine, 76*(4), 390–393. doi:10.1097/00001888-200104000-00021 PMID:11299158

Makoul, G., & Clayman, M. L. (2006). An integrative model of shared decision making in medical encounters. *Patient Education and Counseling, 60*(3), 301–312. doi:10.1016/j.pec.2005.06.010 PMID:16051459

Martin, L. R., & DiMatteo, M. R. (Eds.). (2014). *The Oxford Handbook of health Communication Behavior Change and Treatment Adherence*. Oxford University Press.

Mccamant, K. (2006). Humanistic Nursing, Interpersonal Relations Theory, and the Empathy-Altruism Hypothesis. *Nursing Science Quarterly*, *19*(4), 334–338. doi:10.1177/0894318406292823

McGuire, W. (1968). Personality and attitude change: an information processing theory. In A. Greenwald, T. Brock, & T. Ostrom (Eds.), *Psychological foundation of attitudes* (pp. 171–196). Academic Press. doi:10.1016/B978-1-4832-3071-9.50013-1

McGuire, W. (1989). Theoretical foundations of campaigns. In R. E. Rice & C. K. Atkin (Eds.), *Public communication campaigns* (2nd ed., pp. 43–65). Sage.

McGuire, W. J. (1964). Inducing resistance to persuasion: Some contemporary approaches. In L. Berkowitz (Ed.), Advances in experimental social psychology. Academic Press.

McGuire, W. J., & Papageorgis, W. (1961). The relative efficacy of various types of prior belief-defense in producing immunity against persuasion. *Journal of Abnormal and Social Psychology*, *62*(2), 327–337. doi:10.1037/h0042026 PMID:13773992

Nimmon, L., & Regehr, G. (2018). The complexity of patient health communication social networks: A broadening of physician communication. *Teaching and Learning in Medicine*, *30*(4), 352–366. doi:10.1080/10401334.2017.1407656 PMID:29271662

Nørgaard, B. (2011). Communication with patients and colleagues. An intervention study on the impact of a communication skills training course on health care professionals' ability to communicate with patients and colleagues. *Danish Medical Bulletin*, 1–20.

Ogden, J. (2004). *Psicologia da Saúde*. Climpesi Editores.

Ong, L., de Haes, J. D., Hoos, A. M., & Lammes, F. B. (1995). Doctor-patient communication: A review of literature. *Social Science & Medicine*, *40*(7), 903–918. doi:10.1016/0277-9536(94)00155-M PMID:7792630

Parsons, P. J. (2012). *Beyond Persuasion. Communication Strategies for Healthcare Managers in the Digital Age* (2nd ed.). University of Toronto Press.

Parsons, T. (1951). *The Social System*. Tavistock Publications.

Parvanta, C., & Bass, S. B. (2020). *Health Communication Strategies and Skills for a New Era*. Jones & Bartlett Learning.

Paterson, J. G., & Zderad, L. T. (1976). *Humanistic nursing*. Wiley.

Pawlikowska, T., Leach, C. J., Lavallee, P., Charlton, R., & Piercy, J. (2007). Models of Consultation. In R. Charlton (Ed.), *Learning to Consult*. Radcliffe Publishing.

Pendleton, D., Schofield, T., Tate, P., & Havelock, P. (2003). *The new consultation. Developing doctor–patient communication*. Oxford University Press. doi:10.1093/med/9780192632883.001.0001

Porter, C. M. (2015). Revisiting Precede–Proceed: A leading model for ecological and ethical health promotion. *Health Education Journal*, 1–12.

Porter, M. E. (1985). *The value chain and competitive advantage*. Free Press.

Query, J. L. Jr, & Kreps, G. L. (1996). Testing a relational model for health communication competence among caregivers for individuals with Alzheimer's disease. *Journal of Health Psychology*, *1*(3), 335–351. doi:10.1177/135910539600100307 PMID:22011996

Raingruber, B. (2014). *Contemporary Health Promotion in Nursing Practice*. Jones & Bartlett Learning.

Ranjan, P., Kumari, A., & Chakrawarty, A. (2015). How can doctors improve their communication skills? *Journal of Clinical and Diagnostic Research: JCDR*, *9*(3), JE01–JE04. doi:10.7860/JCDR/2015/12072.5712 PMID:25954636

Ratzan, S. (1994). Health communication as negotiation. *The American Behavioral Scientist*, *38*(2), 224–247. doi:10.1177/0002764294038002005

Ruesch, J. (1956). The observer and the observed: Human communication theory. In R. P. Grinker (Ed.), *Toward a unified theory of human behavior*. Basic Books.

Ruesch, J., & Bateson, G. (1951). *Communication the social matrix of pshychiatry*. WW Norton Company Inc.

Rungapadiachy, D. M. (1999). *Interpersonal communication and psychology for health care professionals: Theory and practice*. Butterworth-Heinemann.

Salter, A. (1949). *Conditioned reflex theory*. Creative Age Press.

Schramm, W. (1954). *Process and effects of mass communication*. University of Illinois Press.

Schramm, W. (1955). How communication works. In W. Schramm (Ed.), *The process and effects of mass communication*. University of Illinois Press.

Sherko, E., Sotiri, E., & Lika, E. (2013). Therapeutic communication. *JAHR*, *4*(7), 457–466.

Silverman, D. (1993). *Interpreting qualitative data: Methods for analyzing talk, text and interaction*. Sage.

Silverman, J., Draper, J., & Kurtz, S. M. (1997). The Calgary-Cambridge approach to communication skills teaching II: The SET-GO method of descriptive feedback. *Education for General Practice*, *8*, 16–23.

Silverman, J., Krutz, S., & Draper, J. (2013). *Skills for communicating with patients*. Taylor & Francis Group.

Sondell, K., & Söderfeldt, B. (1997). Dentist-patient communication: A review of relevant models. *Acta Odontologica Scandinavica*, *55*, 116–126.

Street, R. L. Jr. (1991). Information-giving in medical consultations: The influence of patient's communicative styles and personal characteristics. *Social Science & Medicine*, *32*(5), 541–548. doi:10.1016/0277-9536(91)90288-N PMID:2017721

Szasz, T., & Hollender, M. (1956). A contribution to the philosophy of medicine: The basic models of doctor-patient relationship. *Archives of Internal Medicine*, *97*, 585–592. PMID:13312700

Teixeira, J. C. (2006). Problemas psicopatológicos contemporâneos. Uma perspectiva existencial. *Análise Psicológica*, *24*(3), 405–413. doi:10.14417/ap.181

U.S. Department of Health and Human Services and U.S. Department of Agriculture. (2015). *2015–2020 Dietary Guidelines for Americans* (8th ed.). Available at https://health.gov/dietaryguidelines/2015/guidelines/

Vaz de Almeida, C., & Belim, C. (2021). Health professionals' communication competences decide patients' well-being: Proposal of a communication model. In *A. Tkalac Verčič, R. Tench & S. Einwiller (Eds.), Joy. Using strategic communication to improve well-being and organizational success.* Emerald Publishing.

Vaz de Almeida, C., & Sebastião, S. (2018). A perceção dos profissionais de saúde sobre fontes de informação e sua influência na relação terapêutica. *Journal Observatorio.* Disponível em http://obs.obercom.pt

Watzlawick, P., Beavin, J. H., & Jackson, D. D. (1967). *Pragmática da comunicação humana: Um estudo dos padrões, patologias e paradoxo da interação* (S. Paulo, Ed.). Cultrix.

Webb, R. Jr. (1975). *Interpersonal speech communication: Principles and practices.* Prentice-Hall.

Weick, K. E. (1969). *The social psychology of organizing.* Addison-Wesley.

Weick, K. E. (1979). *The social psychology of organizing* (2nd ed.). Addison Wesley.

Westley, B. H., & MacLean, M. S. (1955). A conceptual model for communications research. *Educational Technology Research and Development, 3*(1), 3–12.

Westley, B. H., & MacLean, M. S. Jr. (1957). A conceptual model for communications research. *The Journalism Quarterly, 34*(1), 31–38. doi:10.1177/107769905703400103

Wiemann, J. M., & Backlund, P. (1980). Current theory and research in communicative competence. *Review of Educational Research, 50*(1), 185–199. doi:10.3102/00346543050001185

Wiemann, J. W. (1977). Explication and test of a model of communicative competence. *Human Communication Research, 3*(3), 195–213. doi:10.1111/j.1468-2958.1977.tb00518.x

Williams, S. J., & Calnan, M. (1996). The "limits" of medicalization? Modern medicine and the lay populace in "late" modernity. *Social Science & Medicine, 42*(12), 1609–1620. doi:10.1016/0277-9536(95)00313-4 PMID:8783424

Windover, A.K., Boissy, A., Rice, T.W., Gillian, T., Velez, V.J., & Merlino, J. (2014). The REDE model of healthcare communication: Optimizing relationships as a therapeutic agent. *Journal of Patient Experience*, 8-13.

Wolpe, J. (1968). Psychotherapy by Reciprocal Inhibition. *Conditional Reflex: A Pavlovian Journal of Research & Therapy, 3*(4), 234-240.

Wright, K. B., Rosenberg, J., Egbert, N., Ploeger, N. A., Bernard, D. R., & King, S. (2013). Communication Competence, social support and depression among college students: A model of Facebook and face-to-face support network influence. *Journal of Health Communication, 18*(1), 41–57. doi:10.1080/10810730.2012.688250 PMID:23030518

Yesilot, S.B., & ÖZ, F. (2016). Nursing Presence: A Theoretical Overview. *Journal of Psychiatric Nursing*, 94–99.

Chapter 4
Mirror, Mirror, on the Wall, Who's the Communicationally Competent One of All? and the Other Side of the Mirror:
Health Professional Communication Competences and Patient Evaluation

Célia Belim
ISCSP, University of Lisbon, Portugal

ABSTRACT

This chapter focuses on health professional competence and consequent evaluation by patients who establish with them a therapeutic relationship. Based on a literature review and proposals of best practices to implement in health encounters, it is concluded that competent communication has to give attention to verbal and non-verbal dimensions and to the patient's expectations. Results reveal that the competences are empathy, respect, inclusion of the patient in choices and decisions, confirmation of understanding, use of plain language, and positivity. On the patients' side, some common expectations are associated with the humanization of relationships, such as the manifestation of patience by professionals to the patients' queries and the adoption of personalized communication. The communication lapses are more related to poor attitudes of health professionals, and the patients' expectations can vary depending on their sociodemographic attributes. Different communication styles of health professionals generate different evaluations and expectations of patients.

DOI: 10.4018/978-1-7998-4396-2.ch004

INTRODUCTION

Doctor-patient communication is a fundamental component of clinical practice communication and is a complex interpersonal interaction that requires an understanding of each party's emotional state (Kee, Khoo & Koh, 2018). In spite of communicating with patients is arguably the most common and important activity in medical practice, this activity receives relatively little attention in graduate medical education (Henry, Holmboe & Frankel, 2019). But it is noted a renewed interest in communication skills in graduate medical education (Kee et al., 2018). It can be said that the status of teaching communication skills has changed from "nice to know" to "need to know" (Brown, 2008).

The literature tends to emphasize the "bottom line": the positive therapeutic rapport that patients enjoy with health professionals depends on mutual expectations and on an aligned communication flow from the patient to a health professional and vice versa (Huntington & Kuhn, 2003, p. 158). Tavakoly Sany, Behzhad, Ferns, and Peyman (2020), for example, state that communication skills training for physicians improves health literacy and medical outcomes in patients with hypertension.

In contrast, a collapse in the medical relationship often reveals unsatisfactory communication as a malpractice claim. Kee et al. (2018) explain that this event can be related to the antagonist visions adopted by patients and doctors on what should be an effective communication: patients prefer a psychosocial model of communication and doctors tend to use the biomedical model. One additional problem is the overestimation by doctors of their communication skills. The doctors overestimate their rapport-building skills, or do not pay great attention to them and thus, assume good knowledge and practice without real application (Albahri, Abushibs & Abushibs, 2018; Alnasser et al., 2017; Ha & Longnecker, 2010). The literature states that there is a different perception by each member of the relationship about the professionals' abilities. For example, a survey shows that 75% of orthopedic surgeons consider they had communicated satisfactorily with their patients and only 21% of patients have that evaluation (Tongue, Epps & Forese, 2005).

"We can all learn to communicate better" (Tongue, Howard, Epps & Forese, 2005, p. 652). Having this idea as orientation, this chapter assumes as focus the health professional competences (the "mirror") and the patient's perceptions, evaluation, and expectations (the "other side of the mirror").

BEING COMMUNICATIONALLY COMPETENT

There is a pattern generating about how knowledge (know), skills (know how to do), and personal attributes (know how to be) lead to broader competences (Tench & Moreno, 2015, p. 43). Gregory (2008) explains that competences are how knowledge and skills are used in performance (p. 216). For a complete version, personal attributes should be included (Tench et al., 2013, p. 17; Tench & Moreno, 2015, p. 44).

Relationally competent communicators are empathetic, committed to the message, and can adapt appropriately to the communication (Feingold, 1977). Wiemann (1977) explains that the competent communicator is empathic, affiliative, supportive, relaxed while interacting, capable of adapting his/her behavior as the situation within an encounter changes and as he/she moves from encounter to encounter.

Communication competence is rule-based and tells subjects how and when to communicate (Shimanoff, 1980). It can be defined as the ability of an interactant to choose among available communicative behaviors in order that he/she may successfully accomplish his/her own interpersonal goals during an encounter while maintaining the face and the line of his/her fellow interactants within the constraints of the situation (Wiemann, 1977, p. 198). Each of the dimensions of communicative competence can be defined according to molecular behaviors, all observable in face-to-face encounters (Table 1):

Table 1. Communicative competence's dimensions and behaviors

Dimension	Behavior
Affiliation/support	Eye contact, the alternation, and co-occurrence of specific speech choices which mark the status and affiliative relationships of the interactants, head nods, duration of speaking time and the number of statements per minute, pleasantness of facial expression – smiling, statements indicating "owning of one's perceptions about another, physical proximity chosen during interaction
Social relaxation	General postural relaxation cues, integrating rocking movements, leg and foot movements, and body lean, rate of speech, speech disturbances, hesitations, and nonfluencies, object manipulations
Empathy	Reciprocity of affect displays (e.g., smiling and other immediacy cues), verbal responses indicating an understanding of and feeling for the other's situation (e.g., "I know how you feel"), perceived active listening as indicated by head nods and verbal listener responses or reinforcers
Behavioral flexibility	Verbal immediacy cues, alternation, and co-occurrence of specific speech choices mark the status and affiliative relationships of interactants
Interaction management	Interruptions of the speaker are not permitted, one interlocutor talks at a time, a speaker turns must interchange, frequent and lengthy pauses should be avoided, an interactant must be perceived as devoting full attention to the encounter

Source: *(Wiemann, 1977, pp. 198-199)*

Argyle (1969) identifies two general interaction management skills that are critical to competence: (1) "the ability to establish and sustain a smooth and easy pattern of interaction"; and (2) the ability to maintain control of the interaction without dominating – "responding in accordance with an internal plan, rather than simply reacting to the other's behavior" (pp. 327-328).

Sptizberg and Hecht (1984) also list the skills linked to communication competence (Table 2).

Table 2. Five common skills regarding relational communication competence

Skill	Description
Immediacy	It is a non-verbal concept related to how psychologically close an interlocutor feels towards the other. This skill is linked to closeness, bonding, affection, and inclusion. An immediate interactant reveals behaviors of interest, attraction, and intimacy.
Social anxiety	It is understood as behaviors that display self and other adaptors, shakiness, sweating, or anxiousness.
Interaction management	It is viewed as the way that subjects respond to each other and take turns communicating with each other.
Expressiveness	It is non-verbal and verbal behaviors that show that the participants are engaged in the interaction.
Other-orientation	It is the ability to be attentive to and interested in the other during the interaction.

Source*: (Sptizberg & Hecht, 1984)*

Clinical communication skills refer to a set of "communication skills" required by a healthcare professional to provide patient-centered care (Elayaperumal, Venugopal & Dongre, 2018, p. 514).

Discussing the competences for the health communication specialist of the 21st century, it was recommended organizing competences considering two factors: a) the degree of competency abstraction, ranging from the theoretical to the applied; and b) the level of analysis to which the competency pertains, varying from the individual to societal (Maibach, Parrott, Long & Salmon, 1994).

MIRROR, MIRROR, ON THE WALL, WHO'S THE COMMUNICATIONALLY COMPETENT ONE OF ALL?

Effective communication between patients and their physicians is "one of the cornerstones of high-quality medical care" (Osch, Dulmen, Vliet & Bensing,

2017; Stewart et al., 2000) and there is strong evidence that it has positive effects, contributing to diagnosis, therapeutic outcomes, patient and provider satisfaction and efficient use of resources (Williams, Weinman & Dale, 1998).

The review of the literature made by King and Hoppe (2013) contains impressive evidence supporting positive associations between physician communication practices and positive patient outcomes (e.g., patient recall, patient understanding, patient adherence to therapy). It is noted a consensus about what is the "best practice" for physician communication in therapeutic encounters: (a) fostering the relationship, (b) gathering information, (c) providing information, (d) making decisions, (d) responding to emotions, and (e) enabling disease – and treatment-related to behavior (self-management).

Being emphatic and inducing positive expectations have distinct and combined effects, demonstrating that both influence patients' outcomes for the best (Osch et al., 2017). Weingarten et al. (2010) conducting an Israelite study, analyze 291 videotaped routine encounters, and made seven focus groups with 56 general practitioners. They identify 40% of consultations with cases of conflicts, of which 21,2% are related to the packages of health services/ rationing. The authors mention that conflictual encounters are characterized by shorter opening and closing phases, that the physician shows a certain duality in the management of problems, because of the health system demands, and that the physicians' training might be relevant in view of adequate managing conflict situations. Conducting a longitudinal study in Holland, Bensing et al. (2006) don't find the differences between both patients' groups regarding sex and age. The most recent data reveal that the general practitioners give more medical information and express less concern about patients' health conditions, and patients are less active (e.g., make fewer questions, and also demonstrate fewer concerns). Showing effects of the contagion of positivity, Street, Gordon, and Haidet (2007) conclude that physicians display more patient-centered communication and more favorably perceived patients who express positive affect, are more involved, and who are less contentious, and physicians might communicate better with patients of certain ethnic groups (possibility of bias).

At a primary-care level, clinical communication skills integrate eliciting a patient history, explaining (e.g., giving information or describing a procedure, test, or risk), exploring (e.g., seeking to ascertain what the patient is thinking, feeling, or expecting), discussing informed consent, breaking a news, and negotiating (e.g., working out a management or treatment plan) (Elayaperumal et al., 2018, p. 514). Elayaperumal et al. (2018) consider communication skills: greet the patient, ask for complaints, tell relevant information, help the patient to make decisions, explain various options, return/follow-up plan, micro-skills in communication (p. 516).

Henry et al. (2013) propose a list of 12 evidence-based communication competences that the residency program can integrate as a practical starting point (Table 3). The researchers explain that implementing communication competences requires a commitment to direct observation, faculty development, and patient safety.

Table 3. 12 evidence-based communication competences for graduate medical education

Skill level	Competency	Assessable performance related to the competency
Basic	Ability to take accurate and complete patient histories	See new patients in clinic, patients admitted with new problems
Basic	Ability to communicate with other doctors	Conduct inpatient handoffs, transitions of care in the emergency department
Basic	Ability to communicate with other members of the healthcare team	Coordinate inpatient procedures, plan patient care with outpatient clinic staff
Basic	Ability to set agendas with patients	Set agendas during clinic visits, manage patients' expectations
Intermediate	Ability to assess and improve patient adherence	Assess adherence to blood pressure medications, adherence to fluid restrictions
Intermediate	Ability to deliver diagnostic and prognostic news	Deliver new inpatient diagnoses, communicate test results
Intermediate	Ability to elicit patients' beliefs, perspectives, and concerns about illness	Elicit whether patients believe medications are working, patients' beliefs about the cause of their illness
Intermediate	Ability to communicate treatment plans	Explain medications during hospital discharge, describe medicine changes in clinical settings; explain the rationale for procedures and operations
Complex	Ability to establish patient rapport and demonstrate empathy	Build rapport during initial surgical consultations, rapport overtime in continuity clinics
Complex	Ability to manage conflict and negotiate with patients	Respond to patient requests for unnecessary tests or medications; negotiate treatment goals for chronic disease management
Complex	Basic patient counseling skills	Promote smoking cessation, weight loss, or medication adherence
Complex	Counseling families and caregivers	Conduct a family meeting; counsel caregivers of an Alzheimer's patient

Source: *(Henry et al., 2013, p. 396)*

Physician communication styles influence patients' outcomes (Schmid Mas, Hall & Roter, 2007). Communication style is conceptualized by Norton (1978, 1983) as "the way one verbally or para verbally interacts to signal how literal meaning should be taken, interpreted, filtered, or understood" in a communication context (1978, p. 99). Buller and Buller (1987) assessed the physician's communication style by using a modified 36-item version of Norton's (1978) communication style measure (Table 4).

Table 4. The physician's communication style

Communication style	Item
Affiliation style: composed of communication behaviors designed to establish and maintain a positive relationship between the physician and patient. This style includes behaviors that communicate interest, friendliness, empathy, warmth, genuineness, candor, honesty, compassion, a desire to help, devotion, sympathy, authenticity, a non-judgmental attitude, humor, and a social orientation	very encouraging; extremely friendly; verbally acknowledges other's contributions; very relaxed; doctor's eyes reflect exactly what he/she is feeling; extremely open; open and honest; usually leaves an impression; leaves me with an impression I usually remember; the way doctor says something really leaves an impression on me; leaves a definite impression; very empathetic; extremely attentive; listens very carefully; deliberately reacts in such a way that I know he/she is listening
Dominance/activity/control: includes behaviors that establish and maintain the physician's control in the medical interaction. The physician-patient interaction is characterized by a difference in control, power, and status stemming from the patient's limited understanding of medical problems and treatments, the patient's heightened anxiety and uncertainty about prognosis and treatment, the physician's control of medical information, and the institutionalized roles prescribed for the physician and the patient	tends to come on strong; dominates conversations; verbally exaggerates to emphasize a point; dramatizes a lot; very argumentative; constantly gestures when communicating
Items dropped	always tactful; generally speaks very frequently; tries to take charge of things; physically and vocally acts out what he/she wants to communicate; tells jokes and stories; insists that people document or present proof for what they are arguing; insists upon very precise definitions; when he/she disagrees with someone he/she is very quick to challenge them; have noticed nervous speech mannerisms; calm and collected when talking; rhythm or flow of speech affected by nervousness; actively uses facial expressions when communicating; very expressive non-verbally; does not tell people very much about him/herself until he/she gets to know them quite well; openly expresses feelings and emotion

Source: *(Buller & Buller, 1987, pp. 376, 380)*

The literature proposes some communication skills to be adopted by health professionals, which are gathered in Table 5.

Table 5. Communication skills

Non-verbal communication skills
Attention to first impressions Pleasant introduction for the patient Eye contact Paralanguage Sitting approximately 2 to 4 ft (0.6 to 1.2 m) from the patient Nodding, reflective facial expressions Scheduled follow-up examinations help to motivate and monitor progress Be present, paying attention to the patient, caring for the patient, and working collaboratively and from strengths Demonstration of active and effective listening by hearing and understanding in a way that the patient feels heard and understood Use of non-verbal cues, such as nodding, pausing, maintaining eye contact A calm and consistent tone of voice, denoting interest and concern Be alert about his/her own non-verbal clues like body language, gestures
Verbal communication skills
Appropriate choice of words Open-ended questions allow the patient the opportunity to define the conversation Use of verbal skills, including back-tracking, reflecting, mirroring Recognition of the patient's preferred (or current) mode of communication and selection of the most effective mode of communication for the situation Assessment of patient's understanding of problem and desire for more information Explanation using words that are easy for the patient to understand Plain language communication as a priority competency for medical professionals in a globalized world Positive language leads to positive wellbeing Written communication skills: design easy-to-read tools, use health-education signs effectively, create a welcoming atmosphere with written material, simplify and identify materials to easier read, assess educational materials and client forms for readability, construct helpful posters and educational materials, write the notes during pauses in the conversation Sentences: make sure each sentence is about one thing or serves one purpose, write short sentences, use pronouns like "you" and "we" where appropriate to speak directly to readers, write in the active voice, make the action of each sentence clear, use examples where appropriate, use the simplest form of verbs, avoid using hidden verbs, use contractions where appropriate, don't use jargon or unnecessary technical terms, use short, simple words, don't cluster a bunch of nouns together, cut unnecessary words, don't use slashes, keep the subject, verb, and object close together, but the main idea before exceptions and conditions, place words carefully
Competences related to the content of information transmitted
Adequate information Quality of information provided Always provide information on what the patient wants to know and promptly respond to the patient's reaction Discuss nature, course, and prognosis (both short term and long term) of the disease, treatment options available, and necessity of the investigations Discuss in detail regarding necessity and feasibility of expensive investigations and drugs and their effect on the main course and outcome of a disease Always comprehend details in simple language. The use of medical jargon and abbreviations can have a negative effect
Attitudes
Empathy Respect for the patient's cultural and ethnic beliefs, practices, and language Acceptance and exploration of the patient's feelings, including negative feelings Construction of a sustainable relationship that allows for repair when mistakes are made and includes authenticity, honesty, admission of, and sorrow for, mistakes Understanding of the patient's perspective, including the patient's individual concerns, beliefs, and expectations Creation of an atmosphere of mutuality and respect through patient participation and involvement in decision-making Inclusion of patient in choices and decisions to the extent he or she desires Collaboratively setting of the agenda for encounters Negotiation of mutually acceptable plans in partnership with the patient Putting additional efforts in motivating patients regarding adherence to lifestyle modifications

Source: *(Kee et al., 2018; Mitchell, 2006; Ranjan, Kumari & Chakrawarty, 2015; Rider & Keefer, 2006; Tavakoly Sany et al., 2020; Tongue et al., 2005, U.S. Department of Health and Human Services – Centers for Disease Control and Prevention Agency for Toxic Substances and Disease Registry, n.d.)*

Weatherspoon, Horowitz, Kleinman, and Wang (2015) gather 17 items concerning the routine use of recommended communication techniques from the literacy experts, the American Medical Association (AMA), and previous studies to assess the use of suggested communicational techniques by Maryland dentists and dental hygienists (Horowitz, Clovis, Wang & Kleinman, 2013; Maybury, Horowitz, Wang & Kleinman, 2013; Rozier, Horowitz & Podschun, 2011; Schwartzberg, Cowett, VanGeest & Wolf, 2007) (Table 6). The researchers mention that the use of simple language is the only technique that nearly all physicians routinely used (family physicians, 91%; pediatricians, 93%). Physicians, who had taken a communications course, use significantly more techniques than those who had not (Weatherspoon et al., 2015).

Table 6. Recommended communication techniques

Communication technique
Interpersonal communication
Limit the number of concepts presented at a time (2 to 3)
Ask patients whether they would like a family member or friend to accompany them in the discussion
Draw pictures or use printed illustrations
Speak slowly
Use simple language
Teach-back method
Ask patients to repeat back information or instructions
Ask patients to tell you what they will do at home to follow instructions
Patient-friendly materials and aids
Use video or DVD
Hand out printed materials
Use models or x-rays to explain
Assistance
Highlight key aspects on print material
Follow-up with patients by telephone to check understanding and adherence
Read instructions out loud
Ask other office staff to follow up with patients for post-care instructions
Write or printout instructions
Patient-friendly practice
Refer patients to the Internet or other sources of information
Use a translator or interpret when needed

Source: *(Weatherspoon et al., 2015)*

Therapeutic communication can be organized considering the components of knowledge, attitudes/behaviors, and skills (Table 7).

Table 7. Therapeutic communication

KNOWLEDGE	ATTITUDES/BEHAVIORS	SKILLS
. Understand the principles of effective communication through various means . Know grammar, spelling, and health care terminology . Understand visual, auditory, and tactile communication . Understand the physiological, psychosocial, spiritual, and cultural influences on effective communication . Describe the impact of one's own communication style on others . Understand the nurse's role and responsibility in applying the principles of verbal and non-verbal communication . Understand the nurse's role and responsibility in applying principles of active listening . Recognize the value of validation in an effective therapeutic relationship . Identify techniques for reducing violent and/or disruptive behavior	. Accept responsibility for communicating effectively . Recognize one's individual responsibility to communicate effectively utilizing a collegial tone and voice . Value different means of communication (auditory, visual, and tactile) . Value mutually respectful communication . Value individual cultural and personal diversity . Respect persons' rights to make decisions in planning care . Value the therapeutic use of self in patient care . Appreciate the dynamics of physical and emotional presence on communication . Appreciate the influences of physiological, psychosocial, developmental, spiritual, and cultural influences on one's own ability to communicate . Acknowledge that acceptance of another person's behaviors will enhance the therapeutic relationship and facilitate communication . Recognize situations where de-escalation techniques are required to prevent violence and aggression levels of validation to minimize conflict and enhance the therapeutic relationship	. Use clear, concise, and effective written, electronic, and verbal communications . Document interventions and outcomes of care according to professional standards . Choose the right setting and time to initiate conversation . Assess the patient's readiness/ willingness to communicate . Assess the patient's ability to communicate . Use patient preferences for visual, auditory, or tactile communication . Assess barriers to effective communication . Make appropriate adaptations in own communication based on patient and family assessment . Assess the impact of the use of self ineffective communication . Establish rapport . Actively listen to comments, concerns, and questions . Demonstrate effective interviewing techniques . Provide an opportunity to ask and respond to questions . Assess verbal and non-verbal responses . Adapt communication as needed based on patient's response . Distinguish between effective and ineffective communication with patients and families . Use selected forms and levels of validation to minimize conflict and enhance the therapeutic relationship . Use selected forms and levels of validation to minimize conflict and enhance the therapeutic relationship . Use verbal and non-verbal communication skills to reduce and manage violent and/or disruptive behavior

Source: *(Massachusetts Department of Higher Education Nursing Initiative, 2016, pp. 32-33)*

Recognizing a gap in the medical education literature on teaching non-verbal detection and expression of empathy, Riess and Kraft-Todd (2014) propose a "novel teaching tool" – E.M.P.A.T.H.Y. This acronym means: E.: eye contact; M: muscles of facial expression; P: posture; A: affect; T: tone of voice; H: hearing the whole patient; Y: your response.

THE OTHER SIDE OF THE MIRROR

Biglu, Nateq, Ghojazadeh, and Asgharzadeh (2017) describe the indicators affecting patients' satisfaction with medical performance: devoting enough time, effective listening, description of diagnosis and treatment process, adequate treatment skills, physician's friendly conduct, understanding patient's feelings, creating the sense of calm and confidence, and careful examination. The results derived from the study conducted by the authors demonstrate that there is a significant correlation between the communication skills of physicians (e.g., devoting the appropriate time for visiting the patients, explaining diagnosis and treatment procedures) and patients' satisfaction. In addition, the physicians' therapeutic skills, their friendly manners, respecting the patients' feelings, and careful examination of patients by a physician, revealed a significant correlation with patient satisfaction. On the contrary, there is no statistical evidence of a strong correlation between effective listening to patients and patient satisfaction.

Various studies have shown the correlations between communication variables and the level of satisfaction of patients. For example, Korsch, Gozzi, and Francis (1968) confirm a significant correlation between the respectful behavior of physicians and the patients' satisfaction. The results of a study conducted by Rezaei and Asgari (2014) reveal the meaningful correlation between the interest showed by a physician for listening to the patient and his/her satisfaction. There are other variables correlated to satisfaction of the patient, such as the warm and friendly communication of physicians (Korsch et al.), explanation of diagnosis and treatment process (Suh & Lee, 2010), devoting enough time for visiting the patient (Gross, Zyzanski, Borawski, Cebul & Stange, 1998), communication styles (Buller & Buller, 1987; Schmid Mast et al., 2007), physician's verbal and non-verbal communication while interacting with the patient (Daly & Hulka, 1975; Korsch et al., 1968; Spiro & Heidrich, 1983).

Different communication styles generate different evaluations and expectations by patients. Assessing the impact of distinct types of physicians' communication styles on people' subsequent evaluation of physician attributes, the results of the study conducted by Bientzle, Fissler, Cress, and Kimmerle (2016) reveal that, in the patient-centered communication (PCC) condition, participants perceive the physician to be more empathetic and more competent than in the doctor-centered communication (DCC) condition. In the DCC condition, participants show less attitude change in comparison to the other conditions; in the patient-centered communication with need-orientation (PCC-N) condition, the physician is perceived as more empathetic and more socially competent than in the other conditions. However, participants acquire less knowledge in the PCC-N condition.

In this line, Buller and Buller (1987) observe that: a) affiliative styles generally generate more favorable evaluations than the dominant/active styles (p. 384), b) it is likely that technical competence is generally high and stable relative to communication competence, due to the medical degree and the position in the health organization may be enough to confer high technical competence on the physician before the visit; c) four social characteristics in the medical visit affect the contribution of the physician's communication style to the patient's evaluation: severity of the patient's illness that reduces the importance of the physician's style of communicating, the age of physicians: communication style appeared to be more important in patients' evaluations of younger physicians than of older physicians, the physician's specialty and frequency of visits.

Sobczak, Leoniuk, Janaszczyk, and Pietrzykowska (2016) observe that it seems that the social matrix of freedom/autonomy or political censorship/ dictatorship influences the quality of relations. The authors exemplify Anglo-Saxon societies, that strongly emphasize the autonomy of individuals, which considerably influences the quality of interpersonal relationships. Consequently, in these societies, there is a smaller asymmetry of amplitude in a physician-patient relationship. In Poland and other countries in the region, the value of autonomy is increasing, distancing from paternalistic axiology, still poses a challenge to physicians, patients, and medical education institutions.

Kee et al. (2018) seek to illuminate the communication lapses made by Singapore's junior doctors during therapeutic encounters through a qualitative analysis of complaints submitted by patients and their families. The authors analyzed 125 cases of complaints against doctors between March 2013 and February 2014, of which 38 were identified as complaints against junior doctors. Guided by the question *what are the communication issues from negative patient-doctor interactions that could be addressed in physician education or training?*, Kee et al. (2018) observe that the most commonly identified theme is poor attitudes (lack of empathy and of respect), followed by content of information transmitted, non-verbal and verbal communication errors. Zengin et al. (2014), analyzing records of all patients made between June 2008 and June 2012 retrieved from the archives of the Quality Improvement Unit, also identify that among the primary causes of complaints received are an inappropriate attitude of the staff (p. 123). Corroborating this pattern in the patient's complaints, Wofford et al. (2004) mention that the most common category is disrespect (36%), followed by disagreement about expectations of care (23%), inadequate information (20%), distrust (18%), perceived unavailability (15%), interdisciplinary miscommunication (4%), and misinformation (4%). Their findings point to important subdomains for improving communication (p. 137).

The health responses should be adjusted to the patient's figures and expectations (Table 8). Analyzing a Danish Hospital's patient-centered communication program, Pors (2016) advocates that market and care are co-existing organizing modes that entail expectations of the patient and that the patient is constructed in six information-seeking patient figures: affective patient; target group patient; citizen with rights; patient as a competent resource; user as an active partner; and consumer.

The patients have some common expectations and patient's expectations can vary depending on the patient sociodemographic attributes. Exploring the public views and expectations about a successful communication process between the healthcare providers/physicians and patients in Penang Island, Malaysia, it is found (Hassali, Shafie & Khan) that a common expectation of most of the sample (N=500) is to focus more on the patient history before prescribing any medicine. The results also show that: a) about 60,0% of the respondents expect that the healthcare providers must show patience to the patient's queries, b) the level of satisfaction with the information shared by the health professionals is higher among the respondents with a higher education level, c) patients with a higher level of education expect that physician should competently understand their views and medical history to prescribe a better therapeutic regimen.

An analysis of a large-scale survey data from a German physician-rating website (PRWs), containing 84,680 surveys of patients that totalize 7038 physicians on 24 service attributes and four overall evaluation measures, show that the patients improve the evaluation of physician's pleasantness and friendliness (Bidmon, Elshiewy, Terlutter & Boztug, 2020). The practices' cleanliness and communication behavior of a physician during a visit have constant returns.

In other research (Schmid Mast et al., 2007, p. 21), it is explored the paradox of a non-necessary and non-direct relation between the tendency of women to show the interaction style patients prefer and the more satisfaction with female doctors. The results stress that this evidence is more associated with differences in expectations patients harbor towards female and male doctors: people expect in general a physician to be a man rather than a woman, playing also the patient sex a role. It means that the triad – doctor sex, patient sex, and physician communication style – affects patient satisfaction. The results also demonstrate that, when female doctors adopt a sex-congruent communication style (high caring), the level of satisfaction, at least for female patients, might be beneficial. For male doctors, it seems that their communication performance influences patient outcomes to a lesser degree. Physician communication training cannot be one size fits all. This training and the health professionals should have in consideration that female and male patients harbor different expectations toward professionals.

Table 8. Patient's expectations

Patient's expectations
Awareness by doctors of their own emotions and of the patient's emotions
Empathy, sympathy, and compassion
Patience
Patient expectations concerning a desirable form of verbal and non-verbal communication with a physician vary to a considerable degree. Relatively universal, however, is the wish that the doctors introduce themselves and apply personalized forms of contact
Respect and empathy from doctors

Source: *(Hassali, Shafie & Khan, 2012; Jeffrey, 2016; Sobczak et al., 2016)*

The interaction/dyad between the health professional and the patient can be summarized as the figure shows (Figure 1).

Figure 1. Therapeutic dyad and communication
Source: (Own elaboration)

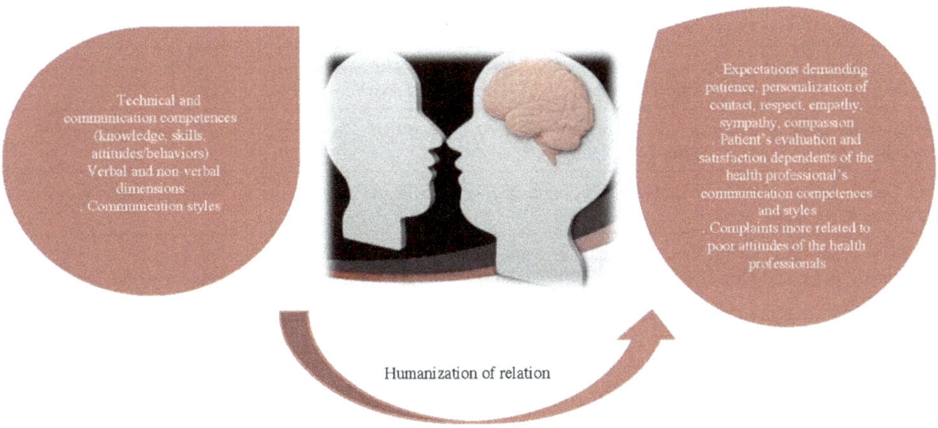

RECOMMENDATIONS AND OPPORTUNITIES

The literature offers some useful recommendations and opportunities that can be emphasized and summarized (Table 9).

Table 9. Some recommendations and opportunities derived from the literature

1. The communication skills curricula should integrate training content related to self-awareness and to how negative emotional spillover affects other parties in the communication skills curricula.
2. Effective interventions to strengthen patient complaints systems need to be comprehensive, integrated within existing systems, context-specific, and cognizant of the information asymmetry and the unequal power relations between the key actors.
3. Facing a hostile or less-than-optimum outcome, the physician should implement a plan of action, considering the guidelines: recognition of the patient's frustration and of his/her possible fear; recognition by a health professional of his/her own feelings of disappointment and anxiety; panic avoidance: to keep lines of communication open; expression of regret that the adverse result occurred but avoidance of finding fault or blaming others; explanation of what happened and of the proposed plan of action in words the patient can decodify; effort in maintaining the patient and family informed and involved in proposed treatment plans and discussions; documentation of the discussion in the medical record.
4. Attention to the cultural identity of the patient: culture is not obvious; we all feel our own culture is best; we misinterpret the actions of others if we do not understand their interpretations of their own observations; if we do not know the culture of the other, we may not know when we are offending; awareness of differences and possible barriers improves our chances for successful interactions; understanding our own "software" or value system is a crucial step in providing culturally competent care.
5. When listening and communicating with each other, patients and healthcare providers are likely to reinforce a shared understanding that may improve future decision-making and the quality of care patients receive.
6. An urgent need is growing to teach non-verbal aspects of communication as medical practices must be reoriented to the increasing cultural diversity represented by patients presenting for care. When the language proficiency may be reduced, non-verbal communication can make a difference and contribute to understanding patients' communications. Subtle non-verbal cues may be the critical entry point for discussions leading to shared medical decisions.
7. It is possible to suggest an order and time frame for the development of communication and professionalism communication competences during medical training. The key competences for clinical communication skills and professionalism are indicated as needing to be achieved sooner.
8. One way to adopt a critical health communication approach is to demystify the discourse and the ways that the use of language in the medical setting acts to perpetuate the interests of some groups over others.
9. The three qualitative themes most important for understanding patients' health beliefs and values as perceived by healthcare providers are education, trust, and culture.
10. Successful communication should be uncomplicated, be specific, use some repetition, minimize jargon, check patient understanding.
12. Task behaviors (e.g., facilitating patient talk, detailing instructions) and affective behaviors (socioemotional exchanges, expressing empathy, and caring) of health professionals show to be positively related to patient satisfaction.
13. A prerequisite for ultimate success will be faculty acceptance of the pertinence of communication skills and a commitment to development. In some scenarios, implementation of learned skills will require system changes to allow sufficient time in encounters for patient-centered approaches to be used.

continues on following page

Table 9. Continued

14. Patients are becoming more consumerist in orientation, and especially the new generation of patients are likely to directly challenge physician authority within the therapeutic encounter. Physicians may be accommodating their patients with a more egalitarian relationship and tolerance for patient participation in decision-making. The implication of these changes is extraordinary and they must be at the center of a completed and serious consideration in conceptualizing how the patient-physician relationship may be articulated in the medical encounter.
15. Patients are more satisfied with their medical encounters when they are given and retain more information about their disease: the teach-back method is efficient.
16. The use of more activated positive emotional words (e.g., lively, vigorous, attentive, humorous) is associated with increased longevity.
17. Literature review has been acknowledging assertive communication as a key strategy for preventing incidents in health care and benefiting patient safety. Researchers have to concentrate on improving healthcare professionals' assertive communication and teamwork skills with some promising results.
18. Healthcare professionals may need to have skills about how to expose information using plain language guidelines. The use of plain language can improve the comprehensibility of complex health information and procedures and instructions, especially for low literacy patients.
19. The balance between scientific-technical and psychosocial elements of patient care is recommended.
20. Conclusion of each medical interview, by reviewing the diagnosis, treatment, and prognosis, is a recommendation. With a sincere and uplifting tone, doctors should say good-bye and, while shaking hands and keeping eye contact, deliberately declare the expectation of a positive result. Expressing hope inspires positively the patient.

Source: *(Bahri, Saljooghi, Noghabi & Moshki, 2018; Bertakis, 1977; Franco, Franco, Lopes, Severo & Ferreira, 2018; Gardenswartz & Rowe, 1999; Grene, Cleary & Marcus-Quinn, 2017; Haug & Lavin, 1983; Howick et al., 2018; Huntington & Kuhn, 2003; Jeffrey, 2016; Kee et al., 2018; Kennedy et al., 2017; King & Hoppe, 2013; Lo, 2011; Lupton, 1994; Lyndon et al., 2012; Mirzoev & Kane, 2018; Omura, Levett-Jones & Stone, 2018; Pressman & Cohen, 2012; Riess & Kraft-Todd, 2012; Roter, Hall & Katz, 1988; Tongue et al., 2005; Vaz de Almeida, 2015, 2016, 2019a, 2019b, 2019c, 2020; Yen & Leasure, 2019)*

CONCLUSION

The literature is unanimous in the recognition that the health professional's adequate communication skills trigger positive effects on the patient. There are arguments in the literature that validate the integration of communication skills in graduate medical education, moving from a "nice to know" phase to a "need to know" one.

An unsatisfactory health professional-patient communication has setbacks in the therapeutic relationship and, consequently and problematically, on the patient's health and well-being. Hence the training and practice of communication skills of health professionals are the keys to better health. The discrepancy in the assessment of health professionals' communication skills by themselves and by patients, tending professionals to exaggerate the assessment of their evaluation, requires careful reflection on the practices and quality of communication in the context of the therapeutic relationship. As Rajashree (2011) says "communication skills are as important as vital needs" and health care professionals have to be aware of their own communication practices.

Communication competence is composed of knowledge (know), skills (know how to do), and personal attributes (know how to be). Researchers have been looking for the ideal formula, the "perfect" model that condenses these skills.

Within an interpersonal relationship, as is the therapeutic relationship, there are dimensions and molecular behaviors that improve the relational quality, such as: immediacy, support, social relaxation, social anxiety, empathy, flexibility, other-orientation, interaction management, expressiveness, reciprocity of affect displays, ability to establish and sustain a smooth and easy pattern of interaction, the ability to maintain control of the interaction without dominating, eye contact, pleasantness of facial expression, reciprocity of affect displays, verbal responses indicating an understanding of and feeling for the other's situation.

Specifically on the communication skills that health professionals should adopt and introduce in the relationships they establish with patients, literature, talking about "best practices" and "communication styles", tends to refer to: empathy; respect, including respect of the patient's cultural and ethnic beliefs, practices and language; abilities to take accurate and complete patient histories, to set agendas with patients, to assess and improve patient adherence, to deliver diagnostic and prognostic news, to elicit patients' beliefs, perspectives, and concerns about illness, to communicate treatment plans, to establish patient rapport and demonstrate empathy, to manage conflict and negotiate with the patient, to provide clarifying information; inclusion of the patient in choices and decisions to the extent he or she desires; confirmation of understanding; concentration on the patient; use of plain language; assertiveness; positivity.

There is some evidence derived from empirical research: doctors were more patient-centered with patients they perceive as better communicators, more satisfied, and more likely to adhere, where plain language is used in interventions, patients understand the information better.

On "the other side of the mirror", there are indicators related to health professionals' performance, that affect patient satisfaction, such as: devoting enough time, description of diagnosis and treatment process, adequate treatment skills, physician's friendly conduct, understanding patient's feelings, creating the sense of calm and confidence, careful examination, respectful behavior of physicians, interest showed by a physician for listening to the patient, the warm and friendly communication of physicians, communication styles, physician's verbal and non-verbal communication while interacting with the patient.

The literature also shows that there are characteristics in the medical visit which affect the contribution of the physician's communication style to the patient's evaluation and that communication lapses are more related to poor attitudes of health professionals.

The patients have some common expectations associated with a humanized contact, such as they expect that the healthcare providers must show patience to their queries and that adopt a personalized style of communication, and patient's expectations can vary depending on the patient sociodemographic attributes (e.g., sex, educational level). Communication styles generate different evaluations and expectations of patients. It can be concluded that being communicationally competent is the *fortune* of a therapeutic relationship.

REFERENCES

Albahri, A. H., Abushibs, A. S., & Abushibs, N. S. (2018). Barriers to effective communication between family physicians and patients in walk-in centre setting in Dubai: A cross-sectional survey. *BMC Health Services Research, 18*(1), 637. doi:10.118612913-018-3457-3 PMID:30107799

Alnasser, Y. S., Bin Nafisah, H. M., Almubarak, Z. A., Aleisa, L. A., El Sarrag, A. I., & Babiker, A. M. (2017). Communication skills between physicians' insights and parents' perceptions in a teaching hospital in KSA. *Journal of Taibah University Medical Sciences, 12*(1), 34–40. doi:10.1016/j.jtumed.2016.09.002 PMID:31435210

Argyle, M. (1969). *Social interaction.* Aldine Atherton.

Bahri, N., Saljooghi, S., Noghabi, A. D., & Moshki, M. (2018). Effectiveness of the teach-back method in improving self-care activities in postmenopausal women. *Przeglad menopauzalny = Menopause review, 17*(1), 5-10. doi:10.5114/pm.2018.74896

Bensing, J. M., Tromp, F., van Dulmen, S., van den Brink-Muinen, A., Verheul, W., & Schellevis, F. G. (2006). Shifts in doctor-patient communication between 1986 and 2002: A study of videotaped General Practice consultations with hypertension patients. *BMC Family Practice, 7*(1), 62. Advance online publication. doi:10.1186/1471-2296-7-62 PMID:17064407

Bertakis, K. (1977). The communication of information from physician to patient: A method for increasing patient retention and satisfaction. *The Journal of Family Practice*, *5*(2), 217–222. PMID:894226

Bidmon, S., Elshiewy, O., Terlutter, R., & Boztug, Y. (2020). What patients value in physicians: Analyzing drivers of patient satisfaction using physician-rating website data. *Journal of Medical Internet Research*, *22*(2), e13830. doi:10.2196/13830 PMID:32012063

Bientzle, M., Fissler, T., Cress, U., & Kimmerle, J. (2016). The impact of physicians' communication styles on evaluation of physicians and information processing: A randomized study with simulated video consultations on contraception with an intrauterine device. *Health Expectations*, *20*(5), 845–851. doi:10.1111/hex.12521 PMID:27860037

Biglu, M., Nateqv, F., Ghojazadeh, M., & Asgharzadeh, A. (2017). Communication skills of physicians and patients' satisfaction. *Materia Socio-Medica*, *29*(3), 192. doi:10.5455/msm.2017.29.192-195 PMID:29109665

Buller, M. K., & Buller, D. B. (1987). Physicians' communication style and patient satisfaction. *Journal of Health and Social Behavior*, *28*(4), 375–388. doi:10.2307/2136791 PMID:3429807

Daly, M. B., & Hulka, B. S. (1975). Talking with the doctor, 2. *Journal of Communication*, *25*(3), 148–152. doi:10.1111/j.1460-2466.1975.tb00617.x PMID:1184777

Elayaperumal, S., Venugopal, V., & Dongre, A. R. (2018). Evaluation of clinical communication skills training program for medical interns at a tertiary care teaching hospital, Puducherry. *International Journal of Medical Science and Public Health*, *7*(7), 514–518. doi:10.5455/ijmsph.2018.0101523032018

Feingold, P. (1977). Toward a paradigm of effective communication: An empirical study of perceived communication effectiveness. *Dissertation Abstracts International*, *37*, 4697A–4698A.

Franco, C., Franco, R., Lopes, J. M., Severo, M., & Ferreira, M. A. (2018). Clinical communication skills and professionalism education are required from the beginning of medical training - a point of view of family physicians. *BMC Medical Education*, *18*(1), 18. doi:10.118612909-018-1141-2 PMID:29558914

Gardenswartz, L., & Rowe, A. (1999). *Managing diversity in health care manual: proven tools and activities for leaders and trainers*. Jossey-Bass.

Gregory, A. (2008). Competencies of senior communication practitioners in the UK: An initial study. *Public Relations Review*, *34*(3), 215–223. doi:10.1016/j.pubrev.2008.04.005

Grene, M., Cleary, Y., & Marcus-Quinn, A. (2017). Use of Plain-Language Guidelines to Promote Health Literacy. *IEEE Transactions on Professional Communication*, *60*(4), 384–400. doi:10.1109/TPC.2017.2761578

Gross, D., Zyzanski, S., Borawski, E., Cebul, R., & Stange, K. (1998). Patient satisfaction with time spent with their physician. *The Journal of Family Practice*, *47*(2), 133–137. PMID:9722801

Ha, J. F., & Longnecker, N. (2010). Doctor-patient communication: A review. *The Ochsner Journal*, *10*(1), 38–43. PMID:21603354

Hassali, M., Shafie, A., & Khan, T. (2012). General public expectation from the communication process with their healthcare providers. *Journal of Young Pharmacists: JYP*, *4*(3), 193–198. doi:10.4103/0975-1483.100028 PMID:23112539

Haug, M., & Lavin, B. (1983). *Consumerism in medicine*. Sage Publications.

Henry, S. G., Holmboe, E. S., & Frankel, R. M. (2013). Evidence-based competencies for improving communication skills in graduate medical education: A review with suggestions for implementation. *Medical Teacher*, *35*(5), 395–403. doi:10.3109/0142159X.2013.769677 PMID:23444891

Horowitz, A. M., Clovis, J. C., Wang, M. Q., & Kleinman, D. V. (2013). Use of recommended communication techniques by Maryland dental hygienists. *Journal of Dental Hygiene*, *87*(4), 212–223. PMID:23986414

Howick, J., Moscrop, A., Mebius, A., Fanshawe, T. R., Lewith, G., Bishop, F. L., Mistiaen, P., Roberts, N. W., Dieninytė, E., Hu, X.-Y., Aveyard, P., & Onakpoya, I. J. (2018). Effects of empathic and positive communication in healthcare consultations: A systematic review and meta-analysis. *Journal of the Royal Society of Medicine*, *111*(7), 240–252. doi:10.1177/0141076818769477 PMID:29672201

Huntington, B., & Kuhn, N. (2003). Communication Gaffes: A Root Cause of Malpractice Claims. *Baylor University Medical Center Proceedings*, *16*(2), 157–161. doi:10.1080/08998280.2003.11927898 PMID:16278732

Jeffrey, D. (2016). Empathy, sympathy and compassion in healthcare: Is there a problem? Is there a difference? Does it matter? *Journal of the Royal Society of Medicine*, *109*(12), 446–452. doi:10.1177/0141076816680120 PMID:27923897

Kee, J. W. Y., Khoo, H. S., Lim, I., & Koh, M. Y. H. (2018). Communication Skills in Patient-Doctor Interactions: Learning from Patient Complaints. *Health Profession Education*, *4*(2), 97–106. doi:10.1016/j.hpe.2017.03.006

Kennedy, B. M., Rehman, M., Johnson, W. D., Magee, M. B., Leonard, R., & Katzmarzyk, P. T. (2017). Healthcare providers versus patients' understanding of health beliefs and values. *Patient Experience Journal*, *4*(3), 29–37. doi:10.35680/2372-0247.1237 PMID:29308429

King, A., & Hoppe, R. B. (2013). "Best practice" for patient-centered communication: A narrative review. *Journal of Graduate Medical Education*, *5*(3), 385–393. doi:10.4300/JGME-D-13-00072.1 PMID:24404300

Korsch, B., Gozzi, E., & Francis, V. (1968). Gaps in doctor-patient communication-I: Doctor-patient interaction and patient satisfaction. *Pediatrics*, *42*, 855–871. PMID:5685370

Lo, L. (2011). *Teamwork and communication in healthcare: A literature review*. Canadian Patient Safety Institute.

Lupton, D. (1994). Toward the development of critical health communication praxis. *Health Communication*, *6*(1), 55–67. doi:10.120715327027hc0601_4

Lyndon, A., Sexton, J. B., Simpson, K. R., Rosenstein, A., Lee, K. A., & Wachter, R. M. (2012). Predictors of likelihood of speaking up about safety concerns in labour and delivery. *BMJ Quality & Safety*, *21*(9), 791–799. doi:10.1136/bmjqs-2010-050211 PMID:22927492

Maibach, E., Parrott, R. L., Long, D. M., & Salmon, C. T. (1994). Competencies for the Health Communication Specialist of the 21st Century. *The American Behavioral Scientist*, *38*(2), 351–360. doi:10.1177/0002764294038002014

Massachusetts Department of Higher Education Nursing Initiative. (2016). *Massachusetts Nurse of the Future Nursing Core Competencies.* Retrieved from: https://www.mass.edu/nahi/documents/NOFRNCompetencies_updated_March2016.pdf

Maybury, C., Horowitz, A. M., Wang, M. Q., & Kleinman, D. V. (2013). Use of communication techniques by Maryland dentists. *The Journal of the American Dental Association*, *144*(12), 1386–1396. doi:10.14219/jada.archive.2013.0075 PMID:24282269

Mirzoev, T., & Kane, S. (2018). Key strategies to improve systems for managing patient complaints within health facilities – what can we learn from the existing literature? *Global Health Action*, *11*(1), 1458938. doi:10.1080/16549716.2018.1458938 PMID:29658393

Mitchell, W. (2016). Positive language leads to positive wellbeing. *BMJ (Clinical Research Ed.)*, *4426*, i4426. Advance online publication. doi:10.1136/bmj.i4426 PMID:27634388

Norton, R. W. (1978). Foundation of a communicator style construct. *Human Communication Research*, *4*(2), 99–112. doi:10.1111/j.1468-2958.1978.tb00600.x

Norton, R. W. (1983). *Communicator style: Theory, applications, and measures*. Sage.

Omura, M., Levett-Jones, T., & Stone, T. E. (2018). Evaluating the impact of an assertiveness communication training programme for Japanese nursing students: A quasi-experimental study. *Nursing Open*, *6*(2), 463–472. doi:10.1002/nop2.228 PMID:30918697

Pors, A. S. (2016). Constructions of the patient in healthcare communications: Six patient figures. *Journal of Health Organization and Management*, *30*(2), 279–298. doi:10.1108/JHOM-12-2014-0216 PMID:27052626

Pressman, S. D., & Cohen, S. (2012). Positive emotion word use and longevity in famous deceased psychologists. *Health Psychology*, *31*(3), 297–305. doi:10.1037/a0025339 PMID:21928902

Rajashree, K. (2011). Training programs in communication skills for health care professionals and volunteers. *Indian Journal of Palliative Care*, *17*(4, Suppl), S12–S13. doi:10.4103/0973-1075.76232 PMID:21811359

Ranjan, P., Kumari, A., & Chakrawarty, A. (2015). How can Doctors Improve their Communication Skills? *Journal of Clinical and Diagnostic Research: JCDR*, *9*(3), JE01–JE4. doi:10.7860/JCDR/2015/12072.5712 PMID:25954636

Rezaei, F., & Asgari, H. (2014). Checking the relationship between physicians' communication skills and outpatients' satisfaction in the clinics of Isfahan Al-Zahra (S) Hospital in 2011. *Journal of Education and Health Promotion*, *28*(3), 105. doi:10.4103/2277-9531.139697 PMID:25250371

Rider, E. A., & Keefer, C. H. (2006). Communication skills competencies: Definitions and a teaching toolbox. *Medical Education*, *40*(7), 624–629. doi:10.1111/j.1365-2929.2006.02500.x PMID:16836534

Riess, H., & Kraft-Todd, G. (2014). E.M.P.A.T.H.Y. *Academic Medicine*, *89*(8), 1108–1112. doi:10.1097/ACM.0000000000000287 PMID:24826853

Roter, D. L., Hall, J. A., & Katz, N. R. (1988). Patient-physician communication: A descriptive summary of the literature. *Patient Education and Counseling*, *12*(2), 99–119. doi:10.1016/0738-3991(88)90057-2

Rozier, R. G., Horowitz, A. M., & Podschun, G. (2011). Dentist-patient communication techniques used in the United States: The results of a national survey. *The Journal of the American Dental Association*, *142*(5), 518–530. doi:10.14219/jada.archive.2011.0222 PMID:21531934

Schmid Mast, M., Hall, J. A., & Roter, D. L. (2007). Disentangling physician sex and physician communication style: Their effects on patient satisfaction in a virtual medical visit. *Patient Education and Counseling*, *68*(1), 16–22. doi:10.1016/j.pec.2007.03.020 PMID:17482418

Schwartzberg, J. G., Cowett, A., VanGeest, J., & Wolf, M. S. (2007). Communication techniques for patients with low health literacy: A survey of physicians, nurses, and pharmacists. *American Journal of Health Behavior*, *31*(Suppl 1), S96–S104. doi:10.5993/AJHB.31.s1.12 PMID:17931143

Shimanoff, S. B. (1980). *Communication rules: Theory and research*. Sage.

Sobczak, K., Leoniuk, K., Janaszczyk, A., & Pietrzykowska, M. (2016). Patients' Expectations as to Doctors' Behaviors During Appointed Visits. *Health Communication*, *32*(4), 517–519. doi:10.1080/10410236.2016.1140285 PMID:27326538

Spiro, D., & Heidrich, F. (1983). Lay understanding of medical terminology. *The Journal of Family Practice*, *17*, 277–279. PMID:6875485

Spitzberg, B. H., & Hecht, M. L. (1984). A component model of relational competence. *Human Communication Research*, *10*(4), 575–599. doi:10.1111/j.1468-2958.1984.tb00033.x

Stewart, M., Brown, J. B., Donner, A., McWhinney, I. R., Oates, J., Weston, W. W., & Jordan, J. (2000). The impact of patient-centered care on outcomes. *The Journal of Family Practice*, *49*(9), 796–804. PMID:11032203

Stewart, M., Brown, J. B., Hammerton, J., Donner, A., Gavin, A., Holliday, R. L., Whelan, T., Leslie, K., Cohen, I., Weston, W., & Freeman, T. (2007). Improving communication between doctors and breast cancer patients. *Annals of Family Medicine*, *5*(5), 387–394. doi:10.1370/afm.721 PMID:17893379

Street, R. L. Jr, Gordon, H., & Haidet, P. (2007). Physicians' communication and perceptions of patients: Is it how they look, how they talk, or is it just the doctor? *Social Science & Medicine*, *65*(3), 586–598. doi:10.1016/j.socscimed.2007.03.036 PMID:17462801

Suh, W., & Lee, C. (2010). Impact of shared-decision making on patient satisfaction. *Journal of Preventive Medicine and Public Health*, *43*(1), 26–34. doi:10.3961/jpmph.2010.43.1.26 PMID:20185980

Tavakoly Sany, S., Behzhad, F., Ferns, G., & Peyman, N. (2020). Communication skills training for physicians improves health literacy and medical outcomes among patients with hypertension: A randomized controlled trial. *BMC Health Services Research*, *20*(60), 60. doi:10.118612913-020-4901-8 PMID:31973765

Tench, R., & Moreno, A. (2015). Mapping communication management competencies for European practitioners. *Journal of Communication Management (London)*, *19*(1), 39–61. doi:10.1108/JCOM-11-2013-0078

Tench, R., Zerfass, A., Verhoeven, P., Moreno, A., Okay, A., & Verčič, D. (2013a). *ECOPSI Benchmarking Report*. Leeds Metropolitan University.

Tongue, J. R., Epps, H. R., & Forese, L. L. (2005). Communication skills for patient-centered care. *Journal of Bone and Joint Surgery*, *87-A*(3), 652–658. doi:10.2106/00004623-200503000-00027

U.S. Department of Health and Human Services – Centers for Disease Control and Prevention Agency for Toxic Substances and Disease Registry. (n.d.). *Your guide to clear writing*. Atlanta, GA: ATSDR. Retrieved from: https://www.cdc.gov/nceh/clearwriting/docs/clear-writing-guide-508.pdf

van Osch, M., van Dulmen, S., van Vliet, L., & Bensing, J. M. (2017). Specifying the effects of physician's communication on patients' outcomes: A randomised controlled trial. *Patient Education and Counseling*, *100*(8), 1482–1489. doi:10.1016/j.pec.2017.03.009 PMID:28318845

Vaz de Almeida, C. (2015, May). *Técnica ACP para melhorar a literacia dos públicos não especializados*. Communication presented at the International Conference Communicating Science - Emerging Publication Models, Beira Interior, Portugal.

Vaz de Almeida, C. (2016, April). *Comunicação e literacia em saúde: Capacitação de profissionais*. Communication presented at the XII Jornadas Associação Portuguesa de Documentação e Informação de Saúde-APDIS, Coimbra, Portugal.

Vaz de Almeida, C. (2019a). Capacitação dos profissionais de saúde. Literacia em saúde e competências de comunicação dos profissionais de saúde. O modelo de comunicação em saúde ACP. *Revista Nephros*, *21*(1), 25–28.

Vaz de Almeida, C. (2019b). Communication determines safety. *Patient Safety & Quality Healthcare*, 1-6.

Vaz de Almeida, C. (2019c). Modelo de comunicação em saúde ACP: As competências de comunicação no cerne de uma literacia em saúde transversal, holística e prática. In *C. Lopes & C. Vaz de Almeida (Coords.), Literacia em saúde na prática* (pp. 43–52). Edições ISPA.

Vaz de Almeida, C. (2020). Modelo de Comunicação em Saúde – ACP. *Revista Enformação*, *10*, 20–22.

Warde, F., Papadakos, J., Papadakos, T., Rodin, D., Salhia, M., & Giuliani, M. (2018). Plain language communication as a priority competency for medical professionals in a globalized world. *Canadian Medical Education Journal*, *9*(2), e52–e59. doi:10.36834/cmej.36848 PMID:30018684

Weatherspoon, D. J., Horowitz, A. M., Kleinman, D. V., & Wang, M. Q. (2015). The Use of Recommended Communication Techniques by Maryland Family Physicians and Pediatricians. *PLoS One*, *10*(4), e0119855. doi:10.1371/journal.pone.0119855 PMID:25856371

Weingarten, M. A., Guttman, N., Abramovitch, H., Margalit, R. S., Roter, D., Ziv, A., Yaphe, J., & Borkan, J. M. (2009). An anatomy of conflicts in primary care encounters: A multi-method study. *Family Practice*, *27*(1), 93–100. doi:10.1093/fampra/cmp082 PMID:19948564

Wiemann, J. M. (1977). Explication and test of a model of communicative competence. *Human Communication Research*, *3*(3), 195–213. doi:10.1111/j.1468-2958.1977.tb00518.x

Williams, S., Weinman, J., & Dale, J. (1998). Doctor-patient communication and patient satisfaction: A review. *Family Practice*, *15*(5), 480–492. doi:10.1093/fampra/15.5.480 PMID:9848436

Wofford, M. M., Wofford, J. L., Bothra, J., Kendrick, S. B., Smith, A., & Lichstein, P. R. (2004). Patient Complaints about Physician Behaviors: A Qualitative Study. *Academic Medicine*, *79*(2), 134–138. doi:10.1097/00001888-200402000-00008 PMID:14744713

Yen, P. H., & Leasure, A. R. (2019). Use and Effectiveness of the Teach-Back Method in Patient Education and Health Outcomes. *Federal practitioner: For the health care professionals of the VA, DoD, and PHS*, *36*(6), 284–289.

Zengin, S., Al, B., Yavuz, E., Kursunköseler, G., Guzel, R., Sabak, M., & Yildirim, C. (2014). Analysis of complaints lodged by patients attending a university hospital: A 4-year analysis. *Journal of Forensic and Legal Medicine*, *22*, 121–124. doi:10.1016/j.jflm.2013.12.008 PMID:24485436

Chapter 5
Eureka:
A Proposal of a Health Communication Model Based on Communication Competences of the Health Professional! The Assertiveness, Clarity, and Positivity Model

Cristina Vaz de Almeida
ISCSP, University of Lisbon, Portugal

ABSTRACT

The health communication model—assertiveness, clarity, and positivity, which in a more synthetic way is called "ACP Model"—allows in an aggregated and interdependent way the use of communication skills in the health relationship, which allow, throughout the consultation, the establishment of a relationship of greater proximity, trust, openness, balanced and with results for health, even after the interaction ends. Among the results obtained in nine focus groups, consisting of 55 participants, of which 25 are specialists in health literacy and the remaining 30 have not previously experienced the ACP model, all are unanimous in the importance of developing communication skills in the therapeutic relationship through assertiveness, clarity, and positivity as a cognitive script of previous skills. It is also confirmed that this aggregate and interdependent group of communication skills increases the level of knowledge and understanding of the patient's health, thus promoting better health outcomes.

DOI: 10.4018/978-1-7998-4396-2.ch005

INTRODUCTION: THE THERAPEUTIC RELATIONSHIP

The therapeutic relationship is developed in a complex microsystem of relationships between professional and patient, in an environment (family, friends, community), with an immediate scenario where this person is integrated (for example, office, home, school, workplace, etc. (Bronfenbrenner, 1977, p. 514).

Having general communication skills is not enough for effective communication in health. It needs models and techniques in order to achieve the best outcomes (Belim & Vaz de Almeida, 2017). Therapeutic communication is concerned with the identification of dyadic communication (and its characteristics) that lead to therapeutic results (Kreps, 1988, p. 345).

Ledingham, Bruning, Thomlison and Lesko in 1997 in a literature review on interpersonal relationships and other disciplines such as marketing, "discovered 18 relational attributes" (Ledindham, 2008, p. 245): investment, commitment, trust, comfort with relational dialectics, cooperation, mutual objectives, interdependence, balance of power, performance satisfaction, comparison of the level of alternatives, adaptation, investment, shared technology, constructions, structural ties, social ties, intimacy and passion. With the debate in small groups, this list of 18 was reduced to five attributes: 1) trust, 2) openness, 3) involvement, 4) investment and 5) commitment (Ledingham, 2009, p. 245) related in a cluster, in a personal, professional and community level (p. 247). Trust refers to what an organization "does what it says it does"; the opening was operationalized in "sharing the organization's plans for the future" with the public; "involvement" refers to "being involved in the well-being of the community"; the investment "extends to the" well-being of the community "and the" organization's commitment to the well-being of the community "(Ledingham, 2009, p. 245).

The therapeutic relationship, rich in multivariate factors related to cognition, emotion, behaviors, social, environmental, economic, and often political factors (regimes influence the way public health is seen), requires that the health professional is endowed of specific communication skills (previous scripts) so that the results of quality in health are even more effective (Vaz de Almeida, 2018; Nutbeam, 1998; Sørensen et al, 2012).

GUIDELINES FOR A BETTER THERAPEUTIC RELATIONSHIP

However, communication, being a central competence of professionals (Williams et al., 2002), is often not understood by patients. There are data (Ong et al., 1995) that indicate that, after leaving the consultation, the patient remembers 50% or less of the information given to him.

Communication used by the professional and other biopsychosocial issues related to the profile of the recipients, such as, people with low socioeconomic strata, ethnic minorities, the elderly, individuals with cognitive disabilities, with chronic illnesses, low levels of education, or poor skills in literacy, they may adversely affect the patient's understanding of his health status, as well as his therapeutic adherence (Kripalani, S., Bentgtzen, R., Henderson, L., Jacobson, T ., 2008).

The health professional has an increased responsibility, which does not mean an assistentialist posture to replace the patient (except if he clearly wants to). Health professionals are required to complete their skills that go beyond "cure" (Greenhalgh, & Heath, 2010). Its intervention is cognitive, emotional and psychological, based on attention, dynamic and endowed with knowledge, skills and attributes (Tench & Konczos, 2013) in order to contribute to the best health results.

In this sense and counting on a "subjective" experience of the consultation (Hulsman, 2009), some postures and attitudes that fall to the health professional as the "strongest side" of this relatioship are highlighted, without intending to be exhaustive (National Action Plan to Improve Health Literacy, 2010; Vaz de Almeida, 2018, p. 33).

Among the various communication skills used in the therapeutic relationship, and as a result of the present investigation, three stand out that, if used properly in an integrated and interdependent manner, produce favorable results in the therapeutic relationship, especially taking into account the patient's need to understand the health instructions. And they are Assertiveness, Clarity of language and Positivity. These skills involve diverse languages, such as verbal and non-verbal language. Also the result of the research initiated in 2012 with several groups of health professionals, it was found that they are simple to understand, need some training to understand each of their specificities and serve as a "previous guide", strengthening the communication skills of health professional and being used throughout the consultation or therapeutic interaction.

HEALTH LITERACY

Health literacy is an evolving dynamic construct that, due to its own dynamics, is related to the development of the skills of individuals to better access, use, evaluate and understand the health system, in order to make informed decisions to maintain health (Sørensen et al., 2012).

It is a critical skill for engaging in healthy behaviors to reduce disease risk and improve health outcomes (National Academies of Sciences, Engineering & Medicine, 2020, p. 1)

From an individual perspective, health literacy is the degree to which individuals have the capacity to obtain, communicate, process, and understand health information, services, and skills needed to make informed health decisions and act (IOM, 2004; Nutbeam, 1998; Ratzan & Parker, 2000).

It is clear from the very definition of health literacy given by the World Health Organization (1998), that this relationship culminates in “reasoned decisions and health management by the individual, through a process of access, use and understanding and evaluation of information in health, which generates health results”. For these results to be efficient, the information content, made available by the sender, the professional (through verbal and non-verbal language), must be understandable by the receiver, the patient, in a clear and accessible way (Silverman et al., 2013, p. 20).

Sørensen and other authors (2012) reviewed the literature on health literacy, identifying 17 definitions and 12 conceptual models. It is common to assume that health literacy, symptomatic of quality of life (Espanha et al., 2016, p. 1034), involves a set of skills, abilities, knowledge of individuals (health professionals and patients) and organizations (Brach et al., 2012).

According to the U.S. Department of Health and Human Services, Office of Disease Prevention and Health Promotion (2010) and Belim & Vaz de Almeida (2018), health literacy depends on individual and systemic factors, such as:

- Patient and professional communication skills
- Non-technical technical and professional knowledge of health topics
- Culture, habits and beliefs
- Health system and public health requirements
- Situation and / or context requirements

In the individual dimension, the concept integrates the skills and knowledge needed to access, understand, evaluate and use health information, “navigate” the health system and make “right” decisions about health care, disease prevention and ways of promoting healthy living (eg Espanha, Ávila & Mendes, 2016, Sørensen et al., 2012).

The data from the European Literacy Questionnaire (HLS - EU-PT, 2014), composed of 47 questions integrating the domains of health care, health promotion and disease prevention, with 4 levels of information processing in the areas of access, understanding, assessment and use of health information, demonstrate that people in Europe have low levels of health literacy. It was assessed that in Portugal, 61% of the surveyed population has a problematic or inadequate level of general health literacy, with the average of the nine countries standing at 49.2% (Pedro et al., 2016; Saboga-Nunes, 2014). These high numbers of people with low health literacy can respond to the lack of understanding that exists on health matters among this population.

In this process, one of the biggest challenges for health professionals is to provide messages to their audiences that are understood, but that are also based on science (Gazmararian, Curran, Parker, Bernahardt & DeBuono, 2005, p. 317).

Figure 1. Acess, understand and use of information and navigation on the health system
Source: (Adapted from Nutbeam, 1998)

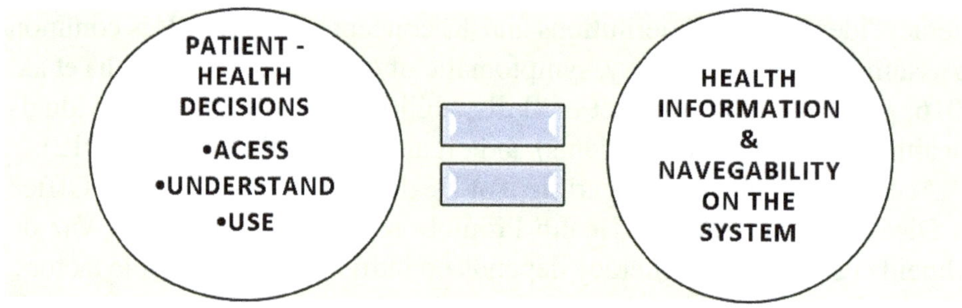

ACP: THE THREE INTERDEPENDENT AND AGGREGATED COMPETENCES

Assertiveness

Assertiveness involves the health professional’s ability to be respectful, encouraging the patient’s participation in the decision-making process and, this continuous health process,based on trust, engagement, involvement (Bruning & Ledingham, 2002) closes a cycle that allows the patient to lead and face his/her problems and needs.

Assertiveness allows an open dialogue process, encouraging the patient to participate and adequately managing all moments of the therapeutic relationship. Assertiveness implies leadership, critical management, the ability to listen and make the necessary silences to produce results in this interaction: perceiving and coordinating the essence of the consultation. Realize what reasons brought the patient to that diadic health meeting.

This is a communication and relational process between the health professional and patient. Relational Theory, originating in Ferguson (1984), emphasizes the construction of a model of relationships, based on interpersonal communication (Bruning & Ledingham, 2002, p. 24; Kim, 2001), "mutually beneficial" (Ledingham & Bruning, 1998), symmetrical and reciprocal (Hon & Grunig, 1999).

Salter (1949) defined six characteristics of an assertive personality. In the first place, an assertive personality has an emotional discourse, that is, it shows feelings openly (Salter, 1949). The second characteristic of assertiveness is being expressive in speech, using precise and spontaneous expressions. Wolpe (1973) also comes to say that it is a manifestation, without anxiety, respecting the characteristics of others. Thirdly, Salter (1949) highlights the ability to have / hear other opinions. Fourth, the assertive person uses the personal pronoun, that is, he assumes what he does and says how "I" say, do, consider ". Fifth, the assertive person accepts praise, not as immodesty, but as self-respect and proper assessment of his strengths and abilities. Finally, and sixthly, the assertive person makes use of improvisation as a spontaneous expression of feelings, needs and daily concerns.

Clarity

During the consultation, it is important to use open and closed questions, through clear and simple language, and have a positive reinforcement of non-verbal language. Literature argues that plain language (clarity) should provide immediate comprehensibility (Kripalani & Weiss, 2006) in a path of simplicity and explanation of technical jargon (Street, 1991, p. 547) and not just make language "simplistic" (Plainlanguage.gov, 2012; WHO, 2013), since it has to be adapted to the interlocutors,

It's necessary to ask the patient is concerns, the ability to clarify and simplify the technical terms (jargon) used during the consultation and making them more understandable to the patient.

When closing the relationship, it's quite important to maintain the clarity of health instructions associated with the positive behavior that the patient must have (efficacy). The U.S. Department of Health and Human Services, Office of Disease Prevention and Health Promotion. (2010), Kripalani and Weiss, 2006 reveals the necessary to train all health care staff in the principles of plain language (p. 30).

Positivity

Emotion has been strongly linked to memory, or retention (Thomas, 2006) and the conversations that doctors and nurses in the social sphere are designed in part to evoke emotions and lead, "more than adherence", to the sharing of decision that implies commitment. The patient's motivation for change is one of the important factors for memorizing health instructions. Some of the aspects of intrinsic motivation are associated with "pleasure" and "mastery or mastery" of information (Baranowski et al. 2008).

Positive language can literally change the brain and assists in good mental and physical health (Corbin, McConnell, Le Masurier, Corbin & Farrar, 2014, 55). Berman, Darryl and Chutka (2016) and Stewart (1995), in this line, reinforce that a positive relationship contributes to a reinforcement of efficiency and professional satisfaction for their profession (p. 243). Reinforcing the positivity of the relationship, Suchman, Roter, Green and Lipkin (1993) emphasize that professional satisfaction unfolds, intrinsically, in the quality of the relationship with the patient and in his cooperative nature and, among the extrinsic factors, in the adequacy of the collection data and the appropriate use of time.

People who think positively are more likely to make changes because they believe that change is possible (Corbin, McConnell, Le Masurier, Corbin & Farrar, 2014, p. 55).

METHOD

A qualitative study with nine focus groups were structured with 55 health professionals, of which 25 are specialists in health literacy and the remaining

30 have not previously experienced the ACP Model. The results show that all particpants are unanimous in the importance of skills development of communication in the therapeutic relationship through Assertiveness, Clarity and Positivity. All agree that these communication skills increase the level of patient health literacy that, through the ACP Communication Model, and stimulate patient to access, understand, process and use health instructions and take better decisions. Among these 55 health professionals, 14 are male and 55 are female with ages between 27 and 68 years old.

The composition of the groups is in accordance with the rate of feminization of health professionals in Portugal. The feminization rate, at national level (Portugal), of nursing staff is 83.4% (SNS, 2016, p. 149). The feminization rate, at national level, of medical personnel (Portugal), is 59.1% (SNS, 2016, p. 149). In this profession, there is a greater numerical balance between the female and male gender than in nursing.

Three exploratory focus groups were previously organized with a diversity of health professionals, in addition to doctors and nurses. Although the results were very similar, we preferred to keep the analysis only with doctors and nurses

All of them give informed consent to participate in this investigation, and the study had previous approval from Ethical Comission of a large hospital in Lisbon (Portugal). The composition of focus Groups is presented in table 1.

The 4 Focus Groups with health professionals who experienced ACP Model (Table 2).

THE ACP HEALTH COMMUNICATION MODEL: ASSERTIVENESS, CLARITY, POSITIVITY

The ACP Model consists of the aggregate and interdependent use of a set of communication skills and competences that integrate Assertiveness, Language Clarity and Positivity by the health professional. This Health Communication Model allows the health professional to immediately choose a model in the therapeutic relationship, managing to be equipped with greater skills to support the patient in understanding health instructions, and for him to also make correct health decisions.

Table 1. Composition of Focus groups- Participants with no knowledge of ACP Model

	Profession	Age	Gender	Years of practice
FOCUS GROUP 2				
A2S	Nurse	49	F	29
B2S	Medical doctor	31	F	9
C2S	Medical doctor	37	F	6
D2S	Medical doctor	47	F	22
E2S	Nurse	52	F	27
F2S	Nurse	45	F	22
FOCUS GROUP 3				
A3S	Nurse	45	F	20
B3S	Nurse	50	F	28
C3S	Nurse	31	M	7
D3S	Nurse	45	F	24
E3S	Nurse	36	F	14
F3S	Nurse	32	F	10
FOCUS GROUP 4				
A4S	Nurse	36	F	11
B4S	Nurse	44	F	21
C4S	Nurse	43	F	21
D4S	Nurse	45	F	22
E4S	Nurse	35	M	11
F4S	Nurse	47	F	24
FOCUS GROUP 5				
A5S	Medical doctor	29	M	5
B5S	Medical doctor	31	M	7
C5S	Medical doctor	67	M	32
D5S	Medical doctor	49	F	24
E5S	Nurse	52	F	30
F5S	Nurse	50	F	27
FOCUS GROUP 6				
A6S	Medical doctor	32	M	9
B6S	Medical doctor	25	M	1
C6S	Medical doctor	52	F	20
D6S	Medical doctor	43	F	10
E6S	Medical doctor	28	F	3
F6S	Medical doctor	27	F	2

Source: (The author with results from the Focus Groups)

Table 2. List of participants in the Focus groups who experienced the ACP Model

FOCUS GROUP com ACP	Profession	Age	Gender	Years of practice
FOCUS GROUP 3				
A3C	Nurse	40	F	12
B3C	Nurse	30	F	3
C3C	Nurse	57	F	28
D3C	Medical doctor	44	M	12
E3C	Nurse	60	F	40
F3C	Nurse	37	F	15
FOCUS GROUP 4				
A4C	Nurse	53	F	30
B4C	Nurse	51	F	28
C4C	Nurse	32	M	10
D4C	Nurse	52	F	29
E4C	Nurse	47	F	24
F4C	Nurse	30	F	5
FOCUS GROUP 5				
A5C	Nurse	61	M	42
B5C	Nurse	68	F	45
C5C	Nurse	59	M	36
D5C	Nurse	56	M	30
E5C	Nurse	62	F	39
F5C	Nurse	60	F	37
FOCUS GROUP 6				
A6C	Nurse	37	M	15
B6C	Nurse	59	F	38
C6C	Nurse	50	F	25
D6C	Nurse	36	M	13
E6C	Nurse	46	F	26
F6C	Nurse	61	F	38
G6C	Nurse	54	F	31

Source: (The author with results from the Focus Groups)

With the ACP Model - Assertiveness, Clarity and Positivity, developed by Vaz dc Almeida (Almeida, 2018, 2019; Belim & Vaz de Almeida, 2018; Vaz de Almeida & Belim, 2021,a, 2021b) health professionals are better able to communicate and stimulate their recipients for better understanding and decision making.

This ACP Model was tested and proven in its effects by a vast group of hundreds of health professionals who benefited between 2012 and 2018, from advanced training at ISPA in Health Literacy, as well as from Postgraduate Studies in Health Literacy: Models, Strategies and Intervention (2017/2018), training in a hospital context in Portugal, as evidenced by 9 focus groups of health professionals from (doctors from general clinic, hospital nurses).

For analysis of Focus groups (n=9) and in-depth interviews (n=3), a qualitative content analysis (ACQ) was carried out. This type of QCA performed is thematic, where the data (Focus groups and depth interviews) are examined to extract the themes. Categories are established in the ACQ. In addition, these categories are the communication skills that make up the ACP model, among others that arise (such as those selected by FG participants in the skills table, listed in descending order) and that may be significant for the model. The generation of initial codes and a coding structure are carried out, informed predominantly by the topics in the discussion guide (1) communication, 2) therapeutic relationship, 3) communication skills, 4) assertiveness, 5) clarity, 6) positivity, although new views expressed by the participants were also captured (trust, holistic view, effectiveness, efficiency).

The data from focus groups and in-depth interviews were coded for this structure, working with paper copies of the transcripts, underlining and writing down the most significant expressions and the codes were organized into possible themes and subthemes, and similarities and differences of views between the target groups and configurations were explored.

The review of topics continued: the data, which were coded into topics, were reviewed and adjusted in order to guarantee the organization of a coherent standard (organization in tables dividing the themes by each category and by profession - doctors and nurses) . Finally, and lastly, a results analysis report was prepared and produced with a comparison between the professional categories, by gender and by theme.

RESULTS: THE HEALTHCARE PROFESSIONAL AS A CONDUCTOR OF THE COMPOSITION OF PATIENT EMOTIONS, FEELINGS AND COGNITIONS

Therapeutic relationship must be endowed with certain requirements that will optimize health results: trust, empathy, understanding, firmness, determination.

Among the participants in the various focus groups carried out in this research and over the years, it is highlighted that health professionals have the responsibility to guide the patient to questions, using clarity, and to invest in patient's self-efficacy, motivating him/her to act (Vaz de Almeida & Belim, 2021a)

There are key components in the relationship associated with cognition, emotion, behaviors. And the combined use of the three communication skills – assertiveness, clarity and posititivity - allows a more effective investment in the results, relieving the health professional of the burden of his responsibility in conducting the therapeutic interaction. The health professional is the conductor, who must allow the patient's emotions and feelings to be transformed into understood and memorized cognitions that lead him to adhere to the instructions.

These requirements can be condensed into a communication model composed of three components: assertiveness, clarity and positivity. But the therapeutic relationship is complex. Following the considerations of the participants in the focus groups, and depth -interviews, we can evaluate this complexity. We summarize the results obtained, on the view that health professionals have of the therapeutic relationship (Table 3).

In the next table (4), we can see some expressions that indicate how doctors and nurses perceive, in the therapeutic relationship, the importance of assertiveness, clear language and positivity, in the dimension of understanding the message.

A table of communication skills associated with communication skills was also distributed. Focus group participants completed the table after the discussion ended. Participants were asked to complete the table according to their own perception of each competency (assertiveness, clarity and positivity).

These 55 participants, all health professionals, selected the expressions that, in their own opinion, sensitivity, understanding and vision, which most corresponded to the components of the ACP Model.

Table 3. The complexity of the therapeutic relationship

1. Evaluate and measure the essence of health consultation
2. Have observation skills
3. Understand the patient's schedule
4. Get agreement on problems and treatment plans
5. Support the identification of needs (conscious and unconscious)
6. Apply non-verbal language (prosody, proxemia, cyesthesias, silences, paraverbal)
7. Apply verbal language with assertiveness, clarity and positivity
8. Work empathy
9. Treat the patient respectfully
10. Facilitate healing: answering patient questions
11. Encourage the patient to participate in the process even if they do not participate in the decision
12. Replace patient if this need is evidente (patients with very low health literacy)
13. Evaluate and anticipate patient reactions
14. Have flexibility in face of the diversity of emotions that the patient presents
15. Use repetition (primacy - in the beginning of conversation; and recency - in the end)
16. Tailored media: writing, drawing, voice, touch according to patient profile
17. Open and closed questions according to theme, timing, context
18. Recognize the limitations, constraints and beliefs
19. Know how to accept the other
20. Know how to listen and have silences
21. Know how to use humor when appropriate
22. Knowing how to distinguish content (health or illness) from context (relationship, culture)
23. Evaluate and guide self-efficacy (know-how)
24. Evaluate the type of visual, audiovisual memory to increase adherence
25. Provide information in parts (chunk & check)
26. Explain procedures, treatments
27. Know how to manage bad news
28. Consider the patient's age, culture and socioeconomic status
29. Use health literacy methods (avoid faint jargon, clear language, teach-back, chunck & check)

Source: (Based on results of 9 Focus Groups and 3 depth interviews; Belim & Vaz de Almeida, 2018; Harrington & Valerio, 2004; Ley, 1989; Ogden, 2004; Pina, 2003; Ranjan et al, 2015; Schwarzer, 1992)

As a result, the 10 main expressions associated with assertiveness integrate the following elements of competence: 1) Conflict management; 2) Leadership; 3) Individual pulse control; 4) Contact Control; 5) Know how to say no; 6) Respect others; 7) Ability to speak openly; 8) Ability to listen; 9) Active behavior; 10) Commitment to the relationship.

As for clarity, the same participants chose as the top 10 references to 1) Plain language; 2) Use of verbs; 3) Simple words; 4) Teach-back method; 5) Use of technical; jargon; 6) Direct language; 7) Ability to speak openly; 8) Clear instructions; 9) Action Orientation; 10) Specific action leading to better health.

Positivity was associated with 1) Motivation; 2) Empathy; 3) Guidance for positive patient behavior; 4) Encouraging Cooperation; 5) Understanding the mistakes of others; 6) Strengthening attitudes in disease prevention and treatment; 7) Guilt and shame (negative); 8) Commitment to the relationship; 9) Courage and 10) Confidence (Table 5).

Table 4. Results of perceptions in the focus groups of assertiveness, clarity and positivity

ASSERTIVENESS
• "Assertiveness allow to improve the relationship and health outcomes" (B3C, D3C) • "Involves the expression of opinion, respecting the limits of the other, in an active listening" (B9S) • "I can think that I am being assertive, but I also have to adapt the language and also be positive" (D3C) • "The professional must also be aware that he can train assertiveness to improve and have more positive results" (A3C) • Assertiveness is an important tool, but it has to be worked on/trained (F3C) • "To act right, taking into account objectification, determination and empathy" (F2S) • "To be consistent" (A4S) • "To have a professional attitude" (E4S) • "To act like an "agent that facilitates the therapeutic relationship" (C4C) • To be "competent, safe, true when transmitting the message and / or information" (F4C) • All of this results in "being correct, being firm" (D4S) • "Has to do with behavior" (E4S)
CLARITY
• "Clear language, being easily understood by others, increases their information and therefore, health literacy, which contributes to improving the therapeutic relationship" (E4C) • "Clarity of language is the simple language used and through which the patient perceives what the professional says" (all FG3C) • "Clear language contributes to increased patient health literacy" (all FG) • "Balance and accuracy of information: The level of information I intend to transmit or receive is exactly what it is to transmit" (A5S, F4C) • "It is more than normal for us to be able to pass on to the patient in a more intelligible language, but it is normal that he cannot reach this citizen" (all FG) • "Communication must be accessible" (A4C, B3C, D4C, F3C) • "Communication must be decoded" (A3C, B3S, B4S, C3S, D4C) • "Language is important as well as the hope placed in this relationship" (D3C).
POSITIVITY
• "Positivity is motivational and allows influencing the patient's self-esteem level" (F3C) • "Positivity is also not creating false expectations. Make the user create the real expectations" (E3C) • "Positivity supports the perception of reality" (E3C) • "Being positive is the safety that the health professional transmits to the patient" (A4C) • "Positivity is the choice of words" (A4C) • "Positivity is the focus on the solution and seeing the way forward" (B4C) • "Positivity involves presenting things in a simpler way" (D4C) • "It means seeing the good side and approaching situations in a practical and easy way and not in a difficult way" (D4C) • "Positivity It is to emphasize the benefits, even though they are difficult to value the "little" (D4C) • "Positivity contributes to the success of the therapeutic relationship. Without positivity, it will be much more difficult to have the user's adherence to the care plan and in maintaining the management of their health or disease" (D4C) • "Being positive is an attribute that can be learned" (A4C) • "Positivity makes the person realize and improve in small things; it is like climbing one step at a time (A4C) • "Positivity allows the person / patient to move forward, involve the person / patient with positive emotions, give a pleasant and beneficial sense to the process in which the relationship takes place" (B4C) • "Is to see the positive aspects of the issues, that is, to be able to remove the good that exists in the change processes" (E5S) • "Is to increase the confidence and motivation of others. (Give an example): when the person says he is sick and with low esteem, reinforcing the positive is showing that there is a good goal that is the one that he still has ahead (A4C)

Source: (Own elaboration based on results of Focus Groups 2018-2019)

Table 5. Assertiveness, clarity and positivity competences choose by the health professionals

ASSERTIVENESS		CLARITY		POSITIVITY	
Conflict management	43	Plain language	47	Motivation	31
Leadership	39	Use of verbs	43	Empathy	28
Individual pulse control	37	Simple words	35	Guidance for positive patient behavior	27
Contact control	34	*Teach-back* method	30	Encouraging Cooperation	26
Know how to say no	33	Use of technical jargon	27	Understanding the mistakes of others	23
Respect for others	31	Direct language	26	Strengthening attitudes in disease prevention and treatment	22
Ability to speak openly	31	Ability to speak openly	25	Guilt and shame	21
Ability to listen	29	Clear instructions	24	Commitment to the relationship	19
Active behavior	28	Action Orientation	20	Courage	17
Commitment to the relationship	27	Specific action leading to better health	16	Confidence	17

Source: (The author, 2019)

All respondents stress that the model, although "intuitive" must be learned. Although these ACP skills are "simple to understand", they are health communication skills that "have to be learned and trained".

Also, the in-depth interviews, made to deepen some questions, reinforced the importance of the ACP Model. We highlight some excerpts from the interviews conclusions about the model. A nurse doing her PhD, a specialist in health literacy (HL1), a doctor who coordinates organ transplantation in a large hospital in Lisbon (Portugal) (HL2) and a professor of psychology, doctorate in health literacy (HL3).

HL1 explains: "I think it is a very useful model: assertiveness involves taking care not to be intrusive, in the clarity of being clear, but not being abrupt and positivity is extremely important because it meets a path and a salutogenic paradigm." HL1 says that positivity "is trying to make people realize that there is still a positive path, that there is still something positive there. And often they are small things. It is necessary to see small gains in health with the patient, which are gains in health results"

Regarding her own learning of the ACP Model, HL2 says that "a few years ago I did not have this awareness of the importance of communication. I didn't have this notion of how technical it is. There are techniques for everything, in fact tools have been developed, and we must think about them because it always improves the relationship". This specialist associate awareness with learning: "It is a learned model. There is always room for improvement when you become aware" And HL2, says: "communication is the basis, it is the instrument par excellence of health literacy". Especifically about positivity, the competence whose definition brought multiple and diverse contributions HL" explains: "[Positivity] bridges the gap between positivity and patient training" and stresses that "the positivity seen in its scope makes an enormous qualitative leap. It is more than the salutogenic paradigm, it is giving hope to the person. It is taking a leap and asking the person: "do you prefer it this way, or do you prefer it in another way?", "How can we do it?"

In 2013, communication specialists Tench and Konczos (2013) consolidated the tripartite competence approach, already listed by the OECD (2005). They emphasize that competencies are foundational skills (p. 43), which allow tasks and responsibilities to be successfully carried out over time and in a stable manner (Tench & Konczos, 2013, p. 43). They are subdivided into knowledge (eg general, theoretical, from other cultures), skills (eg problem solving, persuasion, reading comprehension) and personal attributes (eg honesty, leadership, trust) (Tench & Konczos, 2013). Competence is the combination of skills, knowledge and personal attributes that lead to a superior performance of professionals (Tench & Konczos, 2013, p. 5).

It was also possible, through focus groups and in-depth interviews, the skills associated with the knowledge, skills and attributes of each of the skills of assertiveness, clarity and positivity. The following table presents the summary of this segmentation that seeks to clarify each of the components of each competency (Table 6).

Table 6. Competences: knowledge, skills, and attributes A-C-P

COMPETENCES		
Knowledge **TO KNOW**	**Skills** **TO DO**	**Attributes** **TO BE**
ASSERTIVENESS		
Theorical knowledge Consultation strategies Intercultural domain Planning (script) Understand commitment in the relationship Meets the standards Knows the patient's rights and duties Domain of clinical knowledge Knows conflict management Knows assertive communication	Help the patient to face emotional problems related to his / her condition; Help the patient to express their concerns; To have a respectful behavior: Confirms that the patient understands; Controls enforcement; Controls individual impulses; Controls external factors; Supports the patient (eg "care" conversation instead of "cure" conversation; Encourage the patient to ask questions; Make the patient feel they have time for him / her during the interaction; Generates feelings and emotions for an efficient response; Manage stress; Informs the patient always attentively; Informs the patient respectfully; Leads and negotiates with the patient rationally and positively; Knows how to converse (start, maintain, conduct a conversation); Knows how to say "no"; Knows how to manage moments of tension / sadness; Knows how to influence; Knows how to listen to the patient; Knows self-control; Uses assertive language.	Leader Confident Integral Respectful Self-criticism Self esteem Courageous Disciplined Effective Persuader Resilient Responsible Commited Insurance from you

continues on following page

Table 6. Continued

COMPETENCES		
Knowledge **TO KNOW**	**Skills** **TO DO**	**Attributes** **TO BE**
CLARITY		
Knows the cultural differences and the representation of some languages (verbal and gestural) Knows the dimensions of health literacy (access, understanding and use) Knows the concept of clear language Knows non-verbal language	Helps the patient with simple language to find information; Asks open questions; Confirms that the patient understands everything for their own safety; Knows what said to the patient in previous consultations; Provides information and clarify; Gives clear instructions; Discusses the next steps and follow-up plans with the patient; Demonstrates to the patient how to do it (with graphics, images, drawings, or diagrams); Draws instructions (make graphics, drawings); Writes the instructions to facilitate the patient's memory; Writes clearly; Establishes the relationship with the patient through simple language; Establishes eye contact with the patient; Explains in detail the drugs, treatments and tests; Explains / speaks clearly; Inform the patient about what they want to know, their symptoms and health status; Realizes the information that is given by the patient, to provide quick relief; Prepare the patient about what to expect from healthcare; Translates technical jargon whenever it is used (and not understood); Uses short phrases; Use simple words; Uses of the first person: "I" in the speech; Uses verbs; Uses non-verbal language; Check the information.	Agility of thought Good listener Mental clarity Ethical Flexibility Good evaluator Synthetic Knowing how to ask questions

continues on following page

Table 6. Continued

COMPETENCES		
Knowledge **TO KNOW**	**Skills** **TO DO**	**Attributes** **TO BE**
POSITIVITY		
Understands the mistakes of others Knows positive language Knows the bases of positive relationships (strengths of character) Knows about the human mind (behavior change) Realizes the importance of positive persuasive effects Recognizes the contributions to make the relationship with the patient positive and constructive	Adopts courtesy and care when dealing with the patient; Helps the patient to create positive expectations; Helps the patient cope with health-related emotional problems; Greets cordially; Provides social support (questions on non-clinical issues); Let the patient speak without interruption; Involves the patient in decision making; Avoids using negative words and phrases; Explains situations in a positive way to the patient to perform their daily tasks; Encourages the patient to make decisions; Shows the patient the positive behavior they must have; Shows positive non-verbal communication (posture, eye contact, tone of voice, proximity); Shows emotion and affection; Shows esteem; Smiles; Uses the active voice (subject-predicate - direct complement); Uses positive phrases.	Confident Creative Polite Empathetic Energetic Humorist (in right doses) Motivating Motivator Optimistic

Source: (Own elaboration based on the empirical results and by Cegala, 2003; Gregory, 2008, p. 216; Tench and Konczos, 2013).

DISCUSSION OF RESULTS

The groups were unanimous on the importance of developing health professional's communication skills to improve patients' health literacy following Kickbusch, Wait and Maag (2006) who confirm that professionals need, in this context, to adapt their communication to meet the needs of their patients and see as their responsibility to promote health literacy (2006, p. 16).

Participants also emphasized the importance of verbal and non-verbal language (Kreps, 1988, p. 336). The set of attitudes and behaviors based on communication skills should generate more confidence (Ledingham, 2009; Wiemann, 1977) for the patient and that will allow greater therapeutic adherence as well as a positive consolidation of the therapeutic relationship (Street, 2009).

Participants agreed that a more efficient communication (Nutbeam, 1998), developed through an assertive posture, through clear and positive language, can lead to a better understanding of the receiver / patient and, in turn, to the best health results, individual and societal (meso and macro).

The ACP communication competences model allows the development of a more harmonious and effective therapeutic relationship, with increased awareness and, consequently, the understanding of the patient, memorization and motivation to make better decisions about his health or those who depend on him (Almeida, 2018, 2019; Vaz de Almeida & Belim, 2021a, 2021b). Doctors and nurses in this study know and that a person with greater literacy will know how to take better care of their health and life, but the reality presents us with a rate of more than 50% with problematic or inadequate literacy

In the *Focus groups*, most of the doctors of a large portuguese hospital considered education as "an essential factor", "key- determinant" to improve the level of knowledge of individuals. These results are reinforced by the literature, Tu and Hargraves (2003) claim that education is the key to explaining differences in information demand. Specifically, in the therapeutic relationship, health professionals assume a strategic role, in which communication skills can make a difference. Investment should be centered especially on health professionals' communication skills, which can contribute to motivate the patient to act and be empowered. Communication is a fundamental dimension in the therapeutic relationship (Silverman et al., 2013, p. 7).

Focus groups participants also refer to the importance and difficulties of empowering patients, made possible by communication (Ishikawa & Kiuchi, 2010). It is necessary to give the person a chance and know what he can do, according to the situation of his illness. For therapeutic adherence, people are influenced by various social, economic and cultural determinants of health (Wilkinson and Marmot, 2003).

All the participants agree for strengthening communication skills (Hulsman, 2009) and for considering health literacy not only in terms of the characteristics of individuals, but also in terms of interactional processes (Ishikawa & Kiuchi, 2010) and environmental and educational (Sørensen et al., 2012).

Assertiveness, Clarity, and Positivity

Aiming to fill the gap in the literature and the lack of enunciation of specific and explicit communication skills, the ACP Model could be applied during the consultation process, bringing together a set of three communication skills to be used in the environment of health.

This model of health communication skills provides a simple, aggregate, interdependent, easily recognizable and understandable structure that allows, through learning to provide knowledge, skills and reinforce the attributes of the health professional, with explicit descriptions of its applicability: assertiveness, clarity of language and positivity. For example, and according to the profile of the patient and his "essence" (Egener, & Cole-Kelly, 2004) there may be a weighting of greater incidence of assertiveness and clarity at the beginning, when establishing rapport once it is established. to take the first opening steps and to listen to the patient. The literature also recognizes this selection regarding conflict management and the commitment to the relationship (Alberti & Emmons, 2008; Smith, 1985). In 1973 Lazarus states that the main components of assertive (or emotionally expressive) behaviors fall into four separate and specific patterns, reflecting the ability to 1) say "no", 2) to ask for favors or make requests, 3) to express feelings positive and negative and 4) start, continue or end general conversations (Harris & Brown, 1979, p. 181). Study participants, by considering assertiveness as recognizing their rights and the rights of others, using respect, meet the literature (e.g. Alberti & Emmons, 2008; Smith, 1985). But they go further by involving a deep sense of sharing, emotions and feelings in the therapeutic relationship. In this sense, the use of emotion, positive motivating factors, a controlled and adequate mood provided to the patient, so that he understands and adheres, can contribute to a better understanding and consequent therapeutic adherence (Levinson, Lesser & Epstein, 2010).

During consultation and when is made one physical examination and it is necessary to ask the patient, it is important to use open and closed questions, through clear and simple language, the positive reinforcement of non-verbal language, the ability to clarify and simplify the technical terms used during the consultation, making them more understandable to the patient.

Finally, in closing, the relationship to the clarity of the instructions associated with the positive behavior that the patient must have, the incentive to comply with the guidelines by maintaining respect, encouraging the patient's participation in the decision-making process, closes a cycle that allows comforting the patient and being able to know their initial needs.

With assertiveness, a respectful, balanced relationship is achieved, which moves towards participatory equality, trust, commitment, involvement through mutual respect and transparency.

Through clear language, the content of the instructions flows in an understandable dialogue for both participants who correctly encode and decode the message conveyed and the present needs, considering the levels of health literacy of the interlocutors.

Positivity increases the ability to recognize "active and positive action", contradicting "non-action" and passivity, stimulating behavior for action, motivated behavior change, and understanding of health instructions, which lead to this to better results for the person, for his family, community and system.

CONCLUSION

Health communication models are useful for strengthening health professionals' communication skills. Using the ACP model allows in an aggregate and interdependent way to use assertiveness, clarity and positivity. Just using assertiveness and not being clear or positive does not produce the same results. There may be respect for the patient, but if the language is airtight and complex, the patient does not understand the message. It also does not produce the same results if the conversation is positive, but the health professional dominates the discourse and has a hegemonic attitude. It is necessary to use positivity that encourages positive behavior and action. Thus, in an aggregated form, this model meets the patient, the health professional who also seeks satisfaction from being understood and the results in health, through understanding and better adherence and health and well-being outcomes.

REFERENCES

Alberti, R. E., & Emmons, M. L. (2008). *Your perfect right: Assertiveness and equality in your life and relationships*. Impact Publishers.

Almeida, C. V. (2018). Literacia em saúde – Capacitação dos profissionais de saúde: O lado mais forte da balança. In *C Lopes & C.V. Almeida (Coords), Literacia em saúde: Modelos, estratégias e intervenção* (pp. 33–42). Edições ISPA.

Baranowski, T., Anderson, C., & Carmack, C. (1998). Mediating variable framework in physical activity interventions: How are we doing? How might we do better? *American Journal of Preventive Medicine*, *15*(4), 266–297. doi:10.1016/S0749-3797(98)00080-4 PMID:9838973

Belim, C., & Vaz de Almeida, C. (2017). Healthy thanks to communication: A model of communication competences to optimize health literacy: Assertiveness, clear language, and positivity. In V. E. Papalois & M. Theodospoulous (Eds.), *Optimizing health literacy for improved clinical practices* (pp. 124–152). IGI Global.

Berlo, D. K. (1977). Communication as Process: Review and Commentary. *Annals of the International Communication Association*, *1*(1), 11–27. doi:10.1080/23808985.1977.11923667

Berman, A. C., & Chutka, D. S. (2016). Assessing effective physician-patient communication skills: "Are you listening to me, doc?" *Korean J Med Educ*, *28*(2), 243-249. doi:10.3946/kjme.2016.21

Bronfenbrenner, U. (1977). Toward an experimental ecology of human development. *The American Psychologist*, *32*(7), 513–531. doi:10.1037/0003-066X.32.7.513

Brown, R. F., & Bylund, C. L. (2008). Communication skills training: Describing a new conceptual model. *Academic Medicine*, *83*(1), 37–44. doi:10.1097/ACM.0b013e31815c631e PMID:18162748

Bruning, S. D., & Ledingham, J. A. (2002). Identifying the Communication, Behaviors, and Interaction Patterns of Agency-Client Relationships in Development and Decline. *Journal of Promotion Management*, *8*(2), 21–34. doi:10.1300/J057v08n02_03

Burgoon, K. K., Ster, L. A. S., & Dillman, L. (1995). *Interpersonal adaptation*. Cambridge University Press. doi:10.1017/CBO9780511720314

Cegala, D. J. (2003). Patient communication skills training: A review with implications for cancer patients. *Patient Education and Counseling*, *50*(1), 91–94. doi:10.1016/S0738-3991(03)00087-9 PMID:12767592

Corbin, C. B., McConnell, K. E., Le Masurier, G. C., Corbin, D. E., & Farrar, T. D. (2014). *Health opportunities through physical education*. Human Kinetics.

Council on Linkages between Academia and Public Health Practice. (2014). *Core Competencies for Public Health Professionals*. The Author.

Dance, F. E. X. (1970). The "concept" of Communication. *Journal of Communication, 20*(2), 201–210. doi:10.1111/j.1460-2466.1970.tb00877.x

Deutsch, F., & Madle, R. A. (1975). Empathy: Historic and current conceptualizations and a cognitive theoretical perspective. *Human Development, 18*(4), 267–287. doi:10.1159/000271488 PMID:765261

Egener, B., & Cole-Kelly, K. (2004). Satisfying the Patient, But Failing the Test. *Academic Medicine, 79*(6), 508–510. doi:10.1097/00001888-200406000-00003 PMID:15165968

Engel, G. L. (1981). The clinical application of the biopsychosocial model. *The Journal of Medicine and Philosophy, 6*(2), 101–123. doi:10.1093/jmp/6.2.101 PMID:7264472

Epstein, R. M., & Franks, P. (2005). Patient-centered communication and diagnosis testing. *Annals of Family Medicine, 3*(5), 415–421. doi:10.1370/afm.348 PMID:16189057

Espanha, R., Ávila, P., & Mendes, R. M. (2016). *A literacia em saúde em Portugal*. Lisboa: Fundação Calouste Gulbenkian, CIES – IUL.

Ferguson, M. A. (1984). *Building theory in public relations: Interorganizational relationships*. In Annual Convention of the Association for Education in Journalism and Mass Communication, Gainesville, FL.

Gazmararian, J.A., Curran, J. W., Parker, R.M., Bernahardt, J.M. & DeBuono, A. (2005). Public health literacy I America. An ethical imperative. *AMJ.Prev. Med., 28*(3), 317-322.

Greenhalgh, T., & Heath, I. (2010). *Measuring quality in the therapeutic relationship. An Inquiry into the quality of general practice in England*. The King's Fund.

Gregory, A. (2008). Competencies of senior communication practitioners in the UK: An initial study. *Public Relations Review, 34*(3), 215–223. doi:10.1016/j.pubrev.2008.04.005

Grunig, L. A., Grunig, J. E., & Ehling, W. P. (1992). What is an effective organization? In J. E. Grunig (Ed.), *Excellent public relations and communication management* (pp. 65–90). Lawrence Erlbaum Associates.

Harrington, J., Noble, L.M., & Newman, S.P. (2004). Improving patient's participation with doctors: a systematic review of intervention studies. *Patient Education and Counseling, 52*(1), 7-16.

Harris, T., & Brown, N. (1979). Congruent validity of the rathus assertiveness schedule. *Educational and Psychol. Management*, *39*, 181–186.

Hon, L. C., & Grunig, J. E. (1999). Guidelines for measuring relationships in public relations. Guineville, FL: Institute for Public Relations.

Hulsman, R. L. (2009). Shifting goals in medical communication. Determinants of goal detection and response formation. *Patient Education and Counseling*, *74*(3), 302–308. doi:10.1016/j.pec.2008.12.001 PMID:19135823

Institute of Medicine. (2011). *Clinical Practice Guidelines We Can Trust. Committee on Standards for Developing Trustworthy Clinical Practice Guidelines*. National Academies Press. doi:10.17226/13058

IOM. (2004). Improving Medical Education: Enhancing the Behavioral and Social Science Content of Medical School Curricula. Institute of Medicine. Washington, DC: National Academies Press.

Kaplan, A. (1964). *The conduct of inquiry. Methodology for behavioral science*. Transaction.

Keller, D. B., Sarkar, U., & Schillinger, D. (2014). Health literacy and information exchange in medical settings. In L. R. Martin & M. R. DiMatteo (Eds.), *The Oxford handbook of health communication, behavior change, and treatment adherence* (pp. 23–37). Oxford University Press.

Kim, J.-N., & Grunig, J. E. (2011). Problem solving and communicative action: A situational theory of problem solving. *Journal of Communication*, *61*(1), 120–149. doi:10.1111/j.1460-2466.2010.01529.x

Kreps, G. L. (1988). The pervasive role of information in health and health care: Implications for health communication policy. In J. Anderson (Ed.), *Communication yearbook 11* (pp. 238–276). Sage.

Kripalani, S., Bentgtzen, R., Henderson, L. E., & Jacobson, T. A. (2008). Clinical research in low literacy population: Using teach back to assess comprehension on informed consent and privacy information. *Ethics & Human Research*, *30*(2), 13–19. PMID:18512655

Kripalani, S., & Weiss, B. D. (2006). Teaching about health literacy and clear communication. *Journal of General Internal Medicine*, *21*(8), 888–890. doi:10.1111/j.1525-1497.2006.00543.x PMID:16881953

Lazarus, A. A. (1973). On assertive behavior: A brief note. *Behavior Therapy*, *4*(5), 697–699. doi:10.1016/S0005-7894(73)80161-3

Ledigham, J. A., Bruning, S. D., Thomlinson, D., & Lesko, C. (1997). Toward a theory of relational loyalty: A qualitative approach. *Academy of Managarial Journal.*, *9*, 23–43.

Ledingham, J. A. (2009). A chronology of organization stakeholder relationships with recommendation concerning practitioner adoption of the relational perspective. *Journal of Promotion Management*, *14*(39), 243–262. doi:10.1080/10496490802637846

Ledingham, J. A., & Bruning, S. D. (1998). Relationship Management in Public Relations: Dimensions of an Organization-Public Relationship. *Public Relations Review*, *24*(1), 55–65. doi:10.1016/S0363-8111(98)80020-9

Littlejohn, S. W. (1982). *Fundamentos teóricos da comunicação humana*. Zahar Editores.

National Academies of Sciences, Engineering, and Medicine. (2018). *Community-based health literacy interventions: Proceedings of a workshop*. Washington, DC: The National Academies Press. doi:10.17226/24917

National Action Plan to Improve Health Literacy. (2010). *U.S. Department of Health and Human Services, Office of Disease Prevention and Health Promotion*. Author.

Nutbeam, D. (1998). Health promotion glossary. *Health Promotion International*, *13*(4), 349–364. doi:10.1093/heapro/13.4.349

Ogden, J. (2004). *Psicologia da Saúde*. Climepsi Editores.

Ong, L., de Haes, J. D., Hoos, A. M., & Lammes, F. B. (1995). Doctor-patient communication: A review of literature. *Social Science & Medicine*, *40*(7), 903–918. doi:10.1016/0277-9536(94)00155-M PMID:7792630

Paakkari, L., & Paakkari, O. (2012). Health literacy as a learning outcome in schools. *Health Education, 112*(2), 133–152. doi:10.1108/09654281211203411

Parvanta, C., & Bass, S.B. (2020). *Health Communication Strategies and Skills for a New Era.* Jones & Bartlett Learning.

Pedro, A. R., Amaral, O., & Escoval, A. (2016). Literacia em saúde, dos dados à ação: Tradução, validação e aplicação do European Health Literacy Survey em Portugal. *Revista Portuguesa de Saude Publica, 34*(3), 259–275. doi:10.1016/j.rpsp.2016.07.002

Pendleton, D., Schofield, T., Tate, P., & Havelock, P. (2003). *The new consultation. Developing doctor–patient communication.* Oxford University Press. doi:10.1093/med/9780192632883.001.0001

Pina, A. E. (2003). *A responsabilidade dos médicos* (3rd ed.). Lidel.

Ranjan, P., Kumari, A., & Chakrawarty, A. (2015). How can doctors improve their communication skills? *Journal of Clinical and Diagnostic Research: JCDR, 9*(3), JE01–JE04. doi:10.7860/JCDR/2015/12072.5712 PMID:25954636

Ratzan, S. C. (1994). Health communication as a negotiation. The healthy Amarica act. *The American Behavioral Scientist, 38*(1), 224–247. doi:10.1177/0002764294038002005

Rimal, R. N., & Lapinski, M. K. (2009). Why health communication is important in public health. *Bulletin of the World Health Organization, 87*(4), 247–247. doi:10.2471/BLT.08.056713 PMID:19551226

Ruesch, J. (1963). The role of communication in therapeutic transactions. *Journal of Communication, 13*(3), 132–139. doi:10.1111/j.1460-2466.1963.tb02096.x

Ruesch, J., & Bateson, G. (1951). *Communication The social matrix of psychiatry.* WW Norton & Company.

Saboga-Nunes, L. (2014). Literacia para a saúde e a conscientização da cidadania positiva. *Revista Referência,* (III), 94–99.

Salter, A. (2002). *Conditioned reflex therapy: The classic book on assertiveness that began behavior therapy.* Wellness Institute.

Silverman, J., Krutz, S., & Draper, J. (2013). *Skills for communicating with patients.* Taylor & Francis Group.

Smith, M. J. (1985). *When I say no, I feel guilty*. Bantam Books.

SNS. (2016). *Relatório social do ministério da saúde e do serviço nacional de saúde*. Lisboa: Ministério da saúde.

Sørensen, K., Van den Broucke, S., Fullam, J., Douyle, G., Pelikan, J., Slonska, Z., & Brand, H. (2012). Health literacy and Public health: A systematic review and integration of definitions and models. *BMC Public Health*, *12*(1), 80. doi:10.1186/1471-2458-12-80 PMID:22276600

Street, R. L. Jr. (1991). Information-giving in medical consultation. The influence of patient's communicative styles and personal characteristics. *Social Science & Medicine*, *32*(5), 541–548. doi:10.1016/0277-9536(91)90288-N PMID:2017721

Street, R. L. Jr. (2007). Aiding medical decision making: A communication perspective. *Medical Decision Making*, *27*(5), 550–553. doi:10.1177/0272989X07307581 PMID:17921451

Suchman, A. R., Roter, D. L., Green, M., & Lipkin, M. Jr. (1993). Physician satisfaction with primary care office visits. *Medical Care*, *31*(12), 1083–1092. doi:10.1097/00005650-199312000-00002 PMID:8246638

Teixeira J. A. C. (1999). Comunicação em Saúde. Relação Técnicos de Saúde – Utentes. *Notas Didáticas*, 615-620.

Teixeira, J. A. C. (2004). *Comunicação em saúde: Relação técnicos de saúde – utentes*. Instituto Superior de Psicologia Aplicada.

Tench, R., & Konczos, M. (2013). *Mapping European communication practitioners' competencies: A review of the European communication professional skills and innovation program*. ECOPSI.

Thomas, R. K. (2006). *Health Communication*. Springer.

Thompson, T. L., Dorsey, A. M., Miller, K., & Parrott, R. (Eds.). (2003). *Handbook of Health Communication*. Lawrence Erlbaum Associates.

Tu, H. T., & Hargraves, J. L. (2003). Seeking health care information: Most consumers still on the sidelines. *Issue Brief (Center for Studying Health System Change)*, *61*, 1–4. PMID:12647763

U.S. Department of Health and Human Services, Office of Disease Prevention and Health Promotion. (2010). *National Action Plan to Improve Health Literacy*. Author.

Vaz de Almeida, C., & Belim, C. (2021a). Health professionals' communication competences decide patients' well-being: Proposal of a communication model. In *A. Tkalac Verčič, R. Tench & S. Einwiller (Eds.), Joy. Using strategic communication to improve well-being and organizational success*. Emerald Publishing.

Vaz de Almeida, C., & Belim, C. (2021b). Health Professionals' Communication Competences as a Light on the Patient Pathway: The Assertiveness, Clarity, and Positivity (ACP) Model. *International Journal of Applied Research on Public Health Management*, *6*(1), 14–29. doi:10.4018/IJARPHM.2021010102

Watzlawick, P., Beavin, J. H., & Jackson, D. D. (1967). *Pragmática da comunicação humana: Um estudo dos padrões, patologias e paradoxo da interação* (S. Paulo, Ed.). Cultrix.

WHO. (2009). *Background Note: regional preparatory meeting on promoting health literacy*. UN ECOSOC

Wiemann, J.W. (1977). Explication and test of a Model of Comunicative Competence. *Spring, 3*(3), 195-213.

Wilkinson, R., & Marmot, M. (Eds.). (2003). *Social Determinants of Health. The solid facts*. WHO Europe International Centre for Health and Society.

Williams, M. V., Davis, T., Parker, R. M., & Weiss, B. D. (2002). The role of health literacy in patient-physician communication. *Family Medicine*, *34*(5), 383–389. PMID:12038721

Zarcadoolas, C., Pleasant, A., & Greer, D. S. (2003). Elaborating a Definition of Health Literacy: A Commentary. *Journal of Health Communication: International Perspectives*, *8*(S1), 119–120. https://dx.doi.org/10.1080/713851982

Chapter 6
Better Safe Than Sorry:
Analysis of International Media Campaigns on Cancer Prevention

Célia Belim
ISCSP, University of Lisbon, Portugal

ABSTRACT

This chapter focuses on cancer prevention media campaigns, concretely on the construction of the persuasive message. Methodologically, semiotic analysis is used, exploring the verbal and visual dimension of 19 international ads linked to the five most deadly cancers, in order to understand and deconstruct the message and the communication tactics used. The results reveal the diversity of resources and tactics. In the verbal dimension, it presents the use of rhetorical tactics (e.g., statistical and factual evidence and stimulation of emotions), the popular vocabulary, cues to action/motivational content, the phatic, poetic, and appealing functions, stylistic resources, credibility of the source, evocation of good causes, originality and distinction, anecdotal approach. In the visual dimension, it observes the use of three languages' functions, isotopy, stylistic resources, personalization, symbolical approach, polychrome, diversity of phenotypes, the credibility of the source, a pedagogical component.

DOI: 10.4018/978-1-7998-4396-2.ch006

INTRODUCTION

Cancer is the second leading cause of death in the globe, being responsible for an estimated 9.6 million deaths in 2018 (WHO, 2018). This statistical value means that, globally, about 1 in 6 deaths is due to cancer (WHO, 2018). There are risk factors, such as high body mass index, low fruit and vegetable intake lack of physical activity, tobacco use, and alcohol use (WHO, 2018). These five factors are the cancer deaths' leading behavioral and dietary risks, causing around one-third of mortal victims (WHO, 2018).

Persons often seek and receive cancer information from mass media (Hannon et al., 2009). Mass media can be used to motivate individual behavior change and influence policy, and it can help set the cancer prevention and control agenda (Hornik, 2002). Enough simple and straightforward cancer prevention and early detection messages are needed to ensure adequate exposure to achieve these goals (Hornik, 2002).

Generally, mass media campaigns are widely used to expose high proportions of large populations and can generate positive changes or prevent negative health-related practices across the publics (Wakefield, Loken & Hornik, 2010). The "great promise of mass media campaigns" lies in their power to disseminate well-defined behaviorally focused messages to ample audiences in a repeated, longitudinal, incidental, and cheap manner (Wakefield et al., 2010).

Media interventions can effectively promote cancer-preventing lifestyle changes and screening tests that detect cancer early (Viswanath, 2005). Empirical research shows that media campaigns have been used to promote healthy behavior related to cancer prevention, both in urban and rural settings (Campo et al., 2008; Pasick, Hiatt & Paskett, 2004; Rim et al., 2009; Young, McGloin, Zittleman, West & Westfall, 2007; Zittleman et al., 2009). Studies demonstrated that the utilization of media channels to design interventions can be an effective approach to increase healthy behaviors. For example, the media can be effective in the promotion of sun protection behaviors and in the reduction of the risk of skin cancer among outdoor workers (Borland, Hocking, Godkin, Gibbs & Hill, 1991; Mullein, Gardiner, Roseninan, Zhu & Swanson, 1996).

Public health practitioners have used campaigns as a common tool due to their wide reach (Hornik, 2002; Institute of Medicine, 2002; Randolph & Viswanath, 2004; Salmon & Atkin, 2003). As Hornik (2002) states "there is good evidence that public health communication has affected health behavior" (p. xi).

Some studies (e.g. Campo et al., 2008; Randolph & Viswanath, 2004; Watson et al., 2009) reveal that a theory-driven media campaign is successful in increasing awareness. So, from a starting point in the literature, extracting lessons, this article aimed at perceiving the construction of the message, in both verbal and visual dimensions, of media campaigns focused on cancer prevention.

Little is known to inform best practices (Hannon et al., 2009). So, one of the criteria to compose the corpus of the present analysis was the consideration of the best and powerful ads (e.g., Hillier, 2019; Williamswhittle, n.d.) and the higher number of views in the case of videos.

CANCER PREVENTION IN MEDIA CAMPAIGNS: CONVINCING THAT "IT IS BEST TO BE ON THE SAFE SIDE"

Some studies confirm the media effectiveness (e.g. Anderson, Mullins, Siahpush, Spittal & Wakefield, 2009; Dixon et al. 2015; Logan et al., 2013; Watson, Tomar, Dodd, Logan, and Choi, 2009). Anderson et al. (2009) validate the potential of a mass media campaign, conducted in Victoria, Australia, in 2005, in improving cervical screening (27%) during the campaign period. The "Don't just sit there" campaign featured a series of women's legs in a panoply of situations and a voiceover acknowledging that, although having a Pap test can be uncomfortable, being treated for cervical cancer can be even more uncomfortable (Anderson et al., 2009, p. 869). Data do not expose a differential effect found across socio-economic status (SES) groups in terms of the effectiveness of the mass media campaign in encouraging women to screen (p. 873).

A survey applied to Black women reveals that these women expressed strong desires for rational appeals and communications that will provide information and facts and cognitive intentions, once they want to learn more about risks related to breast cancer (Frisby, 2002, p. 498). The data exposes that the most widely held perception about breast cancer is negative thoughts and feelings associated with death, fear, and loss of breasts and/or hair (p. 500). In order to persuade Black women, messages and advertisements should adopt role models of women with this phenotype (p. 500).

Logan et al. (2013) tested the effectiveness of a media campaign designed to increase intentions to seek an oral and pharyngeal cancer screening and discover that a media campaign successfully increases screening intentions by heightening concerns. Participants (N = 1,790) in the intervention condition received messages on posters, handheld fans, pamphlets, and magnets displayed on the sides of cars or trucks. Additionally, the study by Watson et al. (2009) reveals that a theory-driven media campaign was successful in increasing awareness of the oral cancer exam and interest in the exam among blacks/ African Americans.

Focusing on the rise of the awareness of links between alcohol and cancer and of knowledge of drinking guidelines, the results of Dixon et al. (2015)'s study indicate that a population-based mass media campaign can reach the target audience. However, a single campaign may be insufficient to measurably curb drinking behavior in a culture where pro-alcohol social norms and product marketing are pervasive.

An Australian mass media campaign, aired in Victoria and aimed to increase awareness and encourage identification of the abdominal circumference evolving both sexes (Morley, Wakefield, Dunlop & Hill, 2009), have partial success: the campaign conquers its primary aim of increased awareness of the linkage between obesity and cancer and the concrete waist sizes indicate of risk, as well as increased behavioral intentions regarding weight and cancer; however, there is no effect on self-awareness of weight status, perceived personal risk of cancer or weight-loss behavior.

Evidence also indicates that small media campaigns seem to be effective in terms of increasing screening uptake, particularly cervical cancer screening (Schliemann, 2019) and also indicates that organized programs allow to achieve extensive coverage and to enhance equity of access while maximizing the health impact of screening (Senore, 2015). The few interventions that seem to be informed by behavior change theory used constructs from the Health Belief Model – HBM (Schliemann, 2019). Sundstrom, Brandt, Gray, and Pierce (2018) also emphasize the effective use of HBM as the theoretical framework for an integrated campaign (combining community-based grassroots and social media) – "It's my time" –, whose goal was to decrease cervical cancer by increasing human papillomavirus (HPV) vaccination and screening.

There is a growing body of evidence testing different methods of framing health information presented in cancer prevention and control media messages.

One communicational tactic related to cancer prevention is to incorporate narratives (e.g., stories with connected events and characters that include implicit or explicit cancer-relevant messages) into media messages (Kreuter et al., 2007). Narratives can become a powerful tool with which to relay cancer information, especially as they lend themselves well to mass media channels and could be more effective than traditional didactic messages in helping people understand cancer information and overcoming resistance to cancer prevention and screening behaviors (Kreuter et al., 2007).

Katz et al. (2015) describe process data about exposure and content relevance of county-level campaigns conducted in Appalachian Ohio, USA, to improve colorectal cancer (CRC; intervention) screening and fruit and vegetable (F&V; comparison) consumption. The results indicate certain qualities that a campaign should include: a) material location: individuals who report campaign exposure live closer to billboards, confirming the importance of material location; b) increased campaign exposure: may increase the opportunity for learning the message, improve recognition of message importance, increase message discussion, increase the perception that the behavior is socially acceptable and increase the intention to talk to a doctor/nurse about screening in the next six months; c) clarity of message: most of the respondents report that campaign messages are clear, easy to understand, and important; d) similarity of the characters in the campaign with target public and cultural appropriateness of campaign materials: it was reported that individuals feature in the campaigns look like the public target and look like people they can trust. These additional positive observations are important to consider when planning future community-level health-related campaigns.

Campaigns related to cancer prevention are most effective when are theoretically based, are culturally adjusted, use an integrated strategy, including multiple channels, focus and promote a specific health topic, and achieve reasonable levels of message exposure among the priority population (e.g. Campo et al., 2008; Randolph & Viswanath, 2004).

In the scenario of illness, numerous studies suggest that humor is psychologically beneficial (e.g. Chapple & Ziebland, 2004; Heath & Blonder, 2003; Sullivan et al., 2003). For example, the results of the study by Kuiper et al. (1993) mention that humor contributes to the regulation of negative affect by facilitating cognitive re-appraisals and emotional distancing from stressful situations.

Lessons

There are some lessons related to cancer prevention campaigns that can be gathered (Table 1).

Table 1. Lessons extracted from the literature on cancer prevention campaigns

In some studies, virtually all major types of community-based cancer screening interventions have been shown to be effective. No interventions operate absolutely for all people, screening tests, or in all settings.
Old notions of 'hard-to-reach populations should be discarded: effective interventions can overcome obstacles to screening for diverse race/ethnic and socioeconomic groups who are affected by disparities.
Culture and acculturation are assumed as important target publics distinctions. The literature consistently shows that screening behavior differs by income and level of acculturation; screening may also vary by ethnicity.
Interventions should evolve as screening diffuses across the public.
Each type of setting presents advantages and disadvantages in terms of the public who can be reached and the screening aims that can be achieved.
Interventions to reach specific subgroups in well-defined settings (e.g., churches) have been effective in changing screening behavior.
Screening for both breast and cervical cancer can be effectively promoted through community-based interventions. More research is needed to understand how interventions must be adapted for specific cancer tests.
Assuring that there is access to screening and appropriate follow-up should precede interventions to promote increased use of screening.
Compared with all other interventions, those that reduce or eliminate access barriers are most effective in increasing the use of cancer screening.
In several studies, mass media interventions, in combination with other strategies, have been shown to increase breast and cervical cancer screening. Evidence is insufficient to indicate which combinations are strongest and whether these interventions compare favorably to other multi-component interventions. These resource-intensive campaigns have not been assessed for cost-effectiveness.
The prevalence of small (non-tailored) media in community-based cancer screening interventions indicates the importance of this category of strategies. However, little is known to inform best practices, and contributions to overall results have not been measured.
Most community interventions to promote cancer screening include person-to-person outreach and/or education in some form. Evidence-informed principles are needed to understand better the contribution and advantages of these strategies and their variations.
Multi-component interventions are effective in increasing initial and repeat cervical and breast cancer screening across a wide variety of settings and target populations. Multi-component interventions leave unanswered important questions, however, concerning the contribution of individual components and the effect of variations in intervention combinations. Cost-effectiveness analyses of entire interventions and their components are also needed.
To convince African American women to seek breast cancer screening and mammography and other preventive behaviors, messages and advertisements should employ role models of African American women who survived and continue to lead healthy, productive lives.
Ongoing communication, trust, and a shared vision among members of the partnership are critical to successful community-level campaigns.
Evidence reveals that small media campaigns are effective in terms of increasing screening uptake in Asia.
Our challenge now is to create and disseminate cancer prevention and control information that is equally accessible and usable for everyone.
Current inequalities will be exacerbated by media and marketing efforts that use channels that fail to reach diverse populations, language that is not comprehensible to groups with low health literacy, or messages that are culturally inappropriate.
Interdisciplinary collaboration will be needed to address all of these issues successfully.
Given the complexity of cancer and the potential for competing information, some assessment of the information environment in which a given media campaign will be fielded is critical for determining message content and adequate exposure.

continues on following page

Table 1. Continued

Cancer is a complex topic that may be addressed in the context of other issues including tobacco, nutrition, physical activity, early detection, and treatment.
Audience research can be a useful tool to determine what types of narratives will resonate with the target audience.

Source: *(Frisby, 2002, p. 500; Hannon et al., 2009; Katz, 2015; Pasick, Hatt & Paskett, 2004; Randolph & Viswanath, 2004; Viswanath, 2005)*

DIGITALLY CONVINCING: THE USE OF DIGITAL MEDIA CAMPAIGNS

The internet has become a primary forum within which health information, particularly relating to breast cancer, is simultaneously sought and shared (Quinn et al., 2013). To build a community is the typical digital use by breast cancer entities (Sisco & McCorkindale, 2013, p. 290). Social media are often heralded as a valuable vehicle for expanding the reach of public health campaigns cancer campaigns (Vraga et al., 2018) and there exists a rapidly evolving network of cancer patients engaged in information exchange via Twitter (Sugawara et al., 2012). As in other campaigns, the level of success depends on certain variables, such as the nature of the campaign itself, the type of cancer being referred to, and the digital platform being explored.

The study of Vraga et al. (2018) is a pioneer on the comparison of the social media activity on Twitter and Instagram across three time periods: a) #WorldCancerDay in February, b) the annual month-long campaigns of National Breast Cancer Awareness Month (NBCAM) in October and Movember in November, and c) during the full year outside of these campaigns. The results reveal that, across campaigns and social media platforms, women's reproductive cancers, especially breast cancer, tend to outperform men's reproductive cancer, namely prostate cancer. An overall comparison shows that Twitter induces substantially more activity than Instagram for both cancer campaigns, suggesting Instagram may be an unexplored resource. However, the messaging for both campaigns tends to concentrate on awareness and support rather than on specific behaviors.

Vraga et al. (2018, p. 6) observe a notorious similarity in the top terms used on Twitter and Instagram when addressing breast cancer. But none of these words are explicitly connected with cancer or prevention. Two of the terms – "aware/awareness" and "support" – relate to campaign aims, whereas others match existing criticisms by focusing on the campaign itself ("month") and its visual elements ("pink"). Prostate cancer has better results:

while the "Movember" campaign is the top lexeme for both Twitter and Instagram, the other top lexemes on both social media platforms concentrate on "men," "support", and "health." However, on both platforms, the top terms connected with Movember campaign differ: on Twitter, Movember is associated with men's health and prostate cancer awareness as the top four terms, with "donate" as the final; differentially, on Instagram, the Movember campaign emphasizes only one word ("men") related to the target public, and the remaining focus on facial hair.

Concentrated also on the Movember campaign, findings by Bravo and Hoffman-Goetz (2015) reveal that non-health-related content dominated the Movember conversations, and a few individuals from the USA, Canada, or United Kingdom shared actionable or content-rich health information about prostate cancer, testicular cancer, or men's mental health. Regardless of the geolocation, mustache's growing and community engagement are the focus of Twitter conversations.

Additionally, Diddi and Lundy (2017) explore how four different health-related organizations – Susan G. Komen, U.S. News Health, Woman's Hospital, and Breast Cancer Social Media – used their Twitter accounts to talk about varied aspects of breast cancer during 2014, concretely in October, which is the Breast Cancer Awareness Month. A content analysis of 2916 tweets based on the Health Belief Model and its parameters (perceived susceptibility, perceived severity, perceived benefits, perceived barriers, cues to action, self-efficacy) shows the use of varied theoretical constructs of the framework and, while different organizations shared valuable breast cancer-related content on Twitter, each used the social media platform in a different fashion. Overall, the study demonstrates that, out of all the tweets that represented the theoretical constructs, "perceived barriers" was in the maximum number, followed by "cues to action", "self-efficacy", "perceived benefits", and "perceived threat" (p. 248).

Exploring an organizational approach, Sisco and McCorkindale (2013), studying the top 20 breast cancer charities during January 2011, found a strong relationship between the transparency and credibility of the organization and conclude that most of these organizations are active on both Twitter and Facebook, differing in terms of activity, credibility, and transparency. Organizations that tweeted more had more "likes", more followers, and more overall tweets and were seen to be more transparent and credible by virtue of activity alone.

The verbal and visual material collected from official websites of British and American breast cancer foundations and Russian social media reveals the communicative strategies adopted (Table 2).

Table 2. Communicative strategies in breast cancer prevention discourse

Communicative purposes	Strategies
To inform the public	. providing scientific facts strategy . providing figures and statistics strategy . providing anecdotal evidence of cancer survivor's strategy . providing guidelines on personal prevention strategy . appealing to authority
To urge action	. the direct urge to action . the indirect urge to action or to reflection
To inform + to urge for action	. breast cancer awareness promotion through verbal symbol, images, logo, associated with breast cancer campaign: pink ribbon, think pink, pink awareness . breast cancer awareness promotion through popular film or soap operas characters . breast cancer awareness promotion through "diagnose coming out"

Source: *(Stebletsova & Enkova, 2016)*

The discourse present in breast campaign cancer campaigns is endowed with specific attributes (Table 3).

Table 3. Breast cancer campaign discourse is characterized by

. the **dominant use of common (non-technical) vocabulary**: want to know, stop, chemicals, tiny amounts, rise rapidly; . **wide use verb + noun phrases as markers of colloquial language**: take action, make a change, put pressure, make a difference, do maths; . a **common use of emotionally marked words**: harmful chemicals, trustworthy institutions, fair use, pink abuse; . **limited use of terminology (technical vocabulary)**: cancer cells, metastasis, lymph nodes; . the **dominant use of you and your pronouns for a direct appeal to the audience**: we need your support… we want you to think…. . a **common use of contractions as a marker of colloquial language**: We couldn't do our work without the generous support of members of the public… We don't receive funding from the Government… We're all exposed to synthetic chemicals on a daily basis . **use of direct rhetorical questions as a marker of a direct appeal to the audience:** Do you know what's in your cosmetics? . **a common use of imperative sentences as a marker of the direct urge to take action or strong advice**: Reduce your family's exposure to some of the chemicals in your food and drink that are linked with breast cancer Avoid some of the hazardous chemicals commonly found in household cleaners

Source: *(Stebletsova & Enkova, 2016, p. 7)*

Lessons

Some lessons on the use of digital media campaigns in the benefit of cancer prevention can be synthesized (Table 4).

Table 4. Lessons from the literature on digital media campaigns in benefit of cancer prevention

Health communication efforts need to focus on effective messaging and building engaged communities for cancer communication across social media platforms (Vraga et al. 2018).
Determining how organizations, especially cause nonprofits, are using social media as well as the level of transparency and credibility of the organization is extremely important (Sisco & McCorkindale, 2013, p. 290).
To truly gauge the utility of social media, there has to be some way to measure key indicators (Sisco & McCorkindale, 2013, p. 299).
Organizations need to take advantage of the benefits of digital platforms, which appeal to different audiences. The usage and content need to be consistent and frequently updated. Organizations need to use digital media to not only communicate one-way and disseminate information (e.g. McCorkindale, 2010; Sisco & McCorkindale, 2013; Waters et al., 2009) with their audiences but also engage in dialogue.
As social network sites such as Twitter grow in popularity, it will be important to consider how to engage men in productive conversations and capitalize on this platform to increase awareness about important health concerns for men (Bravo & Hoffman-Goetz, 2015).

Source: *(Bravo & Hoffman-Goetz, 2015; McCorkindale, 2010; Sisco & McCorkindale, 2013; Vraga et al., 2018; Waters et al., 2009)*

METHOD

Semiotic Analysis

Semiotic analysis is an analysis technique that is based on the study of the sign, and a sign is anything that carries information that can be received in different ways by each recipient, depending on his/her cultural repertoire (Poulios & Senteri, 2016). Therefore, it is important to emphasize that semiotic reading is a possibility of receiving and interpreting the message. This type of analysis is one of the first procedural moves towards understanding a text in its entirety, as a whole (Mehawesh, 2014, p. 89). The focus is on the deeper meanings of messages (Neuenforf, 2002, p. 6). The technique intends to explore deep structures, latent meanings, and the signifying process through signs, codes, and binary oppositions (p. 6).

The analysis focuses on the two dimensions of the message – the verbal and the visual ones –, like the study conducted by Stebletsova and Enkova (2016). The application of the technique summoned as elements of analysis: 1) the icons (Joly, 2008), 2) the denotation and the connotation (Barthes, 2001; Guiraud, 1999); 3) the plastic signifiers (Joly, 2008); and 4) the functions of language (Bühler, 2011; Jakobson, 1963). Recognition of icons takes place through denotation, which means what the icon represents in the first degree. Its interpretation is based on the process of connotation (Joly, 2008) or "rhetoric of the image" (Barthes, 1999). Barthes (1977) explains that in the photo, at least, the difference between connotation and denotation is clear: denotation is the mechanical reproduction on a film of the object at the limit the camera captures (it is what is shown), the connotation is the human dimension of the process, being the selection of what to include in the frame, of focus, aperture, camera angle, the quality of the film (how it is shown). In sum, denotation is what is photographed or captured, and the connotation is how it is made (Barthes, 1977, Yan & Ming, 2015, p. 62).

Plastic signifiers, such as shape, color, are considered full and integral signs and not the simple matter of expression of icons (Joly, 2008), this is also explored to optimize the analysis at the level of the meaning of the icons. The most evident are emphasized in the analysis of each spot.

The analytical option for language functions, especially poetic, phatic, and appealing, resides in the idea that the communicative function of a visual message, explicit or implicit, determines its significance (Barthes, 1999).

Corpus – Selection Criteria

To choose which cases to analyze, we first opted to consider the most mortal cancers. Then, we selected the campaign materials based on a) actuality – campaign promotion in the 10th decade of the 21st century, b) the credibility of the promoter, c) the number of views in the case of videos, and d) the ranking as the best awareness ads. The most common causes of cancer death are cancers of (WHO, 2018): lung (1.76 million deaths); colorectal (862 000 deaths); stomach (783000 deaths); liver (782000 deaths); and breast (627000 deaths). The corpus is composed of 19 spots.

RESULTS

Table 5. Lung cancer – cases

Matches:30 I Lung cancer screening Ad Council 2019 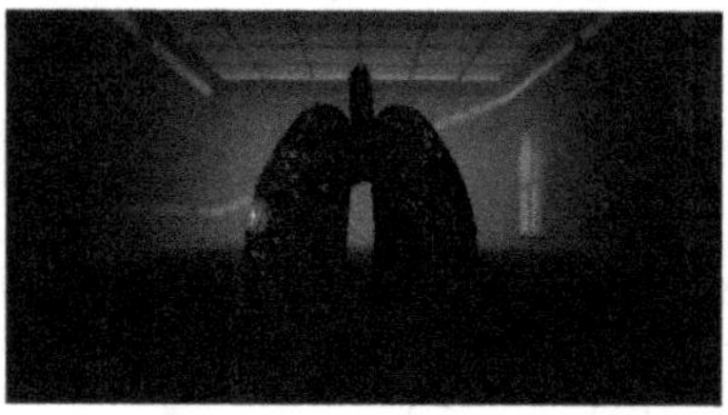	*Verbal dimension* **Antithesis**: "You could smoke and thought that's that" vs. "for the time you see the symptoms it could be too late" Dramatization: "It could be too late" **Appeal approach and cues to action**: "if you smoked get scanned – talk to your doctor or learn more at SavedBytTheScan.org *Visual dimension* **Metaphor**: Two lungs made up of matches and a dark background, representing the imminent danger **Antithesis:** Two lungs, on a black background, made up of matches that light up and fall, representing lung cancer vs. two lungs made up of matches that maintain stability on a light background that seems to be a clinical space
Cat lovers deserve to die Lung Cancer Alliance NoOneDeservesToDie.org 2012 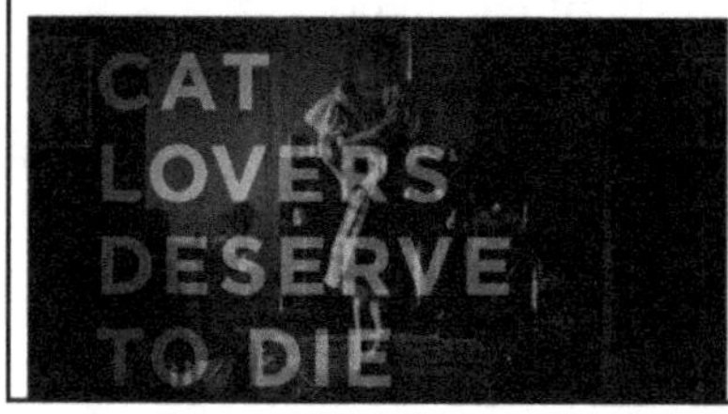	*Verbal dimension* **Phatic approach by shocking**: "Cat lovers deserve to die" … "if they have lung cancer" **Appeal approach**: "Lung cancer doesn't discriminate, neither should you." *Visual dimension* **Personalization and humanization** **Antithesis**: colored images with a car lover and cats vs. images with a black background

DISCUSSING CONCLUSION

The results reveal that, in the verbal dimension, some rhetorical tactics are used, such as statistical and factual evidence (logos) and stimulation of emotions (pathos). Diversity of tactics is a practice. It is observed the use of popular vocabulary; the cues to action; the phatic function (use of a question in order to establish contact with the public) and the appealing function; stylistic resources (poetic function), such as the antithesis, the euphemism, the repetition, the alliteration, the metaphor; tactics associated with the credibility of the communicator/promoter; motivational content; descriptions associated with a pedagogical purpose; musicality/melody; evocation of good causes, originality, and distinction; the descending or ascending use of subtitling; anecdotal approach.

Table 6. Colorectal cancer – cases

Love your butt colon cancer awareness campaign Chris4Life Colon Cancer Foundation 2013 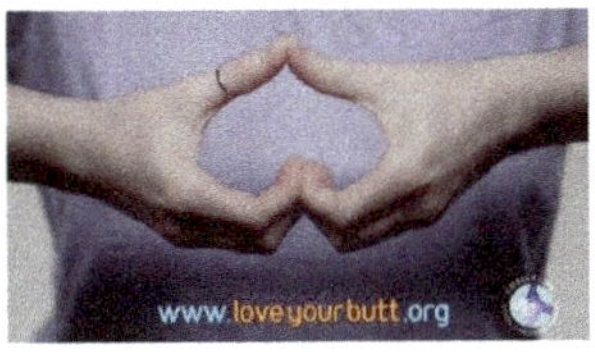 	*Verbal dimension* **Appeal approach and cues to action**: "No matter what you call it. Have it checked.", "love your butt" **Interview style video** **Personalization and humanization**: diverse persons appear sharing how they call the bottom/butt Euphemism: various designations to name the bottom/butt *Visual dimension* **Symbolic approach**: Hands forming hearts were flipped upside down to resemble "butt shapes" **Personalization and humanization**: many persons **Chromatic symbolism**: use of blue that is the color of colorectal cancer
Love your butt colon cancer awareness campaign Chris4Life Colon Cancer Foundation 2014 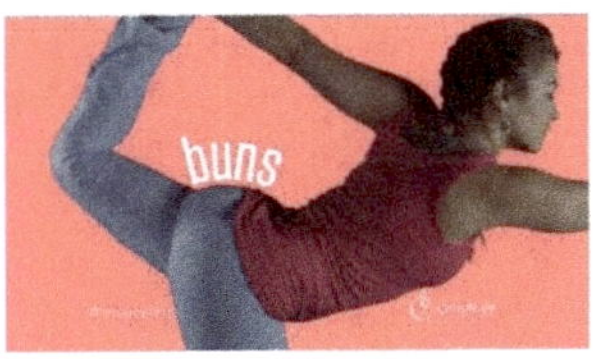 	*Verbal dimension* **Synonyms**: diverse words appear designating the butt ("booty", "bottom", "derrière", "tuchus", "bum", "behind", "tushy", "caboose", "keister", "rump", "buns", "pattoty", "fanny", "money maker", "gluteus maximus" **Euphemism**: various designations to name the bottom/butt **Appeal approach and cues to action**: "No matter what you call it. Have it checked.", "love your butt" **Description**: "March is colon cancer awareness month" **Emotion**: "I love my butt" *Visual dimension* **Personalization and humanization**: many persons, without seeing their heads and faces, appear showing their butt **Symbolic approach**: Hands forming hearts were flipped upside down to resemble "butt shapes". According to popular legend, the heart shape that we know today originated from the shape of the female buttocks. This universal symbol of love was transformed to serve as the icon for the Love Your Butt Colon Cancer Awareness Campaign **Polychrome**: employment of diverse colors in the background scenario

In the visual dimension, there is a variety of creative options to impact the public, such as: the use of bisectional resources; the phatic function of language; the isotopy in the sense of annulling any entropy of the meaning or polysemy of the message; stylistic resources, such as metaphor and antithesis; personalization and humanization, in order to show that the stories are real and create a greater identification with the communicator/character; symbolical approach of icons and colors; polychrome; diversity of phenotypes-totalization/ entirety; visuality; popular platforms and personalities; the presence of elite persons exploring the credibility of the source and the assumptions of the source credibility theory; a pedagogical component with the illustration of how to self-examine.

Table 7. Stomach cancer – cases

No Stomach For Cancer Stomach Cancer Awareness Month www.NoStomachForCancer.org 2018 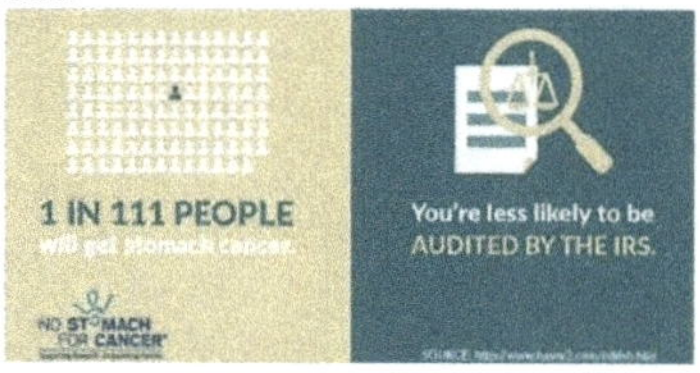	*Verbal dimension* **Statistical evidence**: "1 in 111 people will get stomach cancer." **Factual evidence**: "you're less likely to be audited by the IRS." **Reference to popular vocabulary**: "no stomach for" means to lack the courage, determination, or resolve to do, face, or experience something unpleasant. *Visual dimension* **Bisectional resource**, suggesting being two pages **Chromatic differentiation**: use of different colors to illustrate the 1 in 111 persons who will have stomach cancer **Phatic approach**: use of caps lock or capital letters to emphasize information
No Stomach For Cancer Stomach Cancer Awareness Month www.NoStomachForCancer.org 2017 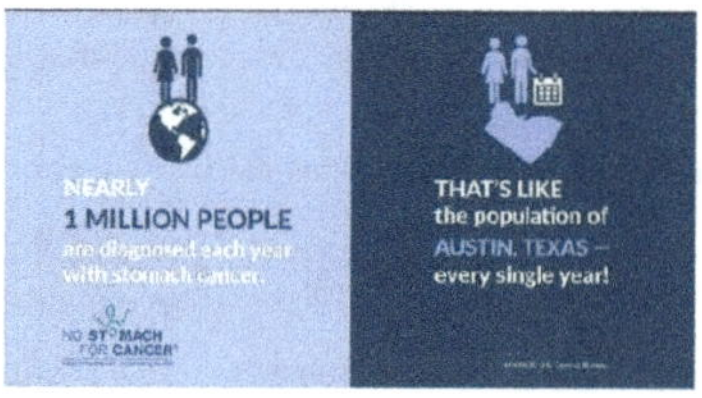	*Verbal dimension* **Statistical evidence**: "1 million people are diagnosed each year with stomach cancer". **Factual evidence**: "That's like the population of Austin, Texas – every single year!" **Reference to popular vocabulary**: "no stomach for" means to lack the courage, determination, or resolve to do, face, or experience something unpleasant. *Visual dimension* **Bisectional resource**, suggesting being two pages **Phatic approach**: use of caps lock or capital letters to emphasize information
Singapore Cancer Society 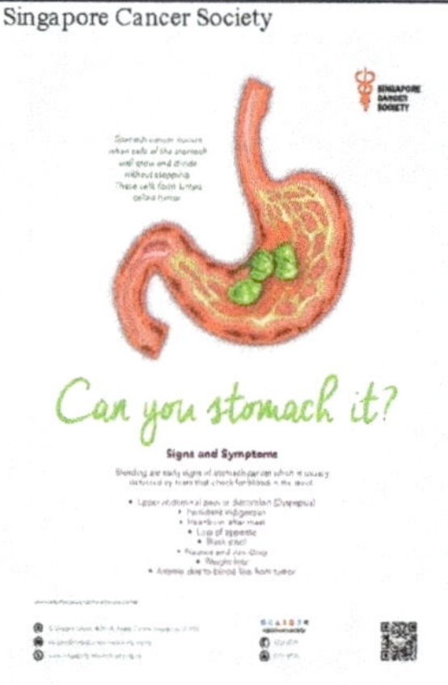	*Verbal dimension* **Factual evidence**: "Stomach cancer occurs when cells of the stomach wall grow and divide without stopping. The cells form lumps called a tumor." **Cues to action**: discrimination of signs and symptoms **Phatic approach**: use of a question mark – "Can you stomach it?" **Wordplay** used with the word "stomach *Visual dimension* **Isotopy**: the image illustrates the text, showing the tumors inside the stomach

The use of repetition and alliteration is beneficial in health contexts, considering the effects this tactic/resource can generate. The literature states that, when stimuli are learned by repetition, they are remembered better and retained longer (Ebbinghaus, 1964; Zhan, Guo, Chen & Yang, 2018).

Table 8. Liver cancer – cases

ALF Statement on Liver Cancer American Liver Foundation (ALF) 2016 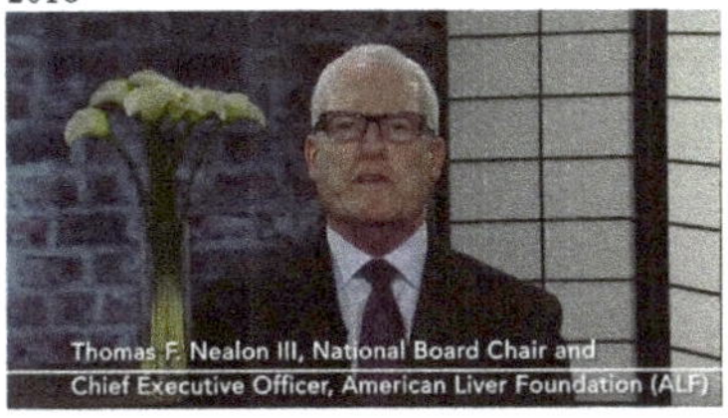	*Verbal dimension* **Credibility**: the spokesperson is the chief executive officer of ALF **Factual evidence**: "the American liver Foundation has made great advances combating liver disease over the past 40 years", "live cancer is one of the few cancers on the rise" **Alert and cues to action**: "we want you to know if you were at risk", "for more information about liver cancer, its risk factors, the importance of early detection", "visit our website" *Visual dimension* **Reference to "elite" persons and humanization**: the chief executive officer of ALF
Deon Bush Liver Cancer PSA ALF 2019 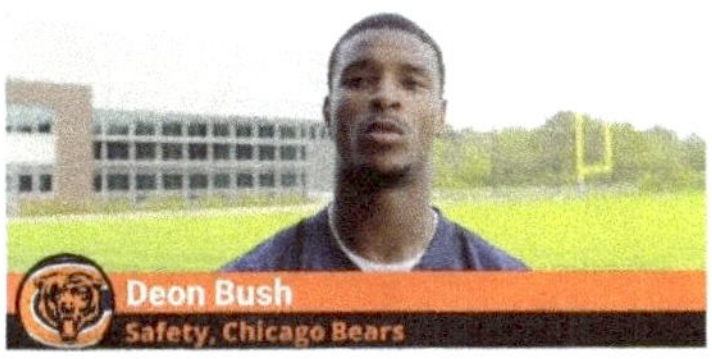	*Verbal dimension* **Credibility**: testimony by Deon Bush, American football safety for the Chicago Bears of the National Football League (NFL) **Factual evidence**: "in 2017, I lost my father to liver cancer" **Inspiration**: "He was a great man who taught me to help others and I'm proud to honor his memory as an ambassador for ALF" **Alert and cues to action**: "early detection of liver cancer can be life-saving, so it's important to know your risks: if you have hepatitis B, hepatitis C, other liver diseases, excessive drinking, certain metabolic conditions, you may be at risk and you should talk to your doctor", for more information go to liverfoundation.org or call *Visual dimension* **Personalization and humanization** **Reference to "elite" persons and humanization**: Deon Bush

Some campaigns follow the suggestion found in the literature to adopt messages and advertisements with role models of Black women's phenotype (Frisby, 2002, p. 498, p. 500), accomplishing the similarity of the characters in the campaign with a target public and cultural appropriateness of campaign materials (Katz et al. 2015).

Since Hovland and Weiss (1951), authors have noted the importance of the source's credibility and authority. For example, Sbaffi and Rowley (2017) conclude that the most widely discussed positive aspect of content features in the literature is the authority of the author, representing the level of expertise of the person or persons writing the information, followed by the credibility or trustworthiness of the information. The source credibility theory explains how the perceived credibility of the source of information influences the communication's persuasiveness (Berlo, Lemert & Mertz, 1969).

Table 9. Breast cancer – cases

<table>
<tr>
<td>Grab Life by the Boobs (2019)
Coppafeel website
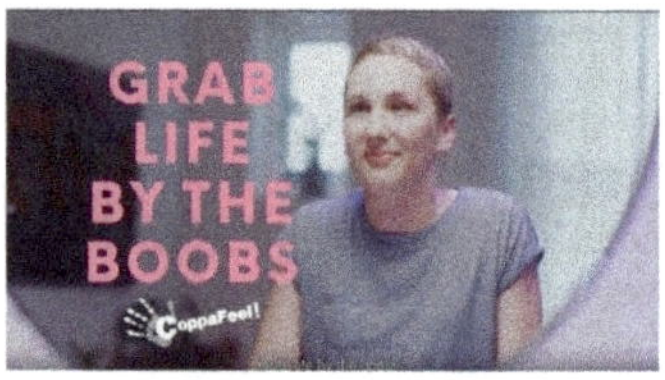
</td>
<td>Verbal dimension
Inspiration: "Life can be a handful. You grab on to everything it has to offer. Your future. Your loved ones. Yourself."

Alert and cues to action: "It could save your life"

Phatic approach: "But what are you going to do? Back down when things get tough? Or confront them, breasts on? Do you let go or grab on for dear life?"
Repetition: "So grab today, grab tomorrow, grab what matters, grab your dreams, grab big and squeeze plenty"

Visual dimension
Totalization: Various female phenotypes, including the black phenotype

Personalization and humanization</td>
</tr>
<tr>
<td>Everyone can help someone (2019)
Marks & Spencer
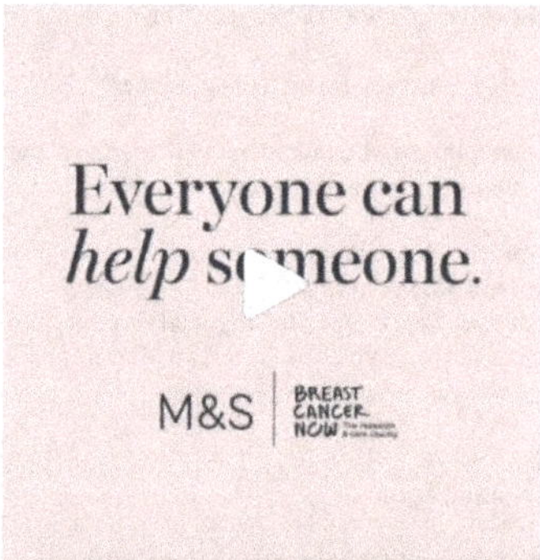
</td>
<td>Verbal dimension
Personalization and humanization: "I never left the house for six months, I lost my confidence to drive, I actually lost my confidence to live."; "Farida and Julie were brought together by their experience of breast cancer."; "you came alone and we both just somehow got through it"

Antithesis: the isolation and demotivation ("darkest times") vs. the proximity of friends who "come forward that you least expect" / mutual support

Inspiration: "Everyone can help someone."; "I knew you'd get through it, I really did."

Cues to action: "Inspired by their experience, they've launched a comedy stage show to help other women"

Visual dimension
Personalization and humanization: Farida and Julie narrate their dyadic and inspirational story

Chromatic symbolism: use of pink, the color associated with cancer breast</td>
</tr>
<tr>
<td>#ITouchMyselfProject (2018)
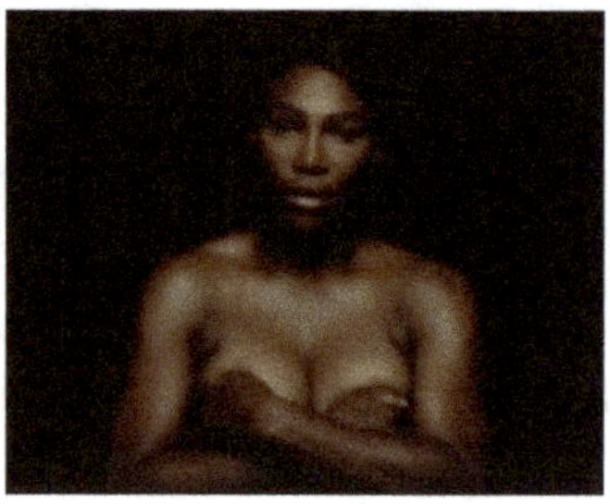</td>
<td>Verbal dimension
Personalization and humanization: "I love myself, I want you to love me
When I feel down, I want you above me
I search myself, I want you to find me
I forget myself, I want you to remind me
I don't want anybody else
When I think about you, I touch myself
Ooh, I don't want anybody else
Oh no, oh no, oh no
Think I would die if you were to ignore me"

Inspiration: "I love myself"

Alert and cues to action: "When I think about you, I touch myself", "Think I would die if you were to ignore me"; ""Touch yourself – A breast health reminder"

Alliteration: "myself", "I want you to"

Musicality: Divinyls' hit "I Touch Myself"

Visual dimension
Presence of "elite persons": the professional tennis player, Serena Williams

Personalization and humanization: focus exclusively on Serena Williams

The presence of the black phenotype
Phatic approach: A topless, singing Serena Williams in a close up are flashy signifiers</td>
</tr>
</table>

continues on following page

Table 9. Continued

#ChangeAndCheck Lorraine 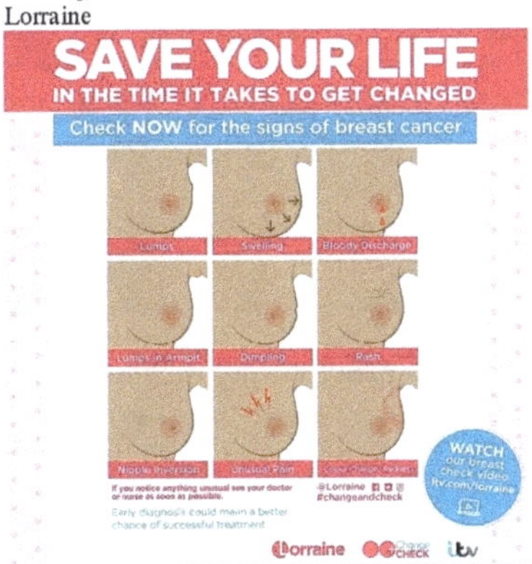 	*Verbal dimension* **Alert and cues to action**: "Save your life in the time it takes to get changed", Check now for the signs of breast cancer", "Early diagnosis could mean a better chance of successful treatment", encouragement to adorn the changing rooms of retail outlets with stickers depicting nine signs of breast cancer **Pedagogical component**: reference to the symptoms *Visual dimension* **Visuality**: the illustration of the breast cancer's symptoms **Use of popular platforms and personalities** to help extend awareness across an ample public
Know your lemons (2017) Knowingyourlemons.com/uk 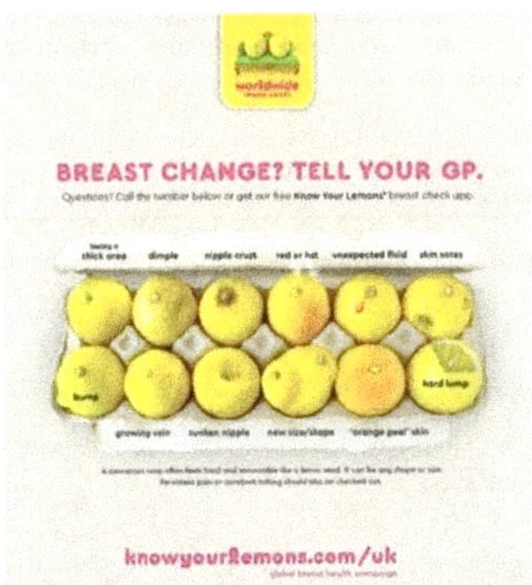 	*Verbal dimension* **Metaphor**: the equivalence between breasts and lemons – "a cancerous lump often feels hard and immovable like a lemon" **Pedagogical component**: the reference to the symptoms – "feeling a thick area", "dimple", "nipple crust", "red or hot", "unexpected fluid", "skin sores", "growing vein", "sunken nipple", "new size/shape" ""orange peel" skin" **Phatic approach**: "Breast change?", "Questions?" *Visual dimension* **Chromatic symbolism**: use of pink, the color associated with cancer breast **Visuality**: the fruit widens the image's reach, as it is more likely to be displayed in public places than a medically precise diagram
Check it before it's removed (2016) The Pink Ribbon Foundation 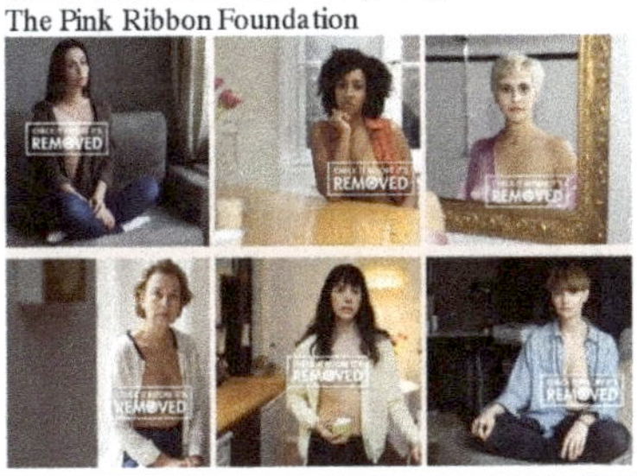 	*Verbal dimension* **Metaphor**: "check it before it's removed" – users were encouraged to share the images through their digital accounts as quickly and far as possible before their inevitable deletion by platform moderators censoring them for violating strict nudity policies. This alludes to the required behavior of self-examine before it is too late and there is a need to extract the breast (delete = remove). *Visual dimension* **Presence of "elite persons"**: several high-profile celebrities and influencers, such as singer Cascada and supermodel Franziska Knuppe, helped spread the campaign to an ampler outreach

continues on following page

Some spots, especially the videos, explore the communication tactic of incorporating narratives (e.g., stories with connected events and characters that include implicit or explicit cancer-relevant messages). This result is in accordance with the findings of Kreuter et al. (2007).

Table 9. Continued

Lux – the soap with a lump 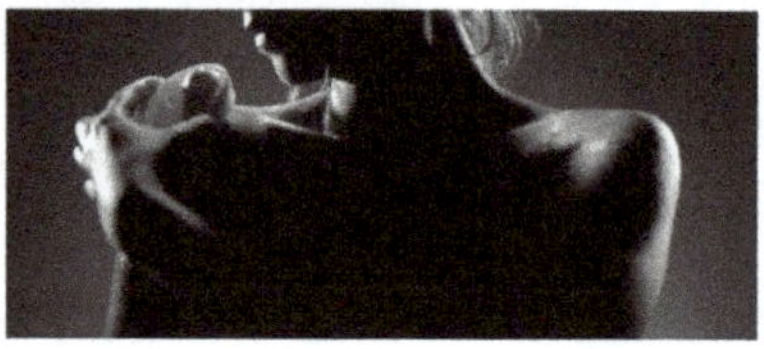	*Verbal dimension* **Alert and cues to action**: "75% of Indian women shy away from self-examination", "until the final use, women are alerted to the fact that they should check their breasts for any deformities", "daily reminder to self-examine" **Reference to statistical data**: "75% of Indian women shy away from self-examination" **Reference to an elite brand and evidence**: "India's leading soap brand, Lux" **Inspiration**: "Beauty is every woman's right. And so is her well-doing" **Metaphor**: the soap with lump alluding to a breast with a lump **Originality and distinction**: change the product – create a soap that has a lump. The added lump has been carefully designed not to dissolve over time with the rest of the soap, prolonging the longevity of its core purpose **Identity of the product**: "keeps you beautiful but best of all can save your life" **Good causes**: "Lux tied up with the Indian Cancer Society and distributed the soap, at their screening camp in Maharashtra, with a helpline in a leaflet to guide the self-examination. Lux's plans include extending this initiative through leading cancer hospitals, awareness workshops, and other community programs across India" *Visual dimension* **Chromatic symbolism:** use of a black and white palette, in order to show the bifurcation of the behavior: to self-examine or not
First haircut (2015) Ulta Beauty-Breast Cancer Research Foundation 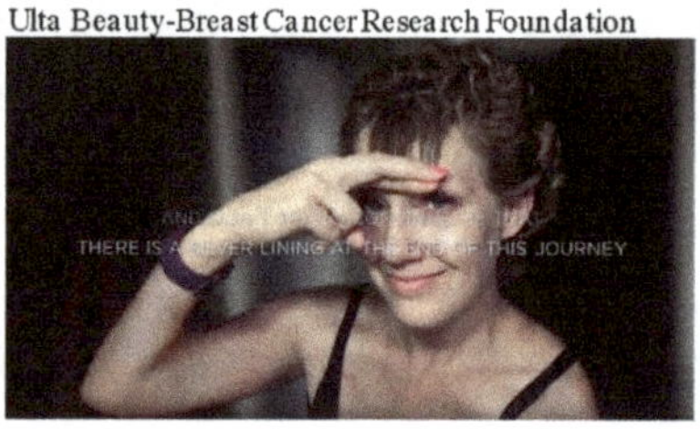	*Verbal dimension* **The descending or ascending use of subtitling** that gains a new signification according to the direction of reading: 'll never forget this feeling This disease is going to take away my beauty And don't try to convince me that There is a silver lining at the end of this journey Because, when you really think about it, Life is unfair Even if Every day is filled with hope My courage won't last And it is not true that I am strong enough Because The fear is too powerful I no longer think I can beat it This Will prevail over My positivity It's all beyond my control And you will never hear me say I am still beautiful **Antithesis**: the discourse is at first negative and depressive, but, reading and listening in an inverse direction, the sense is antagonistic **Inspiration**: the end of the video with an uplifting note, "It's more than just a first haircut, It's a beautiful new beginning" *Visual dimension* **Personalization and humanization**: images of the manifestation of disease, different aspects of hair, of children, post-its, emotions

continues on following page

Table 9. Continued

"The silent couple" Philips India HIM: Husband's Initiated Movement 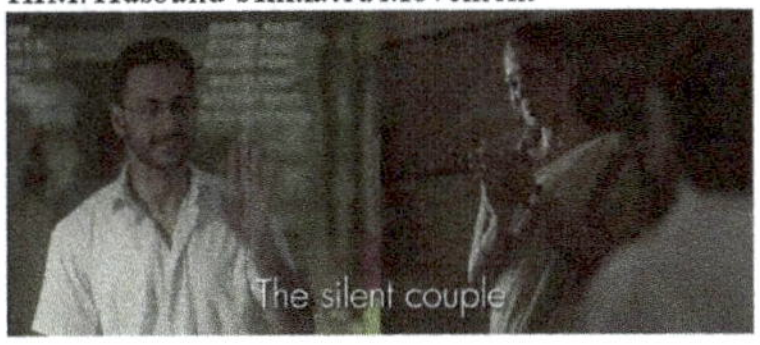 	*Verbal dimension* **Phatic approach**: a silent couple **Antithesis**: silent parents vs. talking daughter; "I will do this" vs. "You do this", silent couple vs. "actions speak louder" **Appeal approach and cues to action**: a husband who made the typically wife's domestic tasks (e.g. cook, wash the dishes) in order to give her "10 minutes to fight breast cancer", "5 steps of breast self-examination: Do one chore your wife does and instead ask her to use the time to do this.", "To the husband who loves his couch" "Because actions speak louder", "Do one chore your wife does", "And instead ask her to practice breast self-examination, help fight breast cancer" **Statistical evidence**: "Every year 1,00,000 women are detected with breast cancer in India" *Visual dimension* **Personalization and humanization** **Chromatic symbolism**: use of pink, the color associated with cancer breast
Your Man Reminder (2011) Rethink Breast Cancer 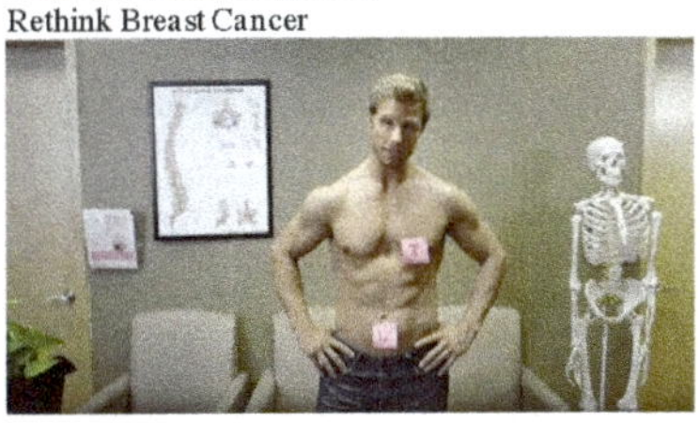	*Verbal dimension* **Credibility**: inside a health center, a doctor, Dr. Rothford Gray, talks directly to the receiver about how many women are not checking regularly for breast cancer; "Isn't that right, doctor? [Anthony]" **Anecdotal approach**: Dr. Gray says that studies have shown that women are more likely to watch videos that feature hot guys, so he presents Anthony, who quickly doffs his shirt to reveal a perfect six-pack. Then, Anthony tells the female viewer about the free "Your Man Reminder" app that sends regular prompts from the hot guy of her choice to tell her to check her breasts. "If Antony isn't your cup of tea, there's Glenn, or Isaac or Christian. That's going to be a tough decision." **Alert and cues to action**: "be on the lookout for anything unusual", "check with your doctor" *Visual dimension* **Pedagogical component**: illustration of how to self-examine

The cues to action stimulate behavior and are a tactic ("direct or indirect urge to action") identified by Stebletsova and Enkova (2016).

The use of metaphors in health communication calls for more mindful and competent use of figurative speech (Michl & Wohlmann, 2019, p. 1). Metaphors are powerful tools that enable alternative ways of thinking about complex issues in health care (p. 1), can also be used in productive ways, and serve as a mode of inquiry into the other and into the self (p. 8). Metaphors are a tool for thinking, explaining, and developing theories, performing specific functions: they can serve as mnemonic tools or provide a safe space for difficult health approaches (p. 1).

Discussing the effects and potential of humor in the health context, Demjén (2016) states that it makes fun of cancer and its consequences, facilitates individual and collective empowerment, and co-created humor builds a sense of community. Similarly, results of some studies (Stebletsova & Enkova, 2016) confirm the use of a humorist tactic in the purpose of cancer prevention and, for example, the research conducted by Greene, Campo, and Banerjee (2010) stress that anecdotal messages are best at altering severity and amount of invested mental effort, but statistical messages overall performed the worst.

Future research can explore the influence of Health Belief Model (HBM) variables on intention, including cues to action and perceived threat.

REFERENCES

Anderson, J. O., Mullins, R. M., Siahpush, M., Spittal, M. J., & Wakefield, M. (2009). Mass media campaign improves cervical screening across all socio-economic groups. *Health Education Research, 24*(5), 867–875. doi:10.1093/her/cyp023 PMID:19342422

Barthes, B. (1977). *Roland Barthes*. Hill and Wang. doi:10.1007/978-1-349-03518-2

Barthes, R. (1999). Rethoric of the image. In J. Evans & S. Hall (Eds.), *Visual culture: The reader* (pp. 33–40). Sage Publications.

Barthes, R. (2001). *Elementos de semiologia*. Edições 70.

Berlo, D. K., Lemert, J. B., & Mertz, R. J. (1969). Dimensions for evaluating the acceptability of message sources. *The Public Opinion Quarterly, 33*(4), 563-576. doi:10.1086/267745

Borland, R. M., Hocking, B., Godkin, G. A., Gibbs, A. F., & Hill, D. J. (1991). The impact of a skin cancer control education package for outdoor workers. *The Medical Journal of Australia, 154*(10), 686–688. doi:10.5694/j.1326-5377.1991.tb121261.x PMID:2034151

Bravo, C. A., & Hoffman-Goetz, L. (2015). Social media and men's health: A content analysis of Twitter conversations during the 2013 Movember campaigns in the United States, Canada, and the United Kingdom. *American Journal of Men's Health, 11*(6), 1627–1641. doi:10.1177/1557988315617826 PMID:26669771

Brouwers, M. C., De Vito, C., Bahirathan, L., Carol, A., Carroll, J. C., Cotterchio, M., Dobbins, M., Lent, B., Levitt, C., Lewis, N., McGregor, S. E., Paszat, L., Rand, C., & Wathen, N. (2011). What implementation interventions increase cancer screening rates? A systematic review. *Implementation Science; IS, 6*(1), 111. doi:10.1186/1748-5908-6-111 PMID:21958556

Bühler, K. (2011). *Theory of language: The representational function of language*. John Benjamins Publishing Company. doi:10.1075/z.164

Campo, S., Askelson, N. M., Routsong, T., Graaf, L. J., Losch, M., & Smith, H. (2008). The green acres effect: The need for a new colorectal cancer screening campaign tailored to rural audiences. *Health Education & Behavior*, *35*(6), 749–762. doi:10.1177/1090198108320358 PMID:18757773

Chapple, A., & Ziebland, S. (2004). The role of humor for men with testicular cancer. *Qualitative Health Research*, *14*(8), 1123–1139. doi:10.1177/1049732304267455 PMID:15359047

Demjén, Z. (2016). Laughing at cancer: Humour, empowerment, solidarity and coping online. *Journal of Pragmatics*, *101*, 18–30. doi:10.1016/j.pragma.2016.05.010

Diddi, P., & Lundy, L. K. (2017). Organizational Twitter Use: Content Analysis of Tweets during Breast Cancer Awareness Month. *Journal of Health Communication*, *22*(3), 243–253. doi:10.1080/10810730.2016.1266716 PMID:28248621

Dixon, H. G., Pratt, I. S., Scully, M. L., Miller, J. R., Patterson, C., Hood, R., & Slevin, T. J. (2015). Using a mass media campaign to raise women's awareness of the link between alcohol and cancer: Cross-sectional pre-intervention and post-intervention evaluation surveys. *BMJ Open*, *5*(3), 1–8. doi:10.1136/bmjopen-2014-006511 PMID:25762231

Ebbinghaus, E. E. (1964). *Memory*. Dover.

Frisby, C. M. (2002). Messages of hope: Health communication strategies that address barriers preventing black women from screening for breast cancer. *Journal of Black Studies*, *32*(5), 489–505. doi:10.1177/002193470203200501

Greene, K., Campo, S., & Banerjee, S. C. (2010). Comparing Normative, Anecdotal, and Statistical Risk Evidence to Discourage Tanning Bed Use. *Communication Quarterly*, *58*(2), 111–132. doi:10.1080/01463371003773366

Guiraud, P. (1999). *A semiologia*. Presença.

Hannon, P., Lloyd, G. P., Viswanath, K., Smith, T., Basen-Engquist, K., Vernon, S. W., … Backinger, C. L. (2009). Mass media and marketing communication promoting primary and secondary cancer prevention. *Journal of Health Communication, 14*(sup1), 30-37. doi:10.1080/10810730902806802

Heath, R. L., & Blonder, L. X. (2003). Conversational humour among stroke survivors. *Humor: International Journal of Humor Research, 16*(1), 91–106. doi:10.1515/humr.2003.007

Hillier, L. (2019, October 21). Nine powerful breast cancer awareness campaigns. *Econsultancy*. Retrieved from https://econsultancy.com/nine-powerful-breast-cancer-awareness-campaigns-marketing/

Hornik, R. (2002). Public health communication: Making sense of contradictory evidence. In R. Hornik (Ed.), *Public health communication: Evidence for behavior change* (pp. 1–19). Lawrence Erlbaum Associates.

Hornik, R. (Ed.). (2002). *Public health communication: Evidence for behavior*. Lawrence Erlbaum Associates. doi:10.4324/9781410603029

Hovland, C. I., & Weiss, W. (1951). The influence of source credibility on communication effectiveness. *Public Opinion Quarterly, 15*(4), 635. doi:10.1086/266350

Institute of Medicine. (2002). *Speaking of health: Assessing health communication strategies for diverse populations*. National Academies Press.

Jakobson, R. (1963). *Essais de linguistique générale*. Editions de Minuit.

Joly, M. (2008). *Introdução à análise da imagem*. Lisboa: Edições 70.

Katz, M. L., Keller, B., Tatum, C. M., Fickle, D. K., Midkiff, C., Carver, S., Krieger, J. L., Slater, M. D., & Paskett, E. D. (2015). Community members' input into cancer prevention campaign development and experience being featured in the campaign. *Progress in Community Health Partnerships, 9*(2), 149–156. doi:10.1353/cpr.2015.0043 PMID:26412757

Katz, M. L., Young, G. S., Reiter, P. L., Pennell, M. L., Plascak, J. J., Zimmermann, B. J., Krieger, J. L., Slater, M. D., Tatum, C. M., & Paskett, E. D. (2016). Process Evaluation of Cancer Prevention Media Campaigns in Appalachian Ohio. *Health Promotion Practice, 18*(2), 201–210. doi:10.1177/1524839916641638 PMID:27178838

Kreuter, M. W., Green, M. C., Cappella, J. N., Slater, M. D., Wise, M. E., Storey, D., Clark, E. M., O'Keefe, D. J., Erwin, D. O., Holmes, K., Hinyard, L. J., Houston, T., & Woolley, S. (2007). Narrative communication in cancer prevention and control: A framework to guide research and application. *Annals of Behavioral Medicine, 33*(3), 221–235. doi:10.1007/BF02879904 PMID:17600449

Kuiper, N. A. (2012). Humor and resiliency: Towards a process model of coping and growth. *Europe's Journal of Psychology*, *8*(3), 475–491. doi:10.5964/ejop.v8i3.464

Logan, H. L., Shepperd, J. A., Pomery, E., Guo, Y., Muller, K. E., Dodd, V. J., & Riley, J. L. (2013). Increasing screening intentions for oral and pharyngeal cancer. *Annals of Behavioral Medicine*, *46*(1), 96–106. doi:10.100712160-013-9480-z PMID:23479338

McCorkindale, T. (2010). Can you see the writing on my wall? A content analysis of the Fortune 50's Facebook social networking sites. *The Public Relations Journal*, *4*(3). https://www.prsa.org/Intelligence/PRJournal/Documents/content_analysis_of_the_fortune_50s_facebook.pdf

Mehawesh, M. (2014). The socio-semiotic theory of language and translation: An overview. *International Journal of Humanities and Social Science*, *4*(8), 87–96.

Michl, S., & Wohlmann, A. (2019). "Hooked up to that damn machine": Working with metaphors in clinical ethics cases. *Clinical Ethics*, *14*(2), 80–86. doi:10.1177/1477750919851064

Morley, B., Wakefield, M., Dunlop, S., & Hill, D. (2009). Impact of a mass media campaign linking abdominal obesity and cancer: A natural exposure evaluation. *Health Education Research*, *24*(6), 1069–1079. doi:10.1093/her/cyp034 PMID:19570919

Mullein, P. B., Gardiner, J. C., Roseninan, K., Zhu, Z., & Swanson, G. M. (1996). Skin cancer prevention and detection practices in a Michigan farm population following an educational intervention. *The Journal of Rural Health*, *12*(4), 311–320. doi:10.1111/j.1748-0361.1996.tb00820.x PMID:10162862

Neuendorf, K. (2002). *The content analysis guidebook*. Sage.

Pasick, R. J., Hiatt, R. A., & Paskett, E. D. (2004). Lessons learned from community-based cancer screening intervention research. *Cancer*, *101*(S5), 1146–1164. doi:10.1002/cncr.20508 PMID:15316912

Poulios, I., & Senteri, E. (2016). Branding Athens at a time of crisis: A semiotic analysis of the current tourism campaign of the historic city. *Phoro*, *21*(1), 37–56.

Quinn, E. M., Corrigan, M. A., McHugh, S. M., Murphy, D., O'Mullane, J., Hill, A. D., & Redmond, H. P. (2013). Who's talking about breast cancer? Analysis of daily breast cancer posts on the internet. *The Breast*, *22*(1), 24–27. doi:10.1016/j.breast.2012.05.001 PMID:22683246

Randolph, W., & Viswanath, K. (2004). Lessons learned from public health mass media campaigns: Marketing health in a crowded media world. *Annual Review of Public Health*, *25*(1), 419–437. doi:10.1146/annurev.publhealth.25.101802.123046 PMID:15015928

Rim, S. H., Zittleman, L., Westfall, J. M., Overholser, L., Froshaug, D., & Coughlin, S. S. (2009). Knowledge, attitudes, beliefs, and personal practices regarding colorectal cancer screening among health care professionals in rural Colorado: A pilot survey. *The Journal of Rural Health*, *25*(3), 303–308. doi:10.1111/j.1748-0361.2009.00234.x PMID:19566617

Salmon, C., & Atkin, C. (2003). Using media campaigns for health promotion. In T. L. Thompson, A. M. Dorsey, K. I. Miller, & R. Parrott (Eds.), *Handbook of health communication* (pp. 449–472). Lawrence Erlbaum.

Sbaffi, L., & Rowley, J. (2017). Trust and credibility in web-based health information: A review and agenda for future research. *Journal of Medical Internet Research*, *19*(6), e218. doi:10.2196/jmir.7579 PMID:28630033

Schliemann, D., Su, T. T., Paramasivam, D., Treanor, C., Dahlui, M., Loh, S. Y., & Donnelly, M. (2019). Effectiveness of mass and small media campaigns to improve cancer awareness and screening rates in Asia: A systematic review. *Journal of Global Oncology: An American Society of Clinical Oncology Journal.*

Senore, C., Inadomi, J., Segnan, N., Bellisario, C., & Hassan, C. (2015). Optimising colorectal cancer screening acceptance: A review. *Gut*, *64*(7), 1158–1177. doi:10.1136/gutjnl-2014-308081 PMID:26059765

Sisco, H. F., & McCorkindale, T. (2013). Communicating "pink": An analysis of the communication strategies, transparency, and credibility of breast cancer social media sites. *International Journal of Nonprofit and Voluntary Sector Marketing*, *18*(4), 287–301. doi:10.1002/nvsm.1474

Stebletsova, A. O., & Enkova, V. V. (2016). *Health discourse in media: The language of breast cancer prevention. The International Conference on Language and Literature in Education and Research*, Prague, Czech Republic.

Sugawara, Y., Narimatsu, H., Hozawa, A., Shao, L., Otani, K., & Fukao, A. (2012). Cancer patients on Twitter: A novel patient community on social media. *BMC Research Notes*, *5*(1), 1–9. doi:10.1186/1756-0500-5-699 PMID:23270426

Sullivan, T., Weinert, C., & Cudney, S. (2003). Management of chronic illness: Voices of rural women. *Journal of Advanced Nursing*, *44*(6), 566–574. doi:10.1046/j.0309-2402.2003.02846.x PMID:14651679

Sundstrom, B., Brandt, H. M., Gray, L., & Pierce, J. Y. (2018). It's My Time: Applying the health belief model to prevent cervical cancer among college-age women. *Journal of Communication Management (London)*, *22*(2), 161–178. doi:10.1108/JCOM-06-2016-0044

Vraga, E. K., Stefanidis, A., Lamprianidis, G., Croitoru, A., Crooks, A. T., Delamater, P. L., Pfoser, D., Radzikowski, J. R., & Jacobsen, K. H. (2018). Cancer and Social Media: A Comparison of Traffic about Breast Cancer, Prostate Cancer, and Other Reproductive Cancers on Twitter and Instagram. *Journal of Health Communication*, *23*(2), 181–189. doi:10.1080/10810730.2017.1421730 PMID:29313761

Wakefield, M. A., Loken, B., & Hornik, R. C. (2010). Use of mass media campaigns to change health behaviour. *Lancet*, *376*(9748), 1261–1271. doi:10.1016/S0140-6736(10)60809-4 PMID:20933263

Waters, R. D. (2009). The use of social media by nonprofit organizations: An examination from the diffusion of innovations perspective. In T. Dumova & R. Fiordo (Eds.), *Handbook of research on social interaction technologies and collaboration software: Concepts and trends* (pp. 473–485). IGI Publishing.

Watson, J. M., Tomar, S. L., Dodd, V., Logan, H. L., & Choi, Y. (2009). Effectiveness of a Social Marketing Media Campaign to Reduce Oral Cancer Racial Disparities. *Journal of the National Medical Association*, *101*(8), 774–782. doi:10.1016/S0027-9684(15)31005-1 PMID:19715040

WHO. (2018). *Cancer*. Retrieved from: https://www.who.int/news-room/fact-sheets/detail/cancer

Williamswhittle-creativity for business. (n.d.). *Top 5 cancer-fighting campaigns*. Retrieved from: https://www.williamswhittle.com/top-5-cancer-fighting-campaigns/

Yan, S., & Ming, F. (2015). Reinterpreting some key concepts in Barthes' theory. *Journal of Media and Communication Studies*, *7*(3), 59–66. doi:10.5897/JMCS2014.0412

Young, W. F., McGloin, J., Zittleman, L., West, D. R., & Westfall, J. M. (2007). Predictors of colorectal screening in rural Colorado: Testing to prevent colon cancer in the high plains research network. *The Journal of Rural Health*, *23*(3), 238–245. doi:10.1111/j.1748-0361.2007.00096.x PMID:17565524

Zhan, L., Guo, D., Chen, G., & Yang, J. (2018). Effects of repetition learning on associative recognition over time: Role of the hippocampus and prefrontal cortex. *Frontiers in Human Neuroscience*, *12*, 277. doi:10.3389/fnhum.2018.00277 PMID:30050418

Zittleman, L., Emsermann, C., Dickinson, M., Norman, N., Winkelman, K., Linn, G., & Westfall, J. M. (2009). Increasing colon cancer testing in rural Colorado: Evaluation of the exposure to a community-based awareness campaign. *BMC Public Health*, *9*(1), 288. doi:10.1186/1471-2458-9-288 PMID:19664277

Chapter 7
It's All About the Heart:
Analysis of Media Campaigns on Cardiovascular Health

Célia Belim
ISCSP, University of Lisbon, Portugal

ABSTRACT

This chapter aimed to provide responses, within the issue of cardiovascular health, to the effectiveness of the relation between the message's content ("what") and form ("how") and the triad of (cognitive-affective-behavioral) effects. The qualitative content analysis, concretely thematic and rhetorical types, was applied to a corpus of five ads from international campaigns (2015-2019) and three static Portuguese ads (2018-2019). One online survey of Portuguese university students (N = 55) was conducted. The findings show that the ads' issues vary from irreparable losses to the encouragement of healthy behaviors. The pathos tends to elicit various reactions (e.g., alarm, call to action, empathy, fear, guilt, hurt, worry). The logos are constructed of discursive devices (e.g., construction of a narrative, use of questions, selection of colors with connotative purposes, descriptions of concepts), evidence, and stylistic devices. Most of the respondents recognize the cognitive and affective influence, but not the behavioral effects.

DOI: 10.4018/978-1-7998-4396-2.ch007

INTRODUCTION

Being healthy and avoiding diseases are goals of joy and are at the center of the satisfaction of any human being. *Can communication be a success factor in achieving these goals? Can health communication improve the quality of life?* This proposal tries to bring and discuss answers to heart disease, the first cause of death in 2000 and 2016 (WHO, 2018), including Portugal, whose disease mortality rate is 29.7% (Sociedade Portuguesa de Cardiologia, 2019). An estimated 17.9 million people died from heart disease n 2016, representing 31% of all global deaths (WHO, 2017). Communication can represent a promising variable, once most cardiovascular diseases (CVDs) can be prevented by avoiding behavioral risk factors, such as tobacco use, unhealthy diet and obesity, physical inactivity, and harmful use of alcohol (WHO, 2017).

Heart disease refers to various types of conditions that can affect heart function (Wedro, 2017), composing a group of disorders of the heart and blood vessels and including coronary heart disease, cerebrovascular disease, peripheral arterial disease, rheumatic heart disease, congenital heart disease and deep vein thrombosis, and pulmonary embolism (WHO, 2017). There is an alarming increase in specific cardiovascular risk factors (CVRF), such as smoking, hypertension, high cholesterol, diabetes, family history of heart problems, bad nutrition habits, obesity (e.g., Wedro, 2017), with a huge impact on the state of health of the population at large. So, we are facing a cardiovascular disease pandemic that has complex multi-factor causes in which different demographic sectors of society are implicated.

Living in societies of consumption and abundance that invite to excesses, individuals indulge in unhealthy habits and there is a need for awareness of the disease and for the prevention of risk behaviors. Cardiovascular health promotion should extend throughout the life of the individual from infancy, when heart-healthy habits are acquired, to old age (Castellano et al., 2014). Exploring the best evidence available, the American Heart Association – AHA (2020) defines the ideal cardiovascular health based on seven factors – "life's simple 7". It is a set of factors that can help to predict and protect the heart health of persons, being composed by four "modifiable behaviors", which consist in actions that can be done to lower chances of developing heart diseases (not smoking, healthy weight, eating healthy, and being physically active), and three measures (blood pressure, cholesterol, and blood sugar).

Pavlik et al. (1993), examining the extent to which exposure to health promotion messages can influence public understanding of heart disease, suggest that exposure to mediated health messages can influence at least two aspects of understanding: breadth and depth of what people know about heart disease. They also reveal that increases in understanding are enhanced by certain aspects of involvement, particularly the belief that lifestyle can affect one's chances of heart disease. Long et al. (2009) observe that women were increasingly aware of heart disease as their leading cause of death and that the rise in awareness was associated with enlarged action to reduce heart disease risk.

In this scenario, the defended argument is that the health campaigns on heart disease lead to positive cognitive, affective, and behavioral effects. Therefore, it is formulated as a starting question: *How do the prevention campaigns on heart disease originate cognitive, affective, and behavioral effects?* The research objectives are: a) to understand the content of the message – "what"; b) to perceive the form and style of the message, concretely the persuasive and argumentative potential – "how"; c) to know the cognitive, affective and behavioral effects, in order to perceive the various forms of communication success.

Designing messages embroils "the selection of substantive material and the creative production of stylistic features" (Atkin & Rice, 2013, p. 9), so we decide to analyze the substance and the style. Methodologically and in order to understand the "what" and the "how" of messages, it is proposed to use qualitative content analysis, namely the thematic analysis, and more formal analysis, concretely the rhetorical analysis. To know the effects and in an exploratory approach, it is intended to concretize an online survey, to be applied to university students.

THE MESSAGE AIMED AT HEART-DISEASE PREVENTION: WHAT AND HOW?

Persuasive messages frequently use a basic expectancy-value mechanism to influence beliefs regarding the subjective likelihood of various outcomes occurring. The operational formula for preventing risky behaviors is susceptibility multiplied by severity, using a loss frame to motivate the public with a high likelihood of suffering painful effects (Atkin & Rice, 2013, p. 9). Atkin and Rice (2013) explain that incentive appeals often build on the existing values of the target public, so the message tends to reinforce the predispositions (p. 9). Murray-Johnson and Witte (2003) explain that the message designers attempt to make the messages salient to the public (p. 475). The authors refer to message content variables, the stimuli, and cues to action. Cues to action are those message features that prompt the public to pay attention to the content (p. 475). Health message designers create the cognitions leading to motivation by choosing those message features, such as vividness, repetition, and placement in the mass media, that communicate "this is important to your health" (p. 475). Repetition can also heighten the motivation to attend to a message (p. 476). Motivational variables, such as ear, threats, perceived severity, perceived susceptibility, are essential to how a message is processed and whether or not action is taken (p. 477).

Focusing on the emotional dimension of the message, Nabi (2014) refers that fear, guilt, and humor are the emotional appeals that have received the most attention (p. 115). On the other hand, O'Keefe (2014) notes that decisions to adopt specific message strategies for use in persuasive health interventions should be evidence-based, just as evidence-based medicine informs health screening and treatment decisions. For example, in deciding to adopt a narrative or a statistical approach, the campaigner should look for evidence in the literature for which will be more effective in influencing attitude, intention, or behavior change.

Lewis (2015) conducted a study that tested the interaction between an individual-level characteristic – identification with other parents – and the effects of persuasive messages based on norms regarding feeding their child healthful foods. The findings show that the parents, who identified with other parents, were more influenced by normatively focused messages than were parents with lower levels of identification.

Discussing the potential of positive and negative messages, Monahan (1995) argues that negative messages foster the use of more elaborate, detail-oriented, and analytical processing strategies (p. 86) and result in more thoughtful processing because negative affect informs the audience that the current situation is problematic (p. 86). On the other hand, positive messages foster good feelings and the use of less elaborate or more heuristic strategies and do not activate feelings of self-protection, but rather engenders feelings of ease or comfort (Monahan, 1995, p. 86). Concretely on preventing cardiovascular disease risk, Bellicha and McGrath (1990) emphasize that a multiplicity of strategies has been developed and tested to encourage adequate actions. Messages have stressed the benefits of adopting healthy habits, such as protecting loved ones, safeguarding one's health, and being around to enjoy the rewards of life. The reverse technique has been used. Focus group testing has indicated that the portrayal of negative effects in a message of mild fear is believable, motivational, and attention-getting (Arkin, 1987). Sharf and Vanderford (2003) also argue that, when personal stories of suffering are constructed, the individual dealing with serious and/or chronic sickness understands a situation that may at first seem not to have a discernible explanation (p. 29). Stories are a way of making sense of an uncertain or chaotic set of circumstances (Bruner, 1990). Narration is also useful in giving order to human experiences, relating those experiences to others, forming communities, and defining one's life (Fisher, 1987).

Rezai et al. (2017) conducted an online survey on regular physical activity through Amazon Mechanical Turk to verify the effectiveness of a particular message-tailoring strategy. The findings demonstrate that among the three different message categories examined, messages that promoted the benefits of performing regular physical activity (promotion-messages) were perceived to be the most persuasive – which is in harmony with previous findings in the literature (Latimer et al., 2008; Pfeffer, 2012). The second most persuasive category of messages was prevention messages Type 2 (messages that highlight physical and mental health problems that can be avoided by performing the regular activity). The least-persuasive category of messages among these three groups was prevention-messages Type 1 (those that stressed the risks and consequences of not engaging in regular activity). Te et al. (2019) conducted a systematic search for health campaigns against sugar-sweetened beverage consumption. Employing content analysis, the authors detect obesity/overweight, diabetes, and CVDs as the most frequently mentioned health messages.

The influential message should have some qualities or appeals, such as (Atkin & Rice, 2013, p. 9): 1. Credibility, by exposing the trustworthiness and competence of the source and convincing evidence; 2. The engaging manner of presenting style and ideas via combination between arousing substance and attractive stylistic execution; 3. The personally involving and relevant selection of content and style, so receivers regard the behavioral recommendation as applicable to their situation and needs; 4. Understandability in the sense that the presentation of content should be simple, explicit, and detailed and consequently comprehensive and comprehensible to receivers; 5. The motivational incentives of the message, that are the gratifications the recipients can get by complying with health recommendations.

The use of rhetoric can significantly influence outcomes that include curing and preventing diseases and longevity (Sharf, 1990, p. 218). Rhetoric seeks to persuade (Aristotle, 2005, p. 23), a goal that is imperative in health messages. Aristotle (2005) enunciates three means of persuasion: a) those derived from the character of the sender/speaker (ethos); b) those derived from the emotion that the speaker arouses in the public (pathos); and c) those grounded on true arguments (logos) (p. 37). Hartelius and Browning (2008) state that ethos is related to the trust and credibility conferred on the speaker by the public (p. 29). Green (2004) argues that the arguments concerning pathos relate to the emotions aroused and can provoke a powerful social action (p. 659). Logos refers to the clarity and utility of an argument, presented on a rational and logical basis (Holt & Macpherson, 2010, p. 26). Ting (2018) says that the use of data/evidence and examples is part of the substance of logical and rational discourse (p. 238). Still, in relation to logos, stylistic devices can make the speaker's thoughts concrete, helping to communicate in a more effective and clear way (Corbett, 2004, p. 143).

EFFECTS OF THE MESSAGE

Wakefield et al. (2014) explain that media health campaigns aim to, directly and indirectly, affect recipients, by invoking cognitive or emotional responses and can help to associate emotions with achieving change, which can strengthen intentions to alter and improve the likelihood of adopting new behaviors. Lancarotte and Nobre (2016), through a literature review on prevention programs for CVDs, observe that, in community interventions, well-designed mass media campaigns are usually successful in rising basic knowledge but unsuccessful for correcting misconceptions.

Bellicha and McGrath (1990) note that the message has changed as awareness and knowledge have grown. From a starting focus on simple awareness of the connection to stroke and heart disease and on emphasis on demonstration of treatment skills, when awareness of adequate treatment has increased messages continue including treatment instructions but as a means of reinforcement. The Stanford Three Community Study demonstrates that certain risk-reduction behaviors, such as improved eating habits, can be learned through media alone concretely when behavior change depended primarily on acquiring new knowledge (Flora et al., 1989). Other risk-reduction behaviors, such as smoking cessation, required media intervention supplemented with skills training, face-to-face communication, social support, and other interventions, reveal to be effective (Flora et al., 1989).

Perry et al. (1992) refer to the effectiveness of school-based programs combined with a community campaign on the smoking, nutrition, and physical activity behavior of adolescents. Campaigns, with mass media components aimed at changing physical activity behaviors, have yielded short-term increases in physical activity, mainly in highly motivated subjects (Cavill & Bauman, 2004; Kahn et al., 2002). Evaluation of campaigns to promote nutrition, physical activity, and tobacco control, demonstrates that short-term changes can be reached, but sustained effects are difficult to maintain after campaigns end (e.g., Cavill & Bauman, 2004; Finlay & Faulkner, 2005; Norman et al., 2007; Pomerleau et al., 2005; Sanigorski et al., 2008).

Koniak-Griffin and Brecht (2015), studying the overweight immigrant Latinas, explain that knowledge is not simply perceived as cognitive content (facts and ideas) by Latinas. Rather, knowledge development includes an interactional process experienced by participants while engaged in dialogue with the promotor and other women. Balcázar, Alvarado, and Ortiz (2011) suggest the use of a new paradigm for public health that integrates Community Health Workers (CHWs)/promotoras into organized community-based prevention efforts. Koniak-Griffin and Brecht (2015) also emphasize the role of CHWs/promotors. Once they are trusted and respected members of communities, constitute "an excellent model" for expanding access to health information that may be helpful in mitigating racial/ethnic disparities in cardiovascular disease knowledge.

METHOD

The techniques used are qualitative content analysis, namely the thematic analysis, and more formal analysis, concretely the rhetorical analysis. Qualitative content analysis is the most prevalent approach to the qualitative analysis of media health messages. It comprises a search out of underlying themes in the materials being analyzed (Bryman, 2012, p. 557). To operate the technique, we adopt the procedures suggested by Altheide (2004): generate a research question (*what are the issues addressed in the media campaigns aimed at heart-disease prevention?*); become familiar with the context within which the messages were/are generated; become familiar with a small number of messages (selected campaigns); generate some categories that will guide the collection of data and draft a schedule for collecting the data in terms of the generated categories. The type of qualitative analysis is mainly thematic. This means that the data is examined to extract core issues.

Rhetorical analysis is the examination of how messages persuade their audiences of their claims (Dysart-Gale, 2010, p. 29). The aim of rhetorical analysis is not simply to describe the claims and arguments advanced within the discourse, but, most importantly, to identify the specific persuasive strategies employed by the speaker to accomplish specific persuasive goals (O'Donohue, 2013). In the analysis operationalized, we use the rhetoric devices referred to by Aristotle.

The corpus is composed of audio-visual ads from international campaigns of reputed entities operating in heart health, launched in the five-year period between 2015 and 2019. There are five ads, each created in each of the years that make up the analysis period (Table 1). Three recent static ads (2018 and 2019) of Portuguese campaigns were added, are also used in the questionnaire (Table 2). In sum, the main selection criteria are recentness, the reputation of the promoters, impact (number of views), and controversy of communication techniques/tactics applied. The number of views on YouTube was updated on March 25, 2020.

The questionnaire was formulated in two sections. In the first section, it is presented three ads of recent (2018 and 2019) Portuguese campaigns aimed at heart-disease prevention and questions about cognitive, affective, and behavioral effects. The second section includes sociodemographic characterization questions.

Table 1. Corpus of international five ads (2015-2019)

Year	Promoter	Selection criteria	Link
2015	British Heart Foundation	More than half a million views on YouTube (557884)	https://www.youtube.com/watch?v=WQtz2wYBFsE
2016	Heart Foundation	More than three thousand views on YouTube (3463)	https://www.youtube.com/watch?v=1gaYfgu4VAM
2017	British Heart Foundation	More than 215 thousand views on YouTube (215113)	https://www.youtube.com/watch?v=k6UK_2xZS_Q
2018	World Health Organization (WHO)	More than 135 thousand views on YouTube (135262)	https://www.youtube.com/watch?v=Fyi-ePw9Qn0
2019	Heart Foundation	Polemical ad removed from YouTube due to the shock tactics used	https://mumbrella.com.au/every-time-i-told-you-i-loved-you-i-was-lying-heart-foundation-campaign-targets-families-581407

Table 2. Corpus of Portuguese ads (2018-2019)

Year	Portuguese Promoter	Slogan	Selection criteria
2018, May	Sociedade Portuguesa de Cardiologia	"Capable heart" ["Coração capaz"]	Campaign's actuality, credibility, and reputation of promoters
2019, February	Sociedade Portuguesa de Cardiologia	"Did not suspect the feeling of fatigue and stopped suddenly in the middle of the trip" ["Não desconfiou da sensação de fadiga e ficou subitamente a meio da viagem"]	
2019, May	Associação Portuguesa de Intervenção Cardiovascular	"Every second counts" ["Cada segundo conta"]	

The online survey was conducted in July 2019 as an exploratory study in a convenience sample of students at the University of Lisbon, concretely at the School of Social and Political Sciences and in the scientific area of Communication Sciences, motivated by: accessibility and proximity of the researcher to the population and the predisposition of the population to be interested in matters related to communication. It was used a non-probability sampling technique, which is the most applicable and widely used technique in clinical research (Elfil & Negida, 2017). In this technique, the investigators enroll subjects according to their availability and accessibility. Therefore, this technique is quick, inexpensive, and convenient. It is called convenient sampling as the researcher selects the sample elements according to his/her convenient accessibility and proximity (Gravetter & Forzano, 2012).

University students were the sociodemographic category selected as they: a) represent almost two-thirds of all young adults in Organization for Economic Co-operation and Development (OECD) countries (2017); b) as potential future leaders, politicians, and managers, their health and well-being are a global public health priority (Stewart-Brown et al., 2000); c) they often report poor health conditions, although they can be seen as a privileged healthy population segment (Montagni et al., 2018); d) have necessarily ample access to digital information devices, being known as "digital natives" or "net generation" (Levine & Dean, 2012). Due to this last factor combined with ease of dissemination, the procedure consisted of disseminating the questionnaire through digital channels, such as Facebook, e-mail.

Data were analyzed using descriptive statistics.

FINDINGS

International Ads

In the 2015's video, the issue is the sudden loss due to heart disease, showing the devastating effects of the disease for a family. The 2016's video focuses on the call to action (e.g., "think of your family", "for heart health information", "Let's keep Australian ♡ beating"). The main issue of the 2017's video is the story of Russell's stroke. In 2018's video, the core issue is to choose health and not tobacco. The 2019's video suggests that people who don't look after their hearts don't care about their families, conveying a heavy message of responsibility and blame.

As all promoters of the ads are reputed in the health field, they have ethos, that is, they are credible and reliable.

In the 2015's video, in terms of pathos, the guilt and fear of leaving children orphans and unprotected, the fear of loss, the shock due to sudden loss, and the empathy are stimulated in the receiver once the narrative focuses on a son (Ben) who loses his father, who experienced a mortal heart disease and, for this reason, does not return home ("I can't come home tonight"). Among parents, the responsibility of having preventive behaviors, so as not to leave their children orphaned and helpless, is raised. The narrative shows how heart disease can be particularly devastating in how it can impact children, forever changing their lives (Figures 1-3). In relation to the logos, the rhetorical devices used are: the construction of a story, although fictitious, with characters who have an intimate relation (father-son) and are victims of fatal and irreversible effects of heart disease, and the use of the personification, by endowing heart disease with human qualities ("heart disease is heartless"), confirming that heart disease is human and a human problem (Figure 4).

Figure 1.

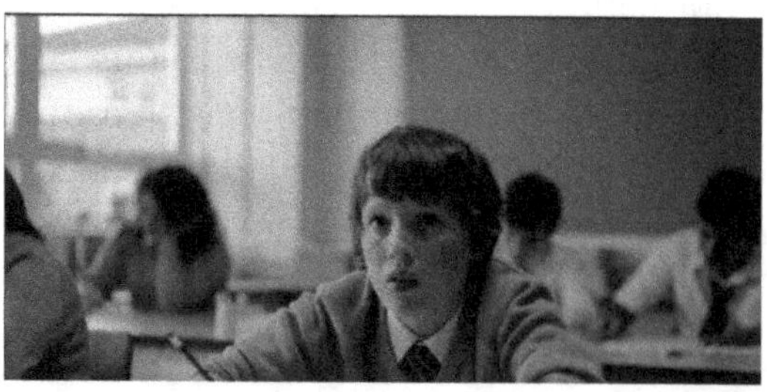

Figure 2.

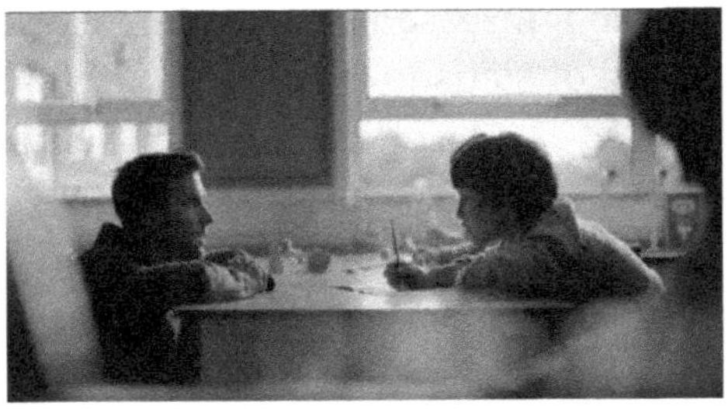

Figure 3.

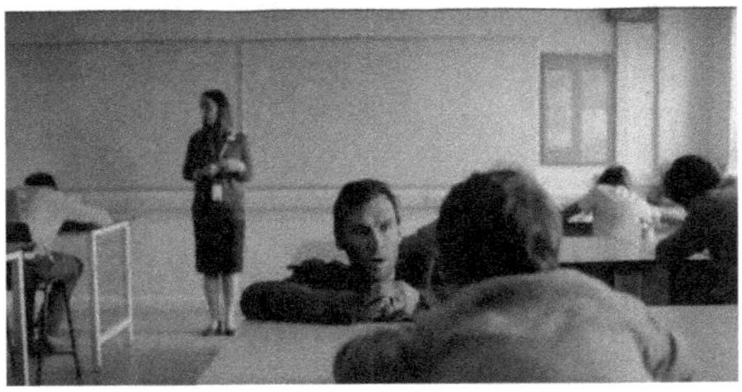

Figure 4.

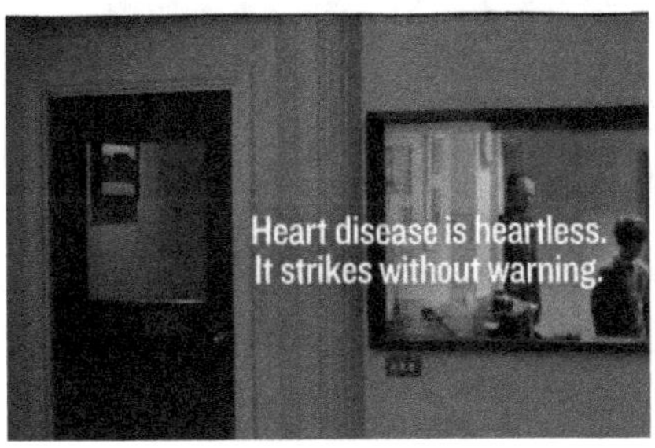

The 2016's video, "Let's keep Australian hearts beating", its depopulated with human images: it only appears icons of a heart (Figure 5), letters-words (Figure 6), and numbers. The color palette is tricolor: red, black, and white. The pathos is present in the questions addressed to the receipt ("Did you hear that?", "But did you know?"), and in the stimulation of emotions, such as: involvement ("that's the sound", "LIFE" – Figure 5), worry ("almost one in three deaths in Australia are caused by cardiovascular disease, that's 1 person every 12 minutes, that's 123 of us every single day" – Figure 7), awareness and consciousness ("Think of your family – (no, really) – think of your family" – Figure 8), alarm ("disease is our leading single cause of death"). The logos are constructed of statistic evidence ("2/3 of our families will be touched by cardiovascular", "123 of us every single day") and of stylistic devices, such as the antithesis ("but while this all seems bleak… we've been working"), the alliteration ("that's"), and the personification ("Let's keep Australian ♡ beating").

Figure 5.

Figure 6.

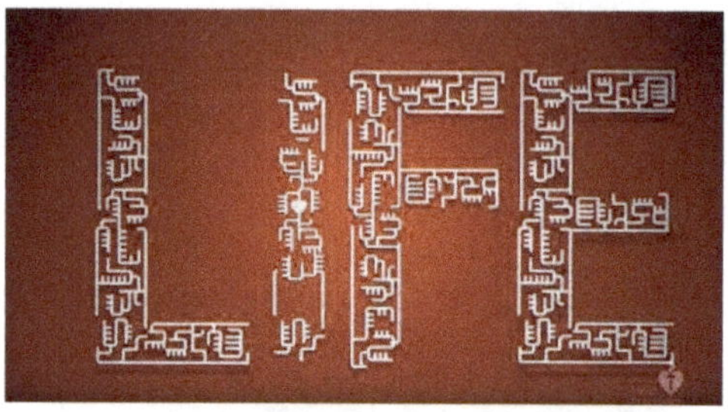

Figure 7.

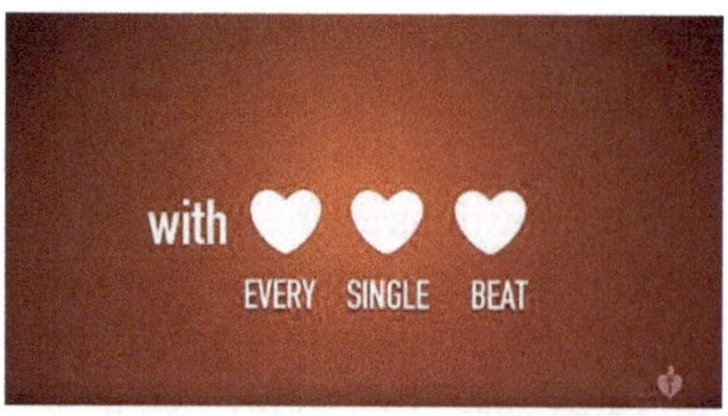

Figure 8.

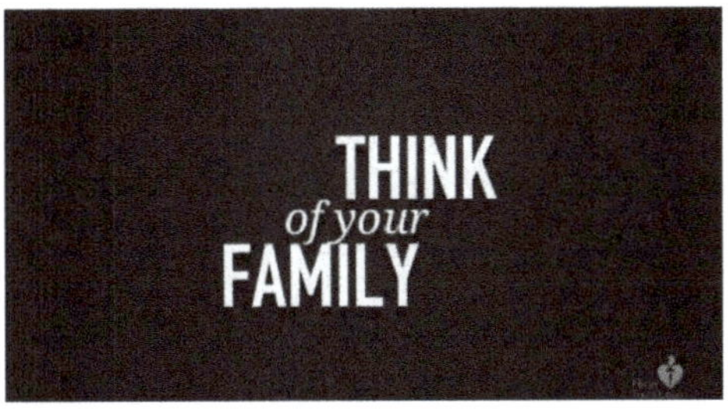

2017's video begins with a close-up shot of a man named Russell (Figure 9). We know his name because the female off-voice says it ("I am Russell") and, speaking voice to Russell, she says that wants to tell us his last conversation. The female voice is broken and tearful, catching Russell. The shot opens and we perceive that Russell is with his wife, Rachel and that she is the speaker (Figure 10). She tells the reason for Russell's muteness: "a stroke robbed me of my voice", "around a quarter of strokes happen to people under 55" (Figure 11).

Figure 9.

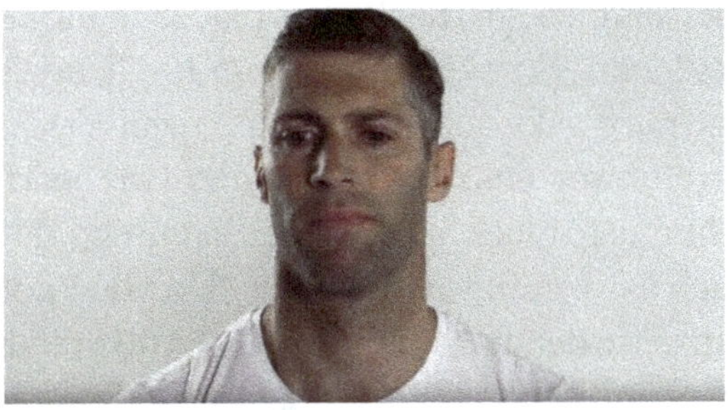

Figure 10.

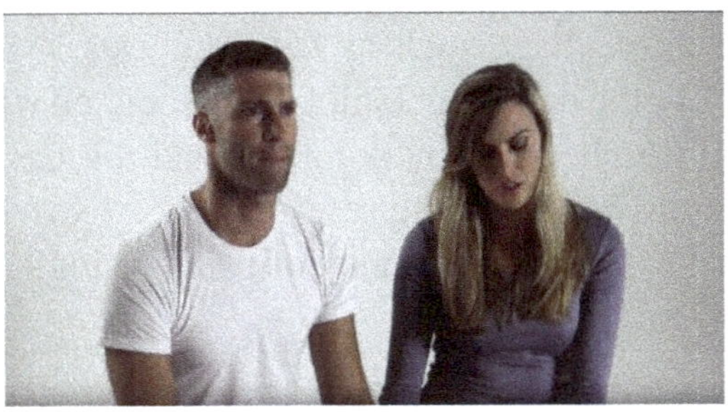

Figure 11.

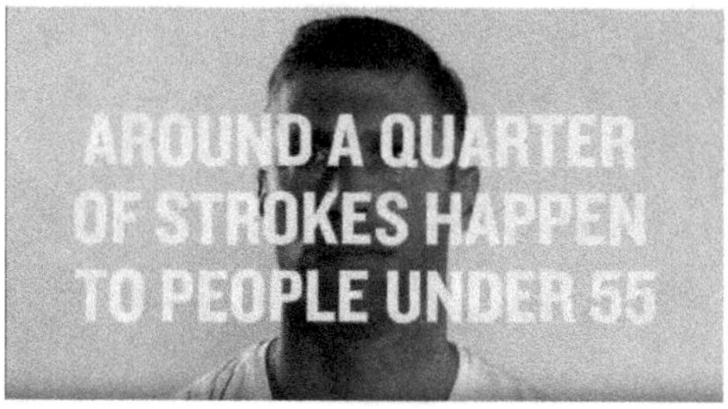

The pathos is visible i: 1. the strangeness that can be caused on the receiver: the contrast and *short circuit* between the off-voice of a woman, who is unseen, and the image of a man who does not speak; 2. the woman's broken and weeping voice and Russell's muteness can cause empathy, transmitting the idea that the stroke can affect any of us; 3. fear, which can be generated from the information that "around a quarter of strokes happen to people under 55"; 3. serenity and confidence ("but our researchers are fighting back"). Logos is present in the use of statistic evidence ("around a quarter of strokes happen to people under 55"), of real characters (personalization and realism of the story), and of stylistic devices, such as the antithesis (the off-voice of a woman, who is unseen *vs.* the image of a man who does not speak; "but").

2018's video focuses on a heart, which is placed in the center of the image and on a red background. Smoke comes from the heart, suggesting that it is smoking. The narrator asks and informs the receiver. As the information provided by the narrator worsens, the appearance of the heart also deteriorates, from red at the beginning to black and diseased at the end. The pathos suggests some reactions, such as: 1 guilt to not know: "Do you know tobacco causes over 1 in 10 heart disease deaths?" (Figure 12), "And breathing second-hand smoke causes strokes and heart attacks?", 2. responsibility of knowing: "But now, you do!", 3. call to action: "Protect your heart and choose health, not tobacco" (Figure 14). The logos anchors in the: 1. statistical evidence (e.g., "Hundreds of millions of tobacco users don't realize tobacco causes heart disease"), 2. stylistic devices, such as the antithesis ("choose health not tobacco" – Figure 14), the metaphor (smoking associated with darkness), and the personification (the heart is smoking), 3. and discursive devices, such as the use of questions to attract the receiver (e.g., "No? Well, you are not alone…" – Figure 13) and the constancy of using a single color, red, which is symbolically the color of the heart.

Figure 12.

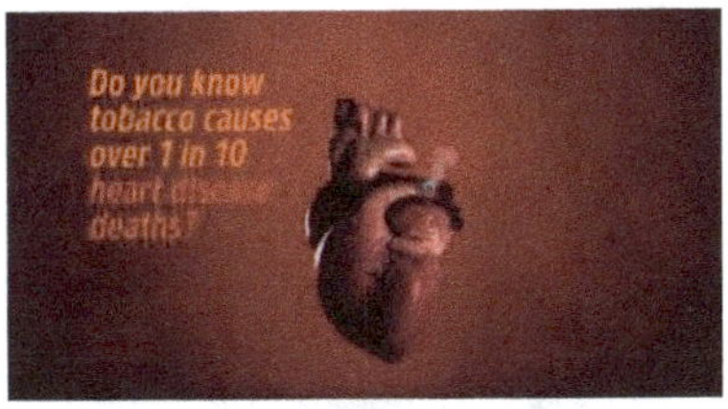

Figure 13.

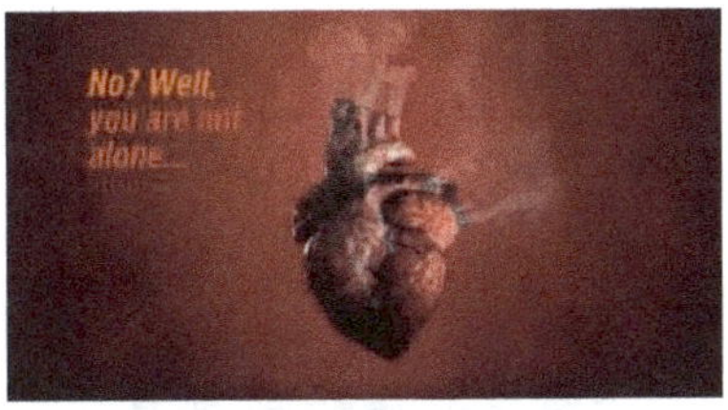

Figure 14.

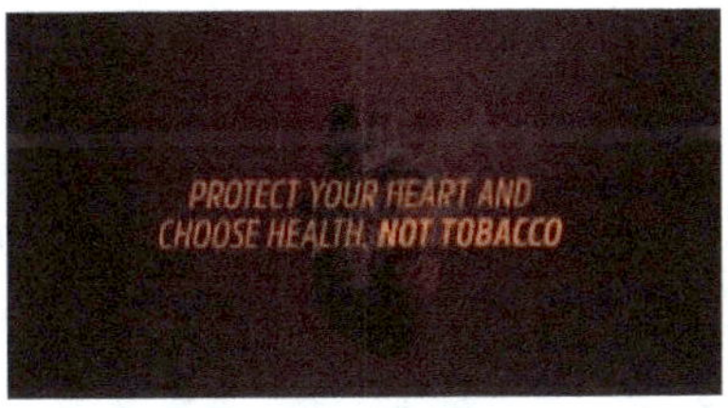

2019's video concentrates on the suggestion that persons who don't look after their hearts don't care about their families. Various scenes are perturbing, because, in normal occasions (washing dishes – Figure 15) or festive occasions (Figure 16), some persons declare shocking statements, such as: "I promise you my heart and I've given it away", "In time, this family will be filled with loss and sadness. But I won't care because I'll be gone", "It's not just my heart, I don't care about it, it's yours". In terms of pathos, the ad can provoke perturbation due to the nature of statements, the guilt of not having healthy behaviors, and even hurt, once some comments in digital platforms accusing the ad to be insensitive and plain ignorant (Stow, 2019). Focusing on logos, statistical evidence is used ("heart disease kills an Australian every 28 minutes"), as well stylistic devices, such as the dysphemism for approaching a problem through shocking statements that are unusual in the chosen contexts.

Figure 15.

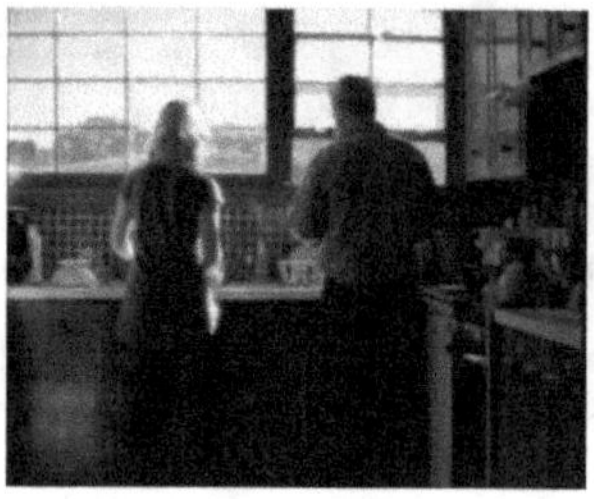

Figure 16.

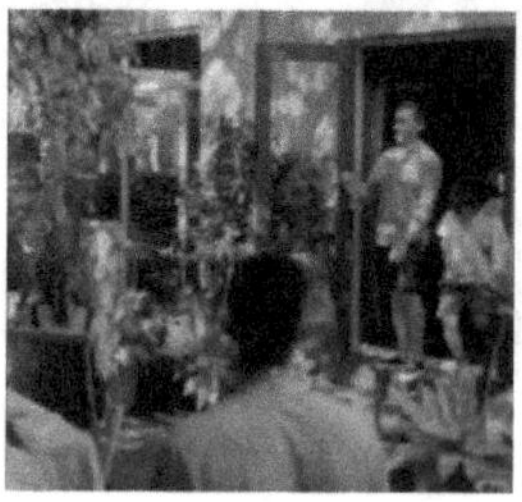

Figure 17.

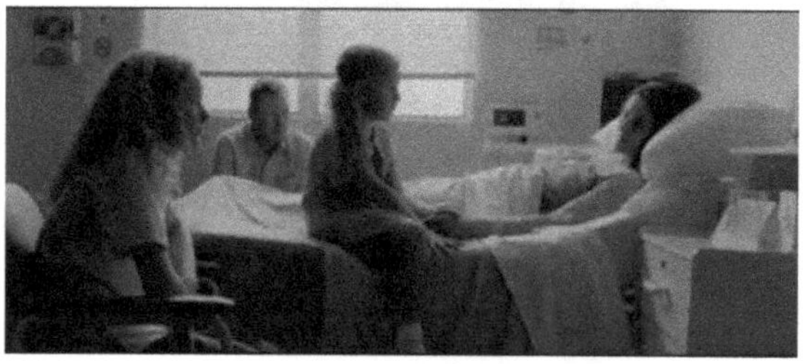

Portuguese Ads

The ad (Figure 18) is about what is a "capable heart". Pathos is evident by the sensibilization to what is a "capable heart" and by the question addressed to the receiver: "Is your heart capable?". Logos is constructed through stylistic devices, such as the antithesis ("a heart that risks for life, but not risks the life" and the anaphor ("a capable heart"), and discursive devices, such as the description of what is a "capable heart" ("is a heart that risks for life, but not risks the life. It is a heart that controls risk factors, seeks help when needs it, and is aware of its rhythm and symptoms. (…) is a heart that wants to live longer and better and always tries to have a healthy life"), the question that retains the attention of the receiver and the use of the red, the color of heart and alarm.

Figure 18. Ad "Capable heart"

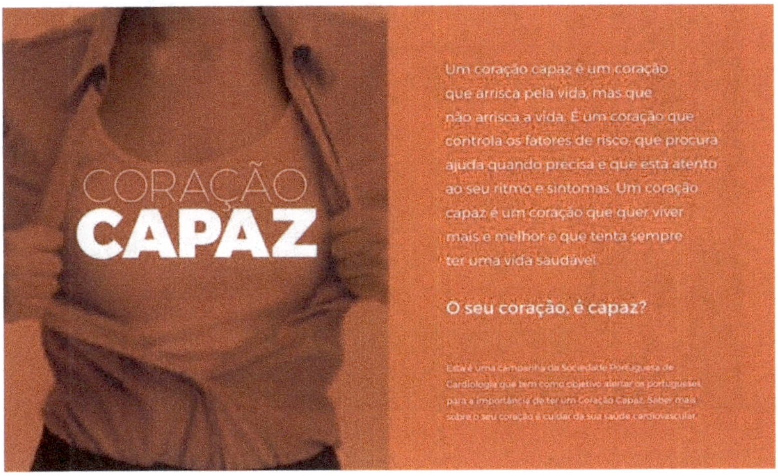
CORAÇÃO
CAPAZ
Um coração capaz é um coração que arrisca pela vida, mas que não arrisca a vida. É um coração que controla os fatores de risco, que procura ajuda quando precisa e que está atento ao seu ritmo e sintomas. Um coração capaz é um coração que quer viver mais e melhor e que tenta sempre ter uma vida saudável.
O seu coração, é capaz?

The ad (Figure 19) highlights a heart, that stayed in the middle of the trip. The pathos is perceptible by the reactions potentially created, such as fear for stopping in the middle he life and call to action ("Pay attention to your heart and recognize the signs of heart failure"). In terms of logos, the ad displays a metaphor (heart is a car that stopped in the middle of the trip) and a personification ("He/she didn't suspect the feeling of fatigue and stopped suddenly in the middle of the trip").

The ad (Figure 20), mainly informative, lays emphasis on acute myocardial infarction, its symptoms, and behavioral proceedings. In terms of pathos, the ad: 1. tries to inject worry and sensibilization to the urgency of time in the receiver ("every second count"); and 2. calls to action, by the enunciation of the advice: "Do not ignore these symptoms. Quickly call to 112. Get treatment". In terms of logos, the ad offers medical evidence ("chest pain, sweating, nausea, vomiting, shortness of breath and anxiety are symptoms of alarm") and, stylistically and visually, it is used as a metaphor: the heart is a clock, validating the idea that every second count, and the red is connotatively linked to heart, danger, and alarm.

We summarize in Table 3 the main rhetorical devices identified.

Figure 19. Ad "He/she didn't suspect the feeling of fatigue and stopped suddenly in the middle of the trip"

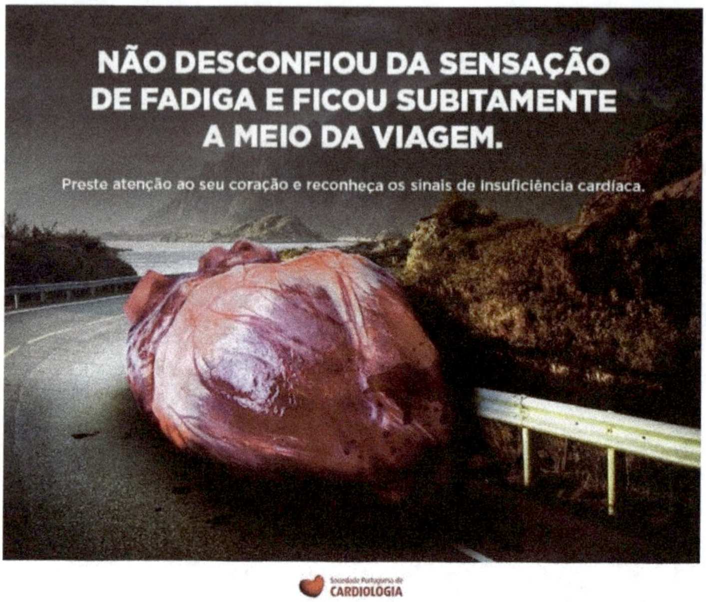
NÃO DESCONFIOU DA SENSAÇÃO DE FADIGA E FICOU SUBITAMENTE A MEIO DA VIAGEM.
Preste atenção ao seu coração e reconheça os sinais de insuficiência cardíaca.
CARDIOLOGIA

Figure 20. Ad "every second count"

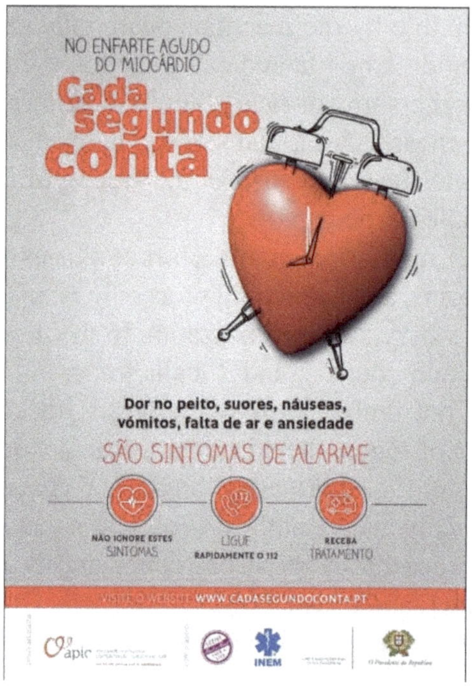
NO ENFARTE AGUDO DO MIOCÁRDIO
Cada segundo conta
Dor no peito, suores, náuseas, vómitos, falta de ar e ansiedade
SÃO SINTOMAS DE ALARME
NÃO IGNORE ESTES SINTOMAS
LIGUE RAPIDAMENTE O 112
RECEBA TRATAMENTO
WWW.CADASEGUNDOCONTA.PT
apic
INEM

Table 3. Rhetorical devices identified in ads

Ethos	Pathos	Logos
. The credibility of the promoter of the ad . Trust in promoter	. alarm . awareness and consciousness . call to action . empathy . fear . guilt . hurt . involvement . perturbation . responsibility of having preventive and healthy behaviors and of knowing . sensibilization . serenity and confidence . shock to a sudden loss . strangeness . worry	. discursive devices: construction of a narrative, use of questions to force the receiver to react, selection of colors with connotative purposes, descriptions-definitions of concepts . medical evidence . statistical evidence . stylistic devices: anaphor, antithesis, dysphemism, metaphor, personification

Effects

Characterization of the Sample

The sample includes 55 individuals, 12 males (21.8%) and 43 females (78.2%). The predominant age range is from 18 to 20 years (40%), followed by 21-25 years (21.8%). The prevalent cycle of studies is the bachelor's degree (52.7%), followed by the master's degree (40%) and, finally, the Ph.D. degree (7.3%). Regarding nationality, Portuguese respondents are the most prevailing (65.5%), followed by Brazilians (32.7%).

Cognitive Effects

42 (76.4%) respondents stated they have gathered knowledge from the three ads. The remaining 13 subjects (23.6%) declare not having learned lessons. Among the knowledge drawn, the symptoms listed in ad 3 stand out.

Effective Effects

23 (41.8%) of university students say they feel "willingness to have preventive care", 16 (29.1%) mention they are afraid of heart disease, 6 (10%) feel discomfort, 5 (9.1%) state they don't feel nothing and 2 (3.6%) feel guilty.

Behavioral Effects

Behavioral effects are not so immediate nor effective. 31 (57.4%) individuals report that they will not have behaviors related to exposure to the three ads, while 23 students (42.6%) commit to ad-inspired behaviors. These behaviors include being more alert to possible symptoms, taking preventive care, and trying to learn more about what to do to ensure optimal and healthy heart functioning.

DISCUSSION

The ads' issues vary from the devastating effects of irreversible and irreparable loss to the encouragement of healthy behaviors. That is, they explore the negative and positive dimensions of messages. Monahan (1995), for example, mentions that negative messages foster the use of more sophisticated, detail-oriented, and analytical processing strategies (p. 86) and provoke more thoughtful processing because negative effect clarifies the public that the current situation is problematic (p. 86). The representation of negative effects in a message of mild fear is believable, motivational, and attention-getting (Arkin, 1987). This is observable by the responses of the university students surveyed who confirm that the negative approach mostly leads to the desire to adopt preventive behaviors and the fear of being a victim of heart disease.

Contrary, positive messages foster good feelings and the use of less elaborate or more heuristic strategies and do not activate feelings of self-protection but rather provoke feelings of ease or comfort (Monahan, 1995, p. 86). Bellicha and McGrath (1990) highlight that a panoply of strategies has been developed and tested to stimulate adequate actions. Messages have stressed the benefits of adopting healthy habits, such as protecting loved ones, safeguarding one's health, and being around to enjoy the rewards of life (e.g., "think of your family", "let's keep Australian ♡ beating", "protect your heart and choose health, not tobacco").

The pathos tends to engender the following reactions: alarm, awareness, and consciousness, call to action, empathy, fear, guilt, hurt, involvement, disturbance, responsibility for having preventive and healthy behaviors and of knowing, sensibilization, serenity and confidence, the shock to a sudden loss, strangeness, and worry.

Focusing on the emotional dimension of the message, Nabi (2014) mentions that fear and guilt are the emotional appeals that have received the most attention (p. 115). Murray-Johnson and Witte (2003) also explain that motivational variables, such as fear, threats, perceived severity, perceived susceptibility, influence how a message is processed and whether or not action is taken (p. 477).

Murray-Johnson and Witte (2003) clarify the potential of the message's salience, that is when it attracts the public (p. 475). The authors mention the stimuli and cues to action, features that prompt the public to pay attention to the content (p. 475). Long et al. (2009) perceive that women were increasingly aware of heart disease as their leading cause of death and that the rise in awareness was associated with enlarged action to reduce heart disease risk. The empathy was recognized by Lewis (2015) in a study whose findings show that the parents who identified with other parents were more influenced by normatively focused messages than were parents with lower levels of identification.

Pavlik et al. (1993) show that increases in understanding are enhanced by certain aspects of involvement, particularly the belief that lifestyle can affect one's chances of heart disease.

There are ads that explore clearly the preventive component of the disease (e.g., 2016's video and Portuguese ad 3), meeting the results found by Rezai et al. (2017) that the second most persuasive category of messages is prevention messages.

The logos are constructed of discursive devices (e.g., construction of a narrative, questions to compel the receiver to react, selection of colors with connotative purposes, descriptions-definitions of concepts), medical evidence, statistical evidence, and stylistic devices (anaphor, antithesis, dysphemism, metaphor, personification).

When personal stories of suffering are constructed, the individual understands a situation that may at first seem not to have a perceptible explanation (Sharf & Vanderford, 2003, p. 29). In this sense, Bruner (1990) explains that stories are a way of making sense of an uncertain or chaotic set of circumstances. So, the narration is also useful in giving order to human experiences, relating those experiences to others, forming communities, and defining one's life (Fisher, 1987).

The use of statistical and medical evidence meets O'Keefe's (2014) recommendation that decisions to adopt specific message strategies for persuasive health interventions should be evidence-based. Ting (2018) says that the use of data/evidence and examples is part of the substance of logical and rational discourse (p. 238). Still, in relation to logos, stylistic devices can make the speaker's thoughts concrete, helping to communicate in a more effective and clear way (Corbett, 2004, p. 143). The anaphor or repetition can also heighten the motivation to assimilate a message (Murray-Johnson & Witte, 2003, p. 476).

All the qualities and appeals referred for Atkin and Rice (2013, p. 9) and the rhetoric advice proposed by Aristotle (2005) are used by the analyzed ads.

Most of the Portuguese university students surveyed recognize cognitive and affective effects derived from the three advertisements. These results confirm the findings of Lancarotte and Nobre (2016) that well-designed mass media campaigns are usually successful for rising basic knowledge. The message has to be designed to reach the target public and to comply with strategical goals. Bellicha and McGrath (1990), in this context, observe that the message has changed as awareness and knowledge have grown. But regarding behavioral effects, most respondents report not adopting health behaviors related to ad exposure. Evaluation of certain health campaigns shows that short-term changes can be reached, but sustained effects, as behavioral, are difficult to maintain after campaigns end (e.g., Cavill & Bauman, 2004; Finlay & Faulkner, 2005; Norman et al., 2007; Pomerleau et al., 2005; Sanigorski et al., 2008).

Although the chapter's purpose is not to discuss the multiple factors that influence health lifestyle and campaign's effects, we recall that there are many social factors simultaneously influencing the outcome of this equation. Hernandez and Blazer (2006) state that several variables, including genetic inheritance, personal behaviors, access to quality health care, and the general external environment (e.g., quality of air, water, and housing conditions), determined health. A crescent set of research has documented associations between health and social and cultural factors (Berkman & Kawachi, 2000; Marmot & Wilkinson, 2006). For example, socioeconomic status, poverty, social networks, and job stress manifest robust evidence of their links to health.

CONCLUSION

The defended argument that health campaigns on heart disease lead to positive cognitive, affective and behavioral effects is confirmed, being the behavioral effects the less evident. The optimization of the relationship between message and effects depends on the encoder/sender's prior knowledge of the content and form/style variables that may be most effective in influencing the target public.

The rhetorical triad and discursive devices are useful for message formulation and maximization of its effects. Respondents reveal that the negative approach leads to the will to adopt preventive behaviors and the fear of being a victim of heart disease.

The survey applied is an exploratory approach on the relationship between the message and effects, knowing that there are more variables that influence the effects of the campaign. In this study, the internal factors of the campaign were explored in order to understand its potential and effectiveness, but it is known, through the literature review, that other external factors influence outcomes.

The use of university students as a convenient sample can be a starting point to develop the survey. However, to understand better responses to health campaigns, differentiated samples should be included.

By learning more about the effects of messages, it will be easier to inform and strategically design more effective health campaigns among the target publics. If the strategical design of messages can produce more positive and controlled effects, this relation will elicit positive social implications regarding heart disease, the world's leading cause of death in 2000 and 2016.

REFERENCES

American Heart Association (AHA). (2020). *Life's simple 7*. Retrieved from https://playbook.heart.org/lifes-simple-7/

Aristóteles. (2005). *Retórica*. Imprensa Nacional-Casa da Moeda.

Arkin, E. B. (1987). *Analysis of high blood pressure target audience and message test reports, 1978-1986*. National Heart, Lung, and Blood Institute.

Atkin, C. K., & Rice, R. E. (2013). Theory and principles of public communication campaigns. In R. R. E. Rice & C. K. Atkin (Eds.), *Public communication campaigns* (pp. 3–20). Sage. doi:10.4135/9781544308449.n1

Balcázar, H., Alvarado, M., & Ortiz, G. (2011). Salud Para Su Corazon (Health for Your Heart) Community Health Worker Model. *The Journal of Ambulatory Care Management*, *34*(4), 362–372. doi:10.1097/JAC.0b013e31822cbd0b PMID:21914992

Bellicha, T., & McGrath, J. (1990). Mass media approaches to reducing cardiovascular disease risk. *Public Health Reports, 105*(3), 245–252. PMID:2113682

Berkman, L., & Kawachi, I. (Eds.). (2000). *Social epidemiology*. Oxford University Press.

Bruner, J. (1990). *Acts of meaning*. Harvard University Press.

Bryman, A. (2012). *Social research methods*. Oxford University Press.

Castellano, J. M., Narula, J., Castillo, J., & Fuster, V. (2014). Promoting cardiovascular health worldwide: Strategies, challenges, and opportunities. *Revista Espanola de Cardiologia*, *67*(9), 724–730. doi:10.1016/j.recesp.2014.01.024 PMID:25172068

Cavill, N., & Bauman, A. (2004). Changing the way people think about health-enhancing physical activity: Do mass media campaigns have a role? *Journal of Sports Sciences*, *22*(8), 771–790. doi:10.1080/02640410410001712467 PMID:15370487

Corbett, E. (2004). Classical rhetoric. In J. Rivkin & M. Ryan (Eds.), Literary theory, an anthology (pp. 142-161). Maiden: Blackwell Publishing.

Dysart-Gale, D. (2010). Techne, technology, and disenchantment in the wind in The Wind in the Willows. In J. C. Horne & D. R. White (Eds.), *Kenneth Grahame's The Wind in the Willows: A children's classic at 100*. Scarecrow Press.

Elfil, M., & Negida, A. (2017). Sampling methods in Clinical Research: *An Educational Review. Emergency (Tehran, Iran)*, *5*(1), e52. PMID:28286859

Finlay, S. J., & Faulkner, G. (2005). Physical activity promotion through the mass media: Inception, production, transmission and consumption. *Preventive Medicine*, *40*(2), 121–130. doi:10.1016/j.ypmed.2004.04.018 PMID:15533520

Fisher, W. R. (1987). *Human communication as narration: Toward a philosophy of reason, value, and action*. University of South Carolina Press.

Flora, J., Maccoby, N., & Farquhar, J. (1989). Communication campaigns to prevent cardiovascular disease: The Stanford Community Studies. In R. Rice & C. Atkin (Eds.), *Public communication campaigns* (pp. 233–252). Sage Publications, Inc.

Gravetter, F., & Forzano, L. (2012). Selecting research participants. *Research Methods Behaviorer Science*, 125-139.

Green, S. Jr. (2004). A rhetorical theory of diffusion. *Academy of Management Review*, *29*(4), 653–669. doi:10.5465/amr.2004.14497653

Hartelius, E., & Browning, L. (2008). The application of rhetorical theory in managerial research. *Management Communication Quarterly*, *22*(1), 13–39. doi:10.1177/0893318908318513

Hernandez, L. M., & Blazer, D. G. (Eds.). (2006). *Genes, behavior, and the social environment: Moving beyond the nature/nurture debate*. National Academies Press.

Holt, R., & Macpherson, A. (2010). Sensemaking, rhetoric and the socially competent entrepreneur. *International Small Business Journal*, *28*(1), 20–42. doi:10.1177/0266242609350822

Kahn, E. B., Ramsey, L. T., Brownson, R. C., Heath, G. W., Howze, E. H., Powell, K. E., Stone, E. J., Rajab, M. W., & Corso, P. (2002). The effectiveness of interventions to increase physical activity. A systematic review. *American Journal of Preventive Medicine, 22*(4), 73-107.

Koniak-Griffin, D., & Brecht, M. L. (2015). Awareness of cardiovascular disease and preventive behaviors among overweight immigrant Latinas. *The Journal of Cardiovascular Nursing*, *30*(5), 447–455. doi:10.1097/JCN.0000000000000181 PMID:25078875

Lancarotte, I., & Nobre, M. R. (2016). Primordial and primary prevention programs for cardiovascular diseases: From risk assessment through risk communication to risk reduction. A review of the literature. *Clinics (São Paulo)*, *71*(11), 667–678. doi:10.6061/clinics/2016(11)09 PMID:27982169

Latimer, A. E., Rivers, S. E., Rench, T. A., Katulak, N. A., Hicks, A., Hodorowski, J. K., Higgins, E. T., & Salovey, P. (2008). A field experiment testing the utility of regulatory fit messages for promoting physical activity. *Journal of Experimental Social Psychology*, *44*(3), 826–832. doi:10.1016/j.jesp.2007.07.013 PMID:19543443

Levine, A., & Dean, D. R. (2012). *Generation on a tightrope: A portrait of today's college student*. Jossey-Bass.

Lewis, N. (2015). Examining normative influence in persuasive health messages: The moderating role of identification with other parents. *International Journal of Communication*, *9*, 3000–3019.

Long, T., Taubenheim, A. M., Wayman, J., Temple, S., & Ruoff, B. A. (2008). The heart truth: Using the power of branding and social marketing to increase awareness of heart disease in women. *Social Marketing Quarterly*, *14*(3), 3–29. doi:10.1080/15245000802279334 PMID:19122892

Marmot, M. G., & Wilkinson, R. D. (Eds.). (2006). *Social determinants of health*. Oxford University Press.

Monahan, J. L. (1995). Thinking positively: Using positive affect when designing health messages. In E. W. Maibach & R. L. Parrott (Eds.), *Designing health messages: Approaches from communication theory and public health practice* (pp. 81–90). Sage. doi:10.4135/9781452233451.n5

Montagni, I., Cariou, T., Feuillet, T., Langlois, E., & Tzourio, C. (2018). Exploring digital health use and opinions of university students: Field survey study. *JMIR mHealth and uHealth*, *6*(3), e65. doi:10.2196/mhealth.9131 PMID:29549071

Murray-Johnson, L., & Witte, K. (2003). Looking toward the future: Health message design strategies. In T. Thompson, A. Dorsey, K. Miller, & R. Parrott (Eds.), *Handbook of health communication* (pp. 473–495). Lawrence Erlbaum Associates.

Nabi, R. L. (2014). Emotional flow in persuasive health messages. *Health Communication*, *30*(2), 114–124. doi:10.1080/10410236.2014.974129 PMID:25470436

Norman, G. J., Zabinski, M. F., Adams, M. A., Rosenberg, D. E., Yaroch, A. L., & Atienza, A. A. (2007). A review of eHealth interventions for physical activity and dietary behavior change. *American Journal of Preventive Medicine*, *33*(4), 336–345. doi:10.1016/j.amepre.2007.05.007 PMID:17888860

O'Donohue, W. (2013). *Clinical psychology and the philosophy of science*. Springer. doi:10.1007/978-3-319-00185-2

O'Keefe, D. J. (2014). Message generalizations that support evidence-based persuasive message design: Specifying the evidentiary requirements. *Health Communication*, *30*(2), 106–113. doi:10.1080/10410236.2014.974123 PMID:25470435

Organisation for Economic Co-operation Development (OECD). (2017). *Education at a glance: OECD indicators*. OECD Publishing.

Pavlik, J. V., Finnegan, J. R. Jr, Strickland, D., Salmon, C. T., Viswanath, K., & Wackman, D. B. (1993). Increasing public understanding of heart disease: An analysis of data from the Minnesota Heart Health Program. *Health Communication*, *5*(1), 1–20. doi:10.120715327027hc0501_1

Perry, C. L., Kelder, S. H., Murray, D. M., & Klepp, K. I. (1992). Communitywide smoking prevention: Long-term outcomes of the Minnesota Heart Health Program and the Class of 1989 Study. *American Journal of Public Health*, *82*(9), 1210–1216. doi:10.2105/AJPH.82.9.1210 PMID:1503159

Pfeffer, I. (2013). Regulatory fit messages and physical activity motivation. *Journal of Sport & Exercise Psychology*, *35*(2), 119–131. doi:10.1123/jsep.35.2.119 PMID:23535971

Pomerleau, J., Lock, K., Knai, C., & McKee, M. (2005). Interventions designed to increase adult fruit and vegetable intake can be effective: A systematic review of the literature. *The Journal of Nutrition*, *135*(10), 2486–2495. doi:10.1093/jn/135.10.2486 PMID:16177217

Rezai, L. S., Chin, J., Bassett-Gunter, R., & Burns, C. (2017). Developing persuasive health messages for a behavior-change-support-system that promotes physical activity. In *Proceedings of the 2017 International Symposium on Human Factors and Ergonomics in Health Care* (pp. 89-95). Santa Monica, CA: Human Factors and Ergonomics Society. 10.1177/2327857917061020

Sanigorski, A. M., Bell, A. C., Kremer, P. J., Cuttler, R., & Swinburn, B. A. (2008). Reducing unhealthy weight gain in children through community capacity-building: Results of a quasi-experimental intervention program, Be Active Eat Well. *International Journal of Obesity*, *32*(7), 1060–1067. doi:10.1038/ijo.2008.79 PMID:18542082

Sharf, B. (1990). Physician-patient communication as interpersonal rethoric: A narrative approach. *Health Communication*, *2*(4), 217–231. doi:10.120715327027hc0204_2

Sharf, B., & Vanderford, M. (2003). Illness narratives and the social construction of health. In T. Thompson, A. Dorsey, K. Miller, & R. Parrott (Eds.), *Handbook of health communication* (pp. 9–34). Lawrence Erlbaum Associates.

Sociedade Portuguesa de Cardiologia. (2019). *As doenças cardiovasculares são a primeira causa de morte em Portugal*. Retrieved from https://spc.pt/web/guest/campanha-coracao-capaz

Stewart-Brown, S., Evans, J., Patterson, J., Petersen, S., Doll, H., Balding, J., & Regis, D. (2000). The health of students in institutes of higher education: An important and neglected public health problem? *Journal of Public Health Medicine*, *22*(4), 492–499. doi:10.1093/pubmed/22.4.492 PMID:11192277

Stow, N. (2019). AD ENOUGH Heart Foundation slammed for ads suggesting people who don't look after their heart don't care about their families. *The Sun*. Retrieved from https://www.thesun.co.uk/news/9173374/heart-foundation-slammed-ad/

Te, V., Ford, P., & Schubert, L. (2019). Exploring social media campaigns against sugar-sweetened beverage consumption: A systematic search. *Cogent Medicine*, *6*(6), 1. doi:10.1080/2331205X.2019.1607432

Ting, S. (2018). Ethos, logos and pathos in university students' informal requests. *Journal of Language Studies*, *18*(1), 234–251.

Wakefield, M. A., Loken, B., & Hornik, R. C. (2010). Use of mass media campaigns to change health behavior. *Lancet*, *376*(9748), 1261–1271. doi:10.1016/S0140-6736(10)60809-4 PMID:20933263

Wedro, B. (2017). Heart disease (Cardiovascular disease, CVD). *MedicineNet*. Retrieved from https://www.medicinenet.com/heart_disease_coronary_artery_disease/article.htm#how_many_people_have_heart_cardiovascular_disease_and_what_is_the_prognosis

WHO. (2017). *Cardiovascular diseases (CVDs)*. Retrieved from https://www.who.int/en/news-room/fact-sheets/detail/cardiovascular-diseases-(cvds)

WHO. (2018). *The top 10 causes of death*. Retrieved from https://www.who.int/news-room/fact-sheets/detail/the-top-10-causes-of-death

Chapter 8
Healthy Together:
Analysis of WHO Guidelines and CDC Guidelines in Developing Countries (The Case of COVID-19)

Cristina Vaz de Almeida
ISCSP, University of Lisbon, Portugal

ABSTRACT

Clinical practice guidelines are procedures, ideas, integrating records, multiple interventions, and decisions that are systematically developed to support professional and patient decisions about healthcare appropriate to specific clinical circumstances. The sudden pandemic that occurred in December 2019 that devastated the world forced reflection and globalized intervention. It was necessary, in a short time, to elaborate and disseminate a set of key rules in order to be able to control the coronavirus pandemic, global information, the protection and safety of people, and the treatment of patients and multiple and complex issues brought up in a communication crisis. In this chapter the author evaluates some of the moments of this global communication led by the World Health Organization and supported by the Centers for Disease Control and Prevention and other entities.

INTRODUCTION

"Guidelines advise people on how something could be done or what course of action can be taken in a particular circumstance (National Health and Medical

DOI: 10.4018/978-1-7998-4396-2.ch008

Research Council Act, *1992)*. The guidelines provide precise instructions on how to provide health care services (Woolf, Grol, Hutchinson, Eccles & Grimshaw 1999, p. 527) and have the potential to improve the care process, especially the results for the patient, although their beneficial effects are related to the success of implementation, being essential the use of a rigorous and transparent process to identify, evaluate, adopt and adapt the guidelines (Graham et al., 2002, p. 608).

According to Graham et at. (2002), "well-developed guidelines have the potential to improve the quality and process of care by our health care professionals and to improve patient health outcomes" (p. 607).

In 2002, WHO announced the importance of a set of approaches (World Health Report, 2002) carried out at the national level that must be implemented to reduce specific risks in health. These approaches included the dissemination of information to the public, especially through the media as it is useful on a large scale of intention to change behaviors (World Health Report, 2002).

A process for implementing the guidelines generally involves a set of entities, the identification of the roles and responsibilities of each, the creation of partnerships, and the implementation at national and local levels, as shown in Figure 1.

Figure 1. Implementation process for health action
Source: (WHO, 2019, p. 188)

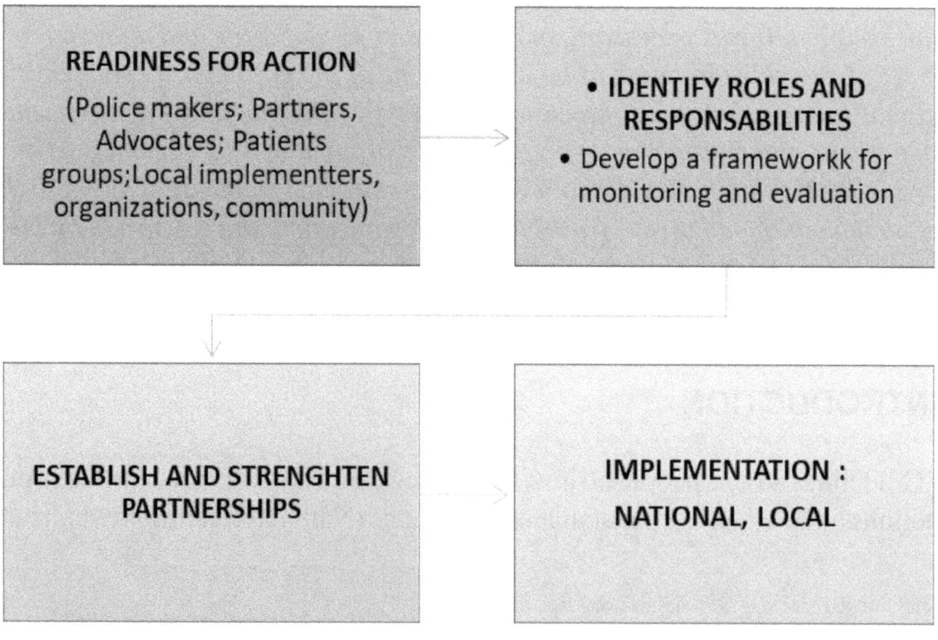

Situations and their contexts are more easily managed if the health professional or other actors (educators and students in learning) are equipped with these previous guidelines.

The World Health Organization has issued, over the years, guidelines that are easy to understand and memorize, with guidelines for individual and public health, just as the CDC provides and makes available to interested parties a collaborative platform of free access with a set of interventions, processes, materials, guidelines with evidence of results (or the lack of them) that currently allow your immediate digital access to know which interventions, campaigns, and most effective solutions exist, through comparative studies carried out by various specialists.

As an example, we present the scheme for implementing guidelines with one of the cases, associated with the dietary guidelines (Figure 2).

Figure 2. Process to implement guidelines: The case of Dietary Guidelines 2015-2020 (WHO)
Source: Own elaboration based on WHO, 2015

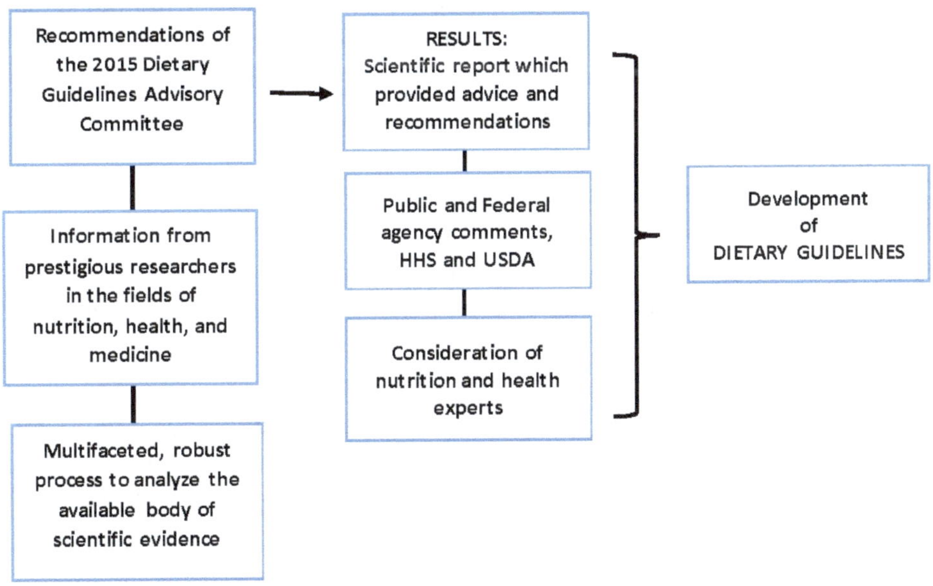

METHOD: QUALITATIVE CONTENT ANALYSIS

For content analysis Ryan and Bernard (2003), propose the following reflection for qualitative analysis (Ryan & Bernard, 2003) (Table 1).

Table 1. Numbering categories to identify themes in qualitative data

1. Repetition of words (quantitative)
2. Indigenous categories or specialized words
3. Words and their context (phrases)
4. Compare and contrast (what is the same and what is different)
5. Social issues (cultural themes)
6. Find the missing information (what is missing from the text?)
7. Metaphors and analogies
8. Transitions, abrupt changes in themes (written / oral)
9. Connectors - words that make connections: why, since, if...
10. Unmarked texts (not associated with the topic discussed) (Humor)

Source: (Author, based on Ryan e Bernard, 2003)

It is an accepted technique in textual research, in which researchers establish a set of categories, and then count the number of expressions that fall within that category, existing as a crucial requirement, that these categories are sufficiently precise to allow coders to arrive the same results when they have the same type of materials (eg newspapers) (Silverman, 2011, p. 64).

According to some authors (eg MacQueen, McLellan, Kay & Milstein, 1998), a good coder guide should include a detailed description of each code, as well as the inclusion and exclusion criteria, and extracts from the actual text for each theme. The development and improvement of coding have been central tasks in ACQ (Berelson, 1952, pp. 147-168; Holsti, 1969, pp. 95-126) and contribute to the construction of concepts (Deese, 1969; Stone et al., 1966, pp. 134-168).

The use of content analysis, in a qualitative approach, aims to understand the objectives of certain messages and contents in their communicative process, allowing through the creation of specific categories, to make inferences, on the one hand, about those who created the texts and messages, that is, its "producers", as well as on the effects felt by its users.

The way in which qualitative research is expressed is through words. These are the words that, extracted from their contents and categorized, are used to understand the contents such as ideas, thoughts, experiences. The repetition of the same words allows a uniformity of terms that can be used in several languages, even though they are written in several and different languages. The aim is to use a common language.

Summarizing the main steps of WHO to design a campaign, we start to exemplify in the following Table 2.

Table 2. Steps Proposed by WHO In "World Days"

1. Recognition of the problem and its background
2. Assessment of causes
3. Consequences for those involved
4. Campaign goals
5. Target population
6. Solutions proposal
7. Commitments

Source: (The authors, based on the WHO campaigns)

THE GUIDE CAMPAIGNS

For WHO, effective communication needs to be proactively integrated and coordinated. WHO (1998) considers communication as a key strategy in the process of disseminating or disseminating health information. Communication is a necessary component of any effort to achieve positive health outcomes (WHO, 2017, p. 10).

Communication is part of the competences of several national (ex. DGS, 2019) and international health organizations, be it accreditation, regulatory guidance, strategic and operational (WHO, 1998). For example, IOM (2004) highlights communication skills as one of its six key domains in its 2004 report, "Improving Medical Education: Enhancing the Behavioral and Social Science Content of Medical School Curricula".

WHO should help countries to understand the importance of health literacy in changing behaviors through comparative data (survey results), or sharing country best policies and practices, as well as advising within a specific national context (Kickbush, 2019). Kickbush (2019) explains that "we don't expect people to make complex calculations of the examples of nutrients in a cereal box, which is why we need to introduce color guidance systems to help them make a healthier decision" (2019, p. 140).

Mikkelsen and Stender (WHO, 2019, p. 136) reflect that the WHO campaigns on these topics can highlight some aspects of greater detail, as happened in the set of rules on the 5 steps of building skills in risk communication (WHO, 2019, p. 134).

Zarfl, Minister of Labor and Social Affairs, Health and Consumer Protection, Austria (WHO, 2019, p. 146) highlights the importance of national policies and guidelines working to improve the quality of health professionals' communication skills in healthcare, which it is considered a critical part of the patient's ability to understand the information provided to him (WHO, 2019, p. 147).

The objectives of this strategic communication are aimed at the effective transmission of information, advice and guidance for a wide range of health issues associated with chronic diseases and emerging and new risks. These WHO guidelines cover specific topics, functions and channels designed to structure strategic communication in 6 regions.

In terms of the variety of topics, we can see that WHO highlights the following themes as essential: Virus (Coronavirus, Adolescent, Health Alert & Response Operations, Bioethics, Antimicrobial Resistance, Cancer, Cholera, Dengue, Diabetes, Essential Medicines, HIV & Stis, Handwashing, Immunization (WHO, 2019). The means used to disseminate these purposes are: Public relation • Health information • Advocacy • Behavior change • Risk communication (emergency / non-emergency). And the channels used most regularly are those that use written, oral, digital media, namely: • Web • Media • Social Media • Print media • Community involvement • Dissemination, and others (Figure 3).

The sequence of information starts from the organization's central services, from its corporate communication, and cascades down to the regional offices in the various countries, to the level of entities that are responsible in each country for this communication and the dissemination of campaigns and other information.

Figure 3. WHO's high Topics
Source: (The author, based on WHO strategic communications framework (2017, WHO global health communication)

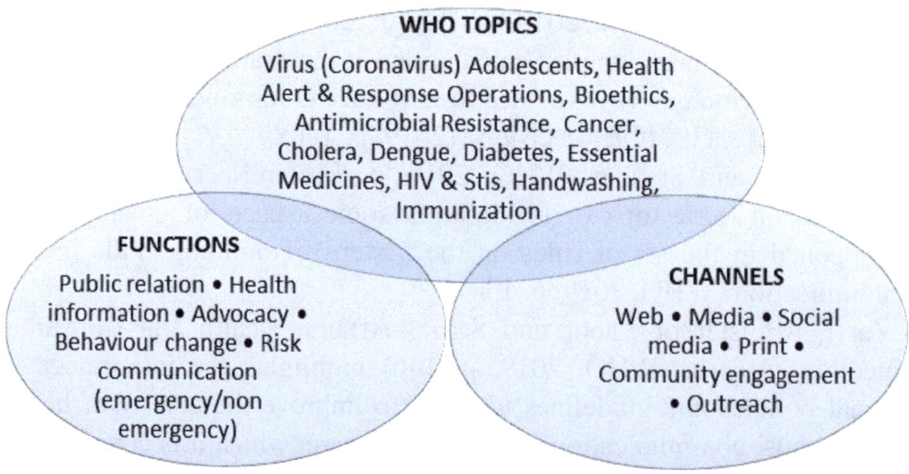

WHO assignments are (2017): 1) Providing information, 2) Advice and 3) Guidance for decision-makers (key audiences) to develop actions that protect the health of individuals, families, communities, and nations (Figure 4).

Figure 4. WHO Strategic Communication
Source: (WHO Strategic Communications Framework, 2017)

Health protection	Providing:	To:
• Individuals • families • Communities • Nations	• Information • Advice • Guidance	• Decicions makers

In the field of public health communication, WHO has over the years developed "global public health days", in which the organization considers that they are an opportunity to "increase awareness and understanding of critical health issues, and mobilize support for action at various levels, whether at the level of families, communities and legislators (WHO, 2019, p. 7).

Figure 5. Framework supports the broad range of communication activities occurring across all parts and levels of WHO
Source: (WHO, 2019)

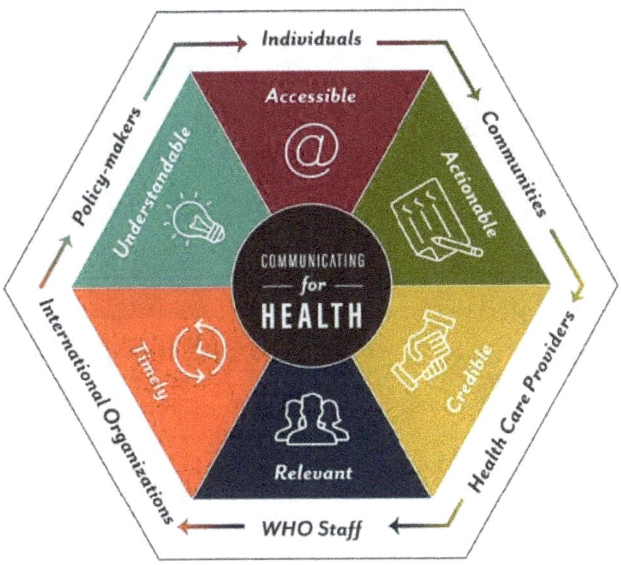

With the basic ecological model, based on the multiple inter-influences of the system (Mcleroy, 1998), WHO understands that mass campaigns aimed at thinking globally and acting locally are important, starting from the interpersonal relationships that interact throughout the cycle of multiple influences (Figure 5).

THE "WORLD DAYS"

Based on morbidity criteria and global trends in health and disease, WHO member states defined the following 7 days and 1 week as global health guidelines (WHO, 2019):

World TB Day, 24 March; World Health Day, 7 April; World Malaria Day, 25 April; World No Tobacco Day, 31 May; World Blood Donor Day, 14 June; World Hepatitis Day, 28 July; World AIDS Day, 1 December and, World Immunization Week, last week of April.

Figure 6. World Days.
Source: ("World Days" https://www.who.int/news-room/campaigns)

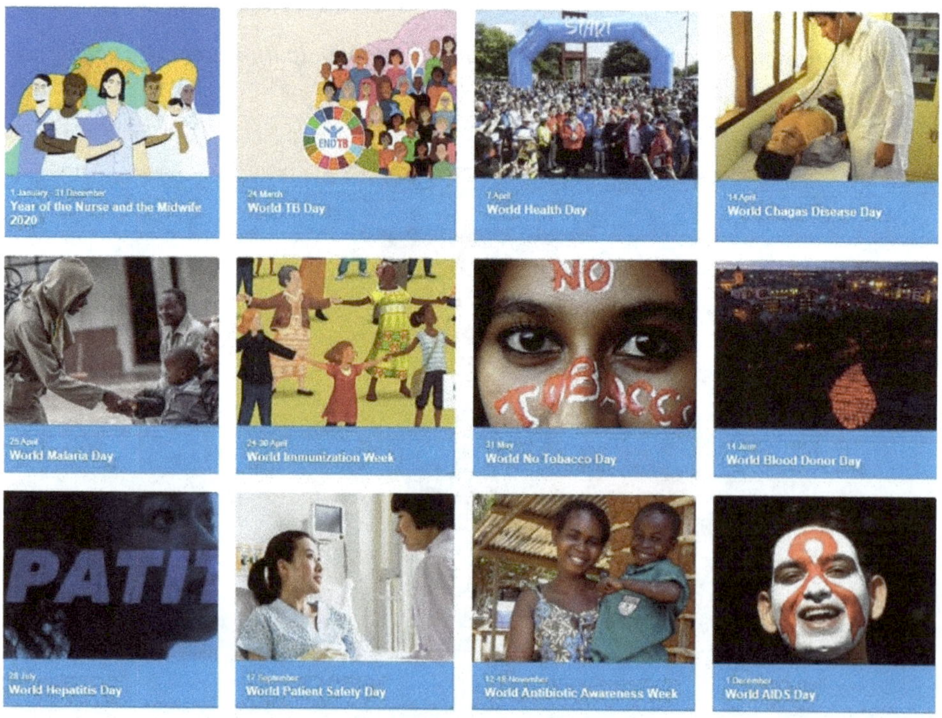
1 January - 31 December
Year of the Nurse and the Midwife 2020
END TB
24 March
World TB Day
7 April
World Health Day
14 April
World Chagas Disease Day
25 April
World Malaria Day
24-30 April
World Immunization Week
NO
TOBACCO
31 May
World No Tobacco Day
14 June
World Blood Donor Day
PATIT
28 July
World Hepatitis Day
17 September
World Patient Safety Day
12-18 November
World Antibiotic Awareness Week
1 December
World AIDS Day

The media and alert campaigns issued by WHO are associated with a strong awareness of issues associated with the health and well-being of citizens worldwide. The so-called "World Days" and involve stakeholders in the health system (Oranizations, entities, health professionals, communities, individuals), who recognize the problem, its cause and the need for a potential solution. (Figure 6).

The "World Days" campaigns urge organizations to disseminate information in an expansive way so that health organizations and other stakeholders participate at the level of countries, regions and locally to act on the issue that is discussed on this "world day". The objective is always to provoke memorization, awareness and intervention on the issue over time and, finally, a change in behavior (Table 3).

Table 3. Steps Proposed by WHO in These Campaigns "World Days"

• Recognition of the problem and its background • Assessment of causes • Consequences for those involved • Campaign goals • Target population • Solutions proposal • Commitments

Source: (The authors, based on the WHO campaigns)

Example: The World Patient Safety Day (WPSD)

The World Patient Safety Day (WPSD), it's a campaign for stakeholders in the health care system to work together to improve patient safety. There is recognition of a problem: the scale of avoidable harm linked with medical errors. It is a global commitment made by all WHO member states to recognize patient safety as an essential health priority and agree to take measures to reduce harm to patients in healthcare settings.

It involves involving global health actors in:

- Extend concerted global action on patient safety
- Implement measures to reduce preventable damage to the patient
- Share and raise awareness about patient safety in the various care environments
- Increase public and media awareness of key issues related to patient safety

Table 4. Principles, meanings and examples of communication campaigns in WHO

Principles	Meaning	Examples
ACCESSIBLE	**WHO's audiences rely on their ability to access the information they need** to protect and improve their health. Communicators should identify all channels that are available and map their comparative capacities to reach priority audiences. Using the right mix of channels helps empower audiences with the information they need to make informed decisions.	**Questions that can be asked:** Which publics are covered? What sociodemographic characteristics? Access to information? What channels? What organizations? Why it's important this information a this moment?
ACTIONABLE	WHO's work is designed to support the adoption of healthy behaviours and the implementation of policies to protect health. Communications is a necessary component of WHO's comprehensive organizational efforts to achieve these goals. **To be successful, communicators must understand target audience knowledge, attitudes and behaviours** in order to create messages that address barriers and encourage decision-makers to take the recommended steps.	Communication adapted to the segments of population. For example, information specifies for health professionals differentiated from information for the rest of the population (COVID - 19)
CREDIBLE AND TRUSTED	WHO's reputation is a key factor for whether individuals will act on the Organization's advice and guidance. The more decision-makers trust WHO, the more likely they will believe, and act on, the information communicated by the Organization. WHO communicators must use every opportunity to reinforce WHO's trustworthiness so that WHO's recommendations become the basis for health decisions	Veronika Skvortsova, Minister of Health of the Russian Federation considering the availability of quality, reliable information in the media and on the internet (WHO, 2019, p. 158) says that in 2018 Russia launched the campaign "You Are Stronger" to promote a healthy lifestyle among the Russian population. *"The campaign was held throughout the Russian Federation. All the main channels of communication were used: federal television, radio, billboards and the internet. The campaign focused on four target areas for improving public health: reducing alcohol consumption; reducing tobacco consumption; responsible nutrition; and responsible reproductive health. The campaign has continued into 2019 and will be extended to 2024 as part of the Federal Project entitled "Strengthening Public Health". (Who, 2019, p. 158)*
RELEVANT	To be relevant, communications **must help decision-makers understand that there is a health risk for themselves** or for those they care about, that the risk could be severe and that they reduce that risk by undertaking recommended actions.	The risk for population and countries (Covid-19) for organizations, Hospitals. • Coronavirus • Hand washing and infections. • Legionella
TIMELY	Across all health issues, WHO must make information, advice, and guidance **available in a timely way,** so audiences have the information they need when they need it in order to make appropriate health decisions.	Communication at the right time? As in the COVID-19 outbreak, communication was daily made by the WHO Director-General and in the countries, sanitary health leaders, and executive government made several communications daily to inform the population (morning, afternoon, and night).
UNDER-STANDABLE	WHO communicates with a wide variety of decision-makers Some have backgrounds in medicine and public health and rely on WHO for technical information. However, many key audiences are not technical experts. They need information that is easy to understand in order to understand health risks and take appropriate actions.	Panorama, 2019, 146-148 Brigitte Zarfl, Minister of Labour, Social Affairs, Health and Consumer Protection, Austria National Guidelines to improve communication and the support to patients to understand health information *"Working to improve the quality of health care communication, including the communication skills of health professionals, which is a critical part of the patient's ability to understand the information they are being provided*" (WHO, Panorama, 2019, p. 147) *"Health care organizations must both train and equip health providers with high quality professional communication and information products in order for them to effectively respond to the needs of patients*", Who -Panorama, 2019, p. 147)

Source: (WHO principles for effective communications https://www.who.int/communicating-for-health/principles/en/)

- Help patients contribute to their own safety

The principles for effective communication are: accessibility, activation, credibility, relevance, the time they are carried out and their understanding. The summary is shown in Table 4.

THE CASE: CORONAVIRUS, A PANDEMIC THAT ALIGNED THE WORLD

In 2002, the General Director of WHO, Brundtland said: "these are dangerous times for the well-being of the world" (World Report, 2002, p. 2). In 2014, Quinn and Kumar (2014) explain that in "today's global society, infectious disease outbreaks can spread quickly across the world, fueled by the rapidity with which we travel across borders and continents" (p. 263). 18 years later, the coronavirus pandemic took people, communities, leaders, organizations, and countries by surprise.

WHO's mission to watch over public health issues worldwide recommends an intervention and a careful and global look at the following processes and events: (1) climate change with effects on citizens' health; 2) uncontrolled epidemics of chronic diseases; 3) increasing resistance of pathogenic microbiological agents to antimicrobials; and 4) the progression of marked inequalities, inequities, and imbalances between communities.

However, his eyes focused on the province of Hubei in December 2019 when what appeared to be a flu contained within a country, quickly became a pandemic with serious worldwide repercussions for both health and the economies of countries.

The spread of influenza through the coronavirus (Covid-19) worldwide, considered a pandemic on March 13, 2020, raises deep issues of an effective cooperation between organizations worldwide supported trough an effective and dayly health communication

The Covid -19 outbreak highlighted the importance of *just in time* communication between national organizations and WHO, as well as cooperation in risk communication between countries.

This virus has infected millions of people worldwide, and originated in China, in the city of Whuwan in December 2019.

The most heard words, repeated by WHO, by national leaders, by organizations, by international media were: COVID - 19, virus, pandemic, solidarity, “heroic” health professionals.

In these words, there was a deep and cascading consultation - WHO - Countries - Health organizations - Media - Communities & other organizations - Individuals.

The number of people infected by the coronavirus worldwide was 197.665.605 millions out of 169 countries. The number of deaths was 4.214.090 million, and people recovered from the disease 178,543,558 (Johns Hopkins website, 31 july, 2021). The number of vaccine doses administered was 4.076.687.867 (31 july, 2021).

In the case of a pandemic (from 100 thousand cases and in more than one country) and therefore with a worldwide scale, WHO made available to the population, through its website and in the daily situation report, a map with the locations where Coronavirus has spread (countries with red spots).

In “crisis” communication, it is important to use credible sources to guarantee the reliability of the information and to control the alarmisms caused by the event.

Among the most credible sources related to the Coronavirus outbreak is John Hopkins University, which daily works on worldwide data on the evolution of the virus.

Figure 7. John Hopkins University data about Coronavirus
Source: (John Hopkins website https://coronavirus.jhu.edu/map.html)

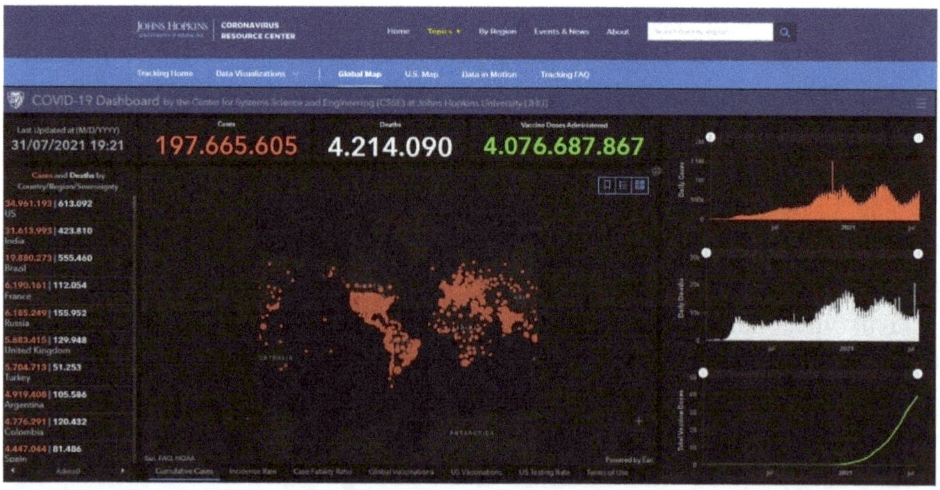

The university itself refers to its direct sources, which are as follows: Data sources: WHO, CDC, ECDC, NHC, DXY, 1point3acres, Worldometers.info, BNO, state and national government health departments, and local media reports. Read more in this blog.

Figure 7 shows the data related to 24 March 2020.

For this worldwide fight against a pandemic, the message conveyed by both WHO and organizations was associated with bringing people together to fight the virus. An idea of "Healthy together" was underlying even though it promoted several partnerships, such as the partnership between WHO and FIFA (World Football Federation) that came together to promote the 5-step campaign. This campaign was led by 28 football players, who gave their voice and testimony in what are considered to be the 5 fundamental virus control steps:

The *"Pass the message to kick out coronavirus"* campaign promotes five key steps for people to follow to protect their health in line with WHO guidance, focused on hand washing, coughing etiquette, not touching your face, physical distance and staying home if feeling unwell . (WHO, website, 23 March 2020)

WHO home page (https://www.who.int/news-room/detail/23-03-2020-pass-the-message-five-steps-to-kicking-out-coronavirus)

WHO, FIFA launch joint campaign to equip football community to tackle COVID-19

23 march 2020

News release

Geneva, 23 March 2020: FIFA, the international governing body of football, and the World Health Organization (WHO) have teamed up to combat the coronavirus (COVID-19) by launching a new awareness campaign led by world-renowned footballers, who are calling on all people around the world to follow five key steps to stop the spread of the disease.

Home Page CDC

Looking at the CDC website (March 2020) the homepage presents the coronavirus image (landscape) with a short text "Coronavirus Disease 2019 CDC is responding to the novel coronavirus outbreak. By clicking on the blue button that says: Learn more about COVID - 19 we enter a 2nd page with small texts and images: "How to protect yourself" and "If you think you are sick" (Figure 8).

Figure 8. Home page of CDC
Source: (Home page – website of CDC, on 20-03-2020)

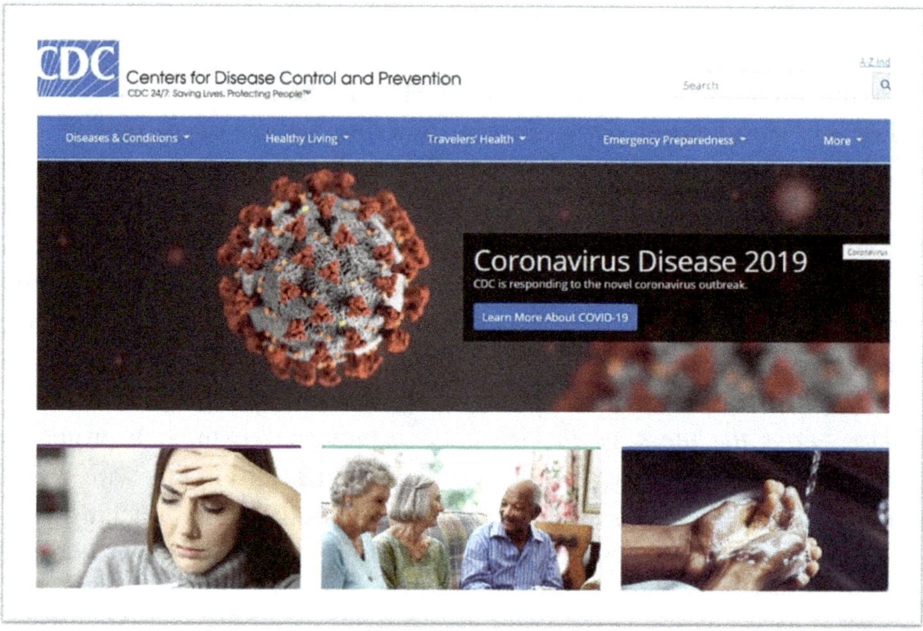

Figure 9. Second link en Coronavirus CDC home page
Source: (Second link, in homepage CDC, about Coronavirus, 20-03-2020).

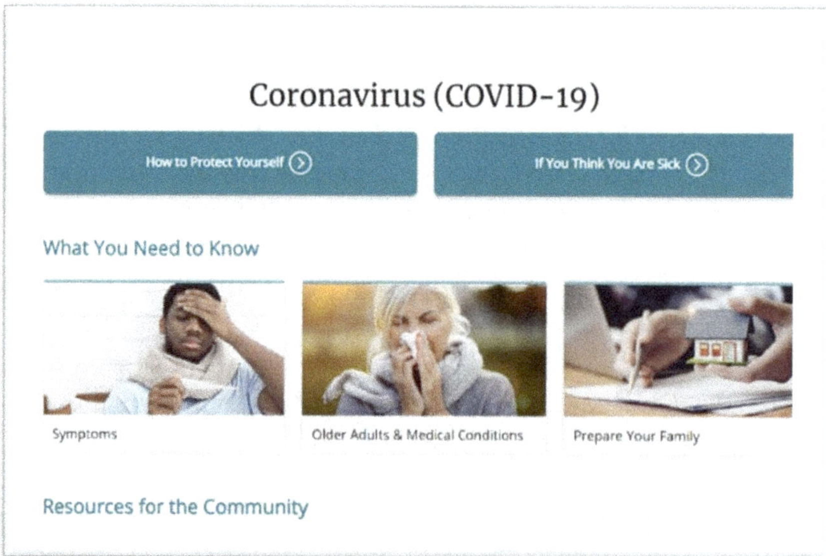

The following guidelines within the CDC webpage and the "Coronavirus" theme are related to: 1) symptoms; 2) older people (elderly) and with chronic conditions (high-risk groups); 3) the family organization. Below are the "community resources (Figure 9).

The rate of progression of the virus led the World Health Organization to declare the "pandemic" on March 13, 2020 and the "state of emergency" in many countries (China, Macau, Singapore, Italy, Portugal, etc.).

The communication process for this disease, which went global in less than a month, required crisis communication measures (Figure 10).

Figure 10. Moment of WHO Director-General speeches
Source: (WHO- website, 2020)

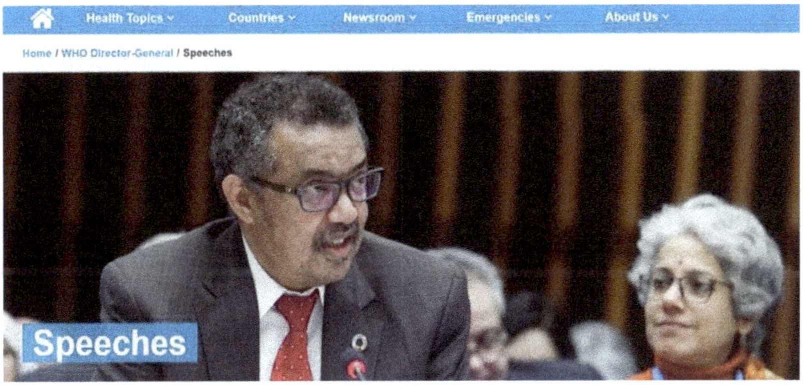

Progression of Information to The Media in The Context of Crisis Communication

On March 2, 2020, the WHO General Diretor's announced the need to monitor the situation and analyze the data:

We appreciate that people are debating whether this is a pandemic or not. We are monitoring the situation every moment of every day, and analyzing the data.

I have said it before and I'll say it again: WHO will not hesitate to describe this as a pandemic if that's what the evidence suggests.

But we need to see this in perspective. Of the 88,913 cases reported globally so far, 90% are in China, mostly in one province.

On March 4, 2020, the WHO General Diretor, in a transversal perspective of the role of this organization, underlines the fight against EBOLA:

Before I get to COVID-19, a few words about Ebola, the other war-front.

We have now had more than two weeks without a case of Ebola, and this is the longest period since the outbreak started, and there are currently no patients receiving treatment.

About COVID - 19 reports that the level of risk assessment of COVID -19 has increased:

But as you know, even as the Ebola outbreak is winding down, the epidemic of COVID-19 is becoming increasingly complex.

There is now a total of 92,943 reported cases of COVID-19 globally, and 3,160 deaths.

As you know, WHO has raised its assessment of the risk of spread and the risk of impact of COVID-19 to very high at the global level.

Regarding the (online) training of people and dissemination media, the WHO DG underlines:

More than 130,000 people have been trained in various aspects of the COVID-19 response through online courses on our OpenWHO.org platform, which are available in 6 UN languages and Portuguese.

At this point and the result of research, a little more is known about the new virus

This virus is not SARS, it is not MERS and it is not influenza. The nature of this virus means we have an opportunity to break the chains of transmission and contain its spread.

On March 5, the WHO General Diretor reports its concern about false information regarding the Corona virus:

The fight against rumours and misinformation is a vital part of the battle against this virus. We rely on you to make sure people have accurate information about the threat they face, and how to protect themselves and others.

On March 11, the WHO General Diretor highlights the concern about the danger of "inaction" and the care with which the term "pandemic" should be used:

WHO has been assessing this outbreak around the clock and **we are deeply concerned both by the alarming levels of spread and severity, and by the alarming levels of inaction.**

We have therefore made the assessment that COVID-19 can be characterized as a pandemic.

Pandemic is not a word to use lightly or carelessly. It is a word that, if misused, can cause unreasonable fear, or unjustified acceptance that the fight is over, leading to unnecessary suffering and death.

Describing the situation as a pandemic does not change WHO's assessment of the threat posed by this virus. It doesn't change what WHO is doing, and it doesn't change what countries should do.

The WHO General Diretor's announcement of the pandemic on 12 March 2020:

As you know, yesterday I said that that the global COVID-19 outbreak **can now be described as a pandemic.**

We have made this assessment for two main reasons: **first,** *because of the speed and* **scale of transmission.**

Almost 125,000 cases have now been reported to WHO, from 118 countries and territories. In the past two weeks, the number of cases reported outside China has increased almost 13-fold, and the number of affected countries has almost tripled.

The second reason *is that despite our frequent warnings, we are deeply concerned that* **some countries are not approaching this threat** *with the level of political commitment needed to control it.*

The Day After - March 13, 2020 - GD of WHO speech the next day

Babies are still being born. Essential surgery is continuing. People still need emergency care after road traffic crashes. People still need treatment for cancer, diabetes, HIV, malaria and many other diseases.

And for all of these, we need health workers.

Today I want to send a personal and sincere thank you to every health worker.

You do a heroic job.

We're encouraged that many countries are now acting on the 8 pillars of WHO's Strategic Preparedness and Response Plan.

Most countries now have a national plan; most are taking a multi-sectoral approach and most have laboratory testing capacity.

Together with the United Nations Foundation and the Swiss Philanthropy Foundation, WHO is today launching the COVID-19 Solidarity Response Fund, to enable individuals and organizations to contribute.

The international guidelines for Coronavirus (WHO, 2020) served as critical guidance for countries, which in turn transposed the rules and guidelines internally.

In Portugal, the General Directorate of Health (DGS) activated the crisis plan, managing information according to WHO guidelines (in cascade), and was daily with the population through the media (television, radio, social media).

The encouragement and motivation of health professionals (involvement and motivation, as mentioned by Kim & Grunig, 2011) was also transversal to health and social and global organizations and entities, reaching even the citizen.

According World health Report (2002), "communication has come to mean much more than the mere passing on of information, as in the older style health education messages. It should also include the promotion of public dialogue between different stakeholders, resolution of conflicts, and agreement on the need for interventions to prevent the risks (p. 39).

Between the 12th and the 13th of March there are differences in the speech of the WHO Director-General. For example. On the day of the announcement of the pandemic, March 12, the top WHO official warned that "we are deeply concerned that some countries are not approaching this threat with the level of political commitment needed to control it". The next day he says "Most countries now have a national plan; most are taking a multi-sectoral approach and most have laboratory testing capacity".

If on the 12th he focuses on the pandemic only on the pandemic issue "outbreak can now be described as a pandemic", the next day he makes reference to the remaining problems in the world, "Babies are still being born. Essential surgery is continuing. People still need emergency care after road traffic crashes "and personally thanks the health professionals calling them heroes": "personal and sincere thank you to every health worker around the world" and highlights nursing "especially nurses and midwives, who we are celebrating this year through the International Year of the Nurse and the Midwife".

Here we see the need to strengthen health professionals and understand the countries, which are making efforts and consider that they already have a national plan (see Appendix for full text of the Director-General's March 12 and March 13 speeches).

Qualitative analysis of speech based on the first speech (13 March 2020) and the speech after pandemic determination of disease (Table 5).

Table 5. Qualitative analysis WHO director general Tedros Adhanom Ghebreyesus speech (12 and 13 March 2020

	"P" DAY When Coronavirus Pandemic is announced. WHO director general Tedros Adhanom Ghebreyesus speech 12 March 2020	**THE DAY AFTER** WHO director general Tedros Adhanom Ghebreyesus speech 13 March 2020
1. Facts/ numbers	*Almost 125,000 cases have now been reported to WHO, from 118 countries and territories. In the past two weeks.* *There are still 77 countries and territories with no reported cases, and 55 countries and territories that have reported 10 cases or less.*	*More than 132,000 cases of COVID-19 have now been reported to WHO, from 123 countries and territories.* *5,000 people have lost their lives, a tragic milestone*
2 Indigenous categories or specialized words	**COVID-19** *This is a controllable pandemic.* *Outbreak* *shift from containment to mitigation* *quarantining their closest contacts* *R&D roadmap* *WHO's Strategic Preparedness and Response Plan* *COVID training courses on OpenWHO.*	**COVID-19** *We have shipped supplies of personal protective* *We've sent almost 1.5 million diagnostic tests to 120 countries.*
3 Words and their context (phrases)	**A GLOBAL CHALLENGE FOR COUNTRIES** *All countries must strike a fine balance between protecting health, preventing economic and social disruption, and respecting human rights.*	**WORDS OF GREAT STIMULATION TO HEALTHCARE PROFESSIONALS WHO GUARANTEE THE SUPPORT, CONTROL AND TREATMENT OF THE DISEASE:** *Today I want to send a personal and sincere thank you to every health worker* *You do a heroic job.* *We know that this crisis is putting a huge burden on you and your families. We know you are stretched to the limit.*
4 Compare and contrast (what is the same and what is different)	**THIS DAY INFORMS THAT COUNTRIES ARE NOT COMMITTED** ***The second reason is** that despite our frequent warnings, we are deeply concerned that some countries are not approaching this threat with the level of political commitment needed to control it.*	**THE NEXT DAY INFORMS THAT COUNTRIES "ARE COMMITTED" AND HAVE PLANS.** *Many countries are now acting on the 8 pillars of WHO's Strategic Preparedness and Response Plan.* ***Most countries now have a national plan; most are taking a multi-sectoral approach** and most have laboratory testing capacity.*
5 Social issues (cultural themes)	**IDEA: THE SPIRIT OF COOPERATION BETWEEN COUNTRIES AND BETWEEN HELP** *In the spirit of solidarity.* *As I keep saying, we're all in this together.*	**OPPORTUNITY TO ANNOUNCE THE THE INTERNATIONAL YEAR OF THE NURSE AND THE MIDWIFE.** *Today I want to send a personal and sincere thank you to every health worker around the world – especially nurses and midwives, who we are celebrating this year through the International Year of the Nurse and the Midwife.* *We're all in this together.*

continued on following page

Table 5. Continued

6 Find the missing information (what is missing from the text?)	**WHO ASSUMES ITS LACK OF KNOWLEDGE OF CORONAVIRUS MATTER:** *This is a new virus and a new situation. We're all learning and we must all find new ways to prevent infections, save lives, and minimize impact* **WHO UNDERLINES THE PROBLEMS (UNIDENTIFIED) THAT COUNTRIES MAY HAVE IF THEY DO NOT CONTROL THE VIRUS** *Countries that decide to give up on fundamental public health measures may end up with a larger problem.*	**WHO GOES BACK TO THEIR LACK OF KNOWLEDGE OF THE CORONAVIRUS MATTER:** *We have never before seen a pandemic sparked by a coronavirus. This is the first pandemic caused by a coronavirus.* *And we have never before seen a pandemic that can be controlled, at the same time.*
7 Metaphors and analogies	**IDEA: LESSONS AS EXPERIENCES** *WHO is working day and night to support all countries.* *All countries have lessons to share*	**IDEA: YOU MUST CONTROL AND ELIMINATE THE VIRUS** *Do not just let this fire burn.* *Every dollar donated is a dollar towards saving lives.*
9 Connectors - words that make connections: why, since, if...	*The second reason is that* ***despite*** *our frequent warnings, we are deeply concerned* ***Because*** *this is a dynamic situation*	***And finally****, you can give (money)* ***Now*** *everyone can contribute.*
10 Unmarked texts (not associated with the topic discussed)	**none**	**IDEA: LIFE GOES ON DESPITE THE VIRUS** *Babies are still being born. Essential surgery is continuing.* . People still need emergency care after road traffic crashes. People still need treatment for cancer, diabetes, HIV, malaria and many other diseases.

Source: (Qualitative content analysis ofgeneral director of WHO, based on Ryan & Bernard, 2003)

CRISIS COMMUNICATION

Based on the WHO guidelines (WHO website, 2020), European countries (and others) aligned their guidelines, transposing the guidelines at national level, as well as the ideas and the words of the WHO Director-General and Kluge, WHO Regional Director for Europe.

There was a cascade alignment of information, ideas and words (these used with great precision and similarity by the chain of actors).

Brundtland (World Health Report, 2002) highlights the importance of communicating risks clearly and openly to the public, and of creating an atmosphere of trust and shared responsibility between the government, the public at large and the media (p. 5). She said "This is essential. We know that most people will choose to adopt healthier behaviours, especially when they receive accurate information from authorities they trust, and when they are supported through sensible laws, good health promotion programmes and vigorous public debate (p. 5).

In this sense, information on the coronavirus in 2020 also followed these guidelines for clarity, openness, generating confidence in reliable information. All decision makers (WHO, CDC, country leaders, and health organizations) announced a global sense of "transparency" in the information conveyed, also assuming the lack of knowledge about the virus, as can be seen in the following WHO expressions, CDC, health entities and the top manager (case of the President of the Republic of Portugal). The reinforcement of transparency in information and the steps that are still being taken to learn about the disease are expressed in various media and announced by country leaders (Table 6).

Table 6. Content of disseminated information

WHO (General Diretor of WHO on 23 March 2020) *More than 300,000 cases of COVID-19 have now been reported to WHO, from almost every country in the world. That's heartbreaking.* *The pandemic is accelerating. It took 67 days from the first reported case to reach the first 100,000 cases, 11 days for the second 100,000 cases and just 4 days for the third 100,000 cases. You can see how the virus is accelerating.* *But we're not prisoners to statistics. We're not helpless bystanders. We can change the trajectory of this pandemic.* ***Numbers matter, because they're not just numbers****. They're people, whose lives and families have been turned upside down.* ***But what matters most is what we do.***
CDC (20 March 2020) - presents doubts about the virus. On the CDC home page: ***How COVID-19 Spreads*** *There is much to learn about the newly emerged COVID-19, including how and how easily it spreads.*
At national level (Portugal) The President of the Portuguese Republic in a communication to the country (Portugal) on March 19, 2020 stated that he would always communicate with Portuguese citizens with "Transparency" and "truth". In this speech, he again reinforced health professionals as "heroes" (also making a bridge with the speech of the WHO **director general on March 13, 2020 when he mentioned: You do a heroic job (2020).**
Media (Portugal case) In the Media, journalists (mainly through television) help spread the information of the WHO DG (on March 13, 20202): *Any country that looks "that won't happen to us" is making a deadly mistake. It can happen to any country.*

Source: (The author based on Media and WHO and CDC websites)

The positioning of constant information, presented in a calm way, with a diverse set of daily information to the population is crucial to the intention of not creating false alarmisms

The application of the problem-solving theory by Kim & Grunig, (2011), which foresees providing greater knowledge of people about the virus, lowering the constraints and barriers (for non-adherence because they consider that mortality is low due to example) and for greater involvement of both individuals and organizations.

In Portugal, the General Directorate of Health (DGS, 2020), following WHO procedures, sought to 1) increase the knowledge of the disease through massive information, using mainly the means of television and radio and the internet 2) to understand the beliefs and people's constraints and trying to control alarmism; 3) to increase people's involvement through precise indications that seek citizens' self-efficacy such as: a) hand hygiene, restraint and social withdrawal; use of health contact numbers (808 24 24 24) available to the population; hiring more doctors and health professionals (those who were already reinforced); increase the population's involvement in the matter.

QUALITATIVE CONTENT ANALYSIS

The following categories were chosen as categories under analysis by WHO as priority (WHO, 2020) and which are the following: Coronavirus - COVID -19 (due to its emergence in 2020 as a pandemic), Handwashing and Healthy life styles (WHO, 2019) (Table 7).

Table 7. Comparison of the contents of the WHO and CDC campaigns.

CORONAVIRUS – COVID – 19 (march 2020)	
WHO	CDC
CORPUS – WHO - CAMPAIGNS REPORTS AND ARTICLES	CORPUS - CAMPAIGNS REPORTS AND ARTICLES
Coronavirus disease (COVID-19) outbreak: Rights, roles, and responsibilities of health workers, including key considerations for occupational safety and health. Numbers matter, because they're not just numbers. They're people, whose lives and families have been turned upside down. But what matters most is what we do.	*CDC works 24/7 protecting America's health, safety, and security. Whether disease start at home or abroad, are curable or preventable, chronic, or acute, or from human activity or deliberate attack, CDC responds to America's most pressing health threats. CDC is headquartered in Atlanta and has experts located throughout the United States and the world.*
Recognition of the problem and its background	**Recognition of the problem and its background**
Coronaviruses are a group of viruses belonging to the family of Coronaviridae, which infect both animals and humans. A new coronavirus that previously has not been identified in humans emerged in Wuhan, China in December 2019. This is a new virus and a new situation. We're all learning, and we must all find new ways to prevent infections	There is currently no vaccine to prevent coronavirus disease 2019 (COVID-19). The best way to prevent illness is to avoid being exposed to this virus. The virus **is thought** to spread mainly from person-to-person. Between people who are in close contact with one another (within about 6 feet). Through respiratory droplets produced when an infected person coughs or sneezes. These droplets can land in the mouths or noses of people who are nearby or possibly be inhaled into the lungs.
Consequences for those involved	**Consequences for those involved**

continued on following page

Table 7. Continued

CORONAVIRUS – COVID – 19 (march 2020)	
WHO	CDC
CORPUS – WHO - CAMPAIGNS REPORTS AND ARTICLES	CORPUS - CAMPAIGNS REPORTS AND ARTICLES
Human coronaviruses **can cause** mild disease like a common cold, while others cause more severe disease (such as MERS - Middle East Respiratory Syndrome and SARS – Severe Acute Respiratory Syndrome).	Older adults and people who have severe underlying medical conditions like heart or lung disease or diabetes **seem to** be at higher risk for developing more serious complications from COVID-19 illness. People **are thought to be most contagious** when they are most symptomatic (the sickest). Some spread **might be possible** before people show symptoms. It **may be possible** that a person can get COVID-19 by touching a surface or object
Solutions proposal	**Solutions proposal**
Health workers are at **the front line** of any outbreak response and as such are exposed to hazards that put them at risk of infection with an outbreak pathogen (in this case COVID-19).	The CDC is closely monitoring an outbreak of respiratory illness caused by a novel (new) coronavirus first identified in Wuhan, Hubei Province, China.
Campaign goals (highlights)	**Campaign goals (highlights)**
WHO has clear advice for governments, businesses and individuals First, prepare and be ready. Second, detect, protect and treat. Third, reduce transmission. And fourth, innovate and learn. And finally, you can give.	The CDC provided a set of critical information for health professionals on its webpage, such as protection strategies, guidance guides, collection of samples from people who died of viruses, infection control, end of isolation, care guide, exposure potential to the virus, guide for patients admitted to obstetrics as in the table
Commitents	**Commitents**
WHO is working closely with global experts, governments and partners to rapidly expand scientific knowledge on this new virus and to provide timely advice on measures to protect people's health and prevent the spread of this outbreak.	CDC is aggressively responding to the global outbreak of COVID-19 and preparing for the potential of community spread in the United States.
Information for health workers	**Information for health workers**
Follow established occupational safety and health procedures, avoid exposing others to health and safety risks and participate in employer-provided occupational safety and health training; Use provided protocols to assess, triage and treat patients; Treat patients with respect, compassion and dignity; • maintain patient confidentiality; Swiftly follow established public health reporting procedures of suspect and confirmed cases; Provide or reinforce accurate infection prevention and control and public health information, including to concerned people who have neither symptoms nor risk; Put on, use, take off and dispose of personal protective equipment properly; Self-monitor for signs of illness and self-isolate or report illness to managers, if it occurs; Advise management if they are experiencing signs of undue stress or mental health challenges that require support interventions; and Report to their immediate supervisor any situation which they have reasonable justification to believe presents an imminent and serious danger to life or health.	CDC's strategies for optimizing the use of eye protection, isolation gowns, facemasks, and N95 respirators. Current Interim Guidance Interim Guidance for Public Health Personnel Evaluating Persons Under Investigation (PUIs) and Asymptomatic Close Contacts of Confirmed Cases at Their Home or Non-Home Residential Settings Interim Guidance for Collection and Submission of Postmortem Specimens from Deceased Persons Under Investigation (PUI) for COVID-19, February 2020 Evaluating and Testing Persons for Coronavirus Disease 2019 (COVID-19) Healthcare Infection Control Guidance Ending Isolation for Immunocompromised Persons Clinical Care Guidance Home Care Guidance Guidance for EMS Healthcare Personnel with Potential Exposure Guidance Inpatient Obstetric Healthcare Guidance

Source: (WHO https://www.who.int/docs/default-source/coronaviruse/who-rights-roles-respon-hw-covid-19.pdf?sfvrsn=bcabd401_0*and CDC website* – https://www.cdc.gov/coronavirus/2019-ncov/hcp/index.html*)*

MAIN STEPS IN CRISIS COMMUNICATION

Emergency risk reporting requires efforts from several countries in cooperation with global (WHO and CDC) and national (Directorate general of health and others) entities.

In a case presented by Frost, Li, Moolenaar, Mao, & Xie (2019), the authors report that during the ten years between the 2003 SARS outbreak and the 2013 H7N9 outbreak China demonstrated a significant improvement in pre-event risk communication capabilities during the event in the H7N9 event responses when compared to the SARS response in 2013.

According to the authors (Frost et al,. 2019), the improvement of communication in emergency conditions improved through the following factors and interventions: 1) preparation: 2) the availability of personnel and resources dedicated to risk communication; 3) internal and clear mechanisms; 4) standardized operational procedures, with external national response; 5) adequated management of rumors; 6) communication with international agencies; 7) creation and dissemination of messages consistent with health care and the private sectors; 8) community involvement as a critical function in any outbreak scenario.

Efforts to strengthen long-term risk communication capacity, which includes collaborations, are not common according to the authors (Frost et

Table 8. Steps and key-factors in crisis communication

1 - Alignment of content issued by WHO, CDC and health organizations in each country: the information has been "cascaded" to countries and to entities and audiences
2 - Transparency of information with simple but careful words to explain what the virus is, how it spreads and how it can limit the spread
3 - Assumption of the lack of information about the virus and its spread that WHO and CDC have at this time with words such as: "Human coronaviruses can cause mild disease" (WHO), "The virus is thought to spread" (CDC), "Like heart or lung disease or diabetes seem to be at higher risk" (CDC), "Some spread might be possible before people show symptoms" (CDC), "It may be possible that a person can get COVID-19" (CDC)
4 - Constant daily communication through the mass media
5 - Focus on positive reinforcement ("the heroes") in health professionals, the first front line to fight the virus
6 - Spirit of "solidarity" from countries, organizations and appeal for financial support by organizations
7 - Involvement of credible international partners (FIFA, Google, Bill Gates, etc.)
8 - Fighting *fake news* by both WHO and national organizations
9 - Organization of daily press conferences to inform the population and prepare credible information
10 - Monitor public opinion and evaluate potential adaptations of the strategy

Source: Own elaboration based on Frost et al (2019; WHO 2021; CDC 2021.

al, 2019), because these lessons can benefit others, the above all low and medium-yielding in building their national emergency risk communication communication capacity (Frost et al, 2019).

From the sample of key texts published by WHO and the CDC in March 2020, we can see in the crisis communication made by these two organizations that lead world information (Table 8)

These factors allowed the level of perceived confidence that the public had to rise.

CONCLUSION

Planning, organizing, involving teams, boosting, and disseminating risk communication is a highly complex process when it engages the whole world.

Communication to promote global health for the world population is done in conjunction with the reference entities. Information and campaigns cascade from WHO or CDC to different countries and then to health organizations and from there to the population. In "crisis" communication, information has to be very well articulated, constant, clear, assertive to generate the population's trust and support.

This was seen in the information disseminated after the coronavirus pandemic in the world. Even the specific words used by the WHO director general were transferred to organizations, countries, and population leaders, such as the word "hero" associated with health professionals who are at the forefront of diseases and in this case, this pandemic.

In a few days, guides, guidelines, campaigns were organized, organizations were moved, countries were financed for recovery, all the mass media were used to convey the message carefully, transparently, and correctly. It was also possible to achieve the adhesion of millions of people around the world, contributing through their confinement to their homes / homes, to the more effective control of the pandemic.

Although the evaluation of this intervention was limited to the period of the announcement of the COVID 19 pandemic (March 2020), the first steps were decisive in the production of credible, transversal and global information, where the factor of humanization and motivation to action focused on the recognized rosbusta capacity of health professionals, who, when called upon to intervene as "heroes" managed to give the best expected human response. The Pandemic crisis is still active despite the protective effect that is beginning to be observed of group immunity through vaccination. The challenges that are to be faced will require concertation, a commitment between countries, a sharing of good practices, the involvement of governments and health authorities and a strengthening of the work of health professionals (human, emotional, and financial support).

Health professionals are "heroes"

REFERENCES

Berelson, B. (1952). *Content analysis in communication research.* Free Press.

CDC. (2020). *Coronavirus Disease 2019 (COVID-19).* Retrieved on 24 of march, https://www.cdc.gov/media/dpk/diseases-and-conditions/coronavirus/coronavirus-2020.html

Deese, J. (1969). Conceptual categories in the study of content. Academic Press.

DGS. (2019). *Plano de ação para a literacia em saúde 2019-2021 - Portugal.* Direção-Geral da Saúde.

Field, M. J., & Lohr, K. N. (1990). *Clinical practice guidelines: Directions for a new program.* Institute of Medicine, National Academy Press. doi:10.17226/1626

Frost, M., Li, R., Moolenaar, R., Mao, Q., & Xie, R. (2019). Progress in public health risk communication in China: Lessons learned from SARS to H7N9. *BMC Public Health, 19*(3), 475–484. doi:10.118612889-019-6778-1 PMID:32326919

Gagliardi, A. R., Brouwers, M. C., & Bhattacharyya, O. K. (2015). The development of guideline implementation tools: A qualitative study. *CMAJ Open, 3*(1), E127–E133. doi:10.9778/cmajo.20140064 PMID:25844365

Gagliardi, A. R., Marshall, C., Huckson, S., James, R., & Moore, V. (2015). Developing a checklist for guideline implementation planning: Review and synthesis of guideline development and implementation advice. *Implementation Science; IS, 10*(1), 1–9. doi:10.118613012-015-0205-5 PMID:25884601

Graham, I. D., Harrison, M. B., Brouwers, M., Davies, B. L., & Dunn, S. (2002). Facilitating the Use of Evidence in Practice: Evaluating and Adapting Clinical Practice Guidelines for Local Use by Health Care Organizations. *JOGNN*, *31*(5), 599–611. doi:10.1111/j.1552-6909.2002.tb00086.x PMID:12353740

Grimshaw, J. M., Schunemann, H. J., Burgers, J., Cruz, A. A., Heffner, J., Metersky, M., & Cook, D. (2012). Disseminating and implementing guidelines: Article 13 in Integrating and coordinating efforts in COPD guideline development. An official ATS/ERS workshop report. *Proceedings of the American Thoracic Society*, *9*(5), 298–303. doi:10.1513/pats.201208-066ST PMID:23256174

Holsti, O. R. (1969). *Content Analysis for the Social Sciences and Humanities. Reading*. Addison-Wesley.

Hulsman, R. L. (2009). Shifting goals in medical communication. Determinants of goal detection and response formation. *Patient Education and Counseling*, *74*(3), 302–308. doi:10.1016/j.pec.2008.12.001 PMID:19135823

Institute of Medicine. (2011). *Clinical Practice Guidelines We Can Trust. Committee on Standards for Developing Trustworthy Clinical Practice Guidelines*. National Academies Press. doi:10.17226/13058

IOM. (2004). Improving Medical Education: Enhancing the Behavioral and Social Science Content of Medical School Curricula. Institute of Medicine. Washington, DC: National Academies Press.

IOM. (2011). *Clinical practice guidelines we can trust*. The National Academies Press., doi:10.17226/13058

Johns Hopkins. (2021). *Coronavirus map*. https://coronavirus.jhu.edu/map.html

Kickbush, I. (2019). Health promotion 4.0. *Health Promotion International*, *34*(2), 179–181. doi:10.1093/heapro/daz022 PMID:30939200

Kickbush, I. (2019). Interview with Ilona Kickbusch, Director of the global health programme at the graduate institute of international and development studies. *Panorama,* 140 – 142.

Kim, J.-N., & Grunig, J. E. (2011). Problem solving and communicative action: A situational theory of problem solving. *Journal of Communication*, *61*(1), 120–149. doi:10.1111/j.1460-2466.2010.01529.x

MacQueen, K. M., McLellan, E., Kay, K., & Milstein, B. (1998). Codebook development for team-based qualitative research. *Cultural Anthropology Methods Journal, 10*(2), 31–36.

Miles, M. B., & Huberman, A. M. (1994). *Qualitative data analysis: An expanded sourcebook* (2nd ed.). Sage Publications, Inc.

National Health and Medical Research Council (NHMRC). (2014). *Australian Clinical Practice Guidelines 2014 Annual Report*. NHMRC.

National Institute for Health and Care Excellence (NICE). (2014). *Developing NICE guidelines: the manual*. NICE.

Quinn, S. C., & Kumar, S. (2014). Health inequalities and infectious disease epidemics: A Challenge for global health security. *Biosecurity and Bioterrorism, 12*(5), 263–273. doi:10.1089/bsp.2014.0032

Quinn, S. C., & Kumar, S. (2014). Health inequalities and infectious disease epidemics: A challenge for global health security. *Biosecurity and Bioterrorism, 12*(5), 263–273. doi:10.1089/bsp.2014.0032 PMID:25254915

Ryan, G. W., & Bernard, H. R. (2000). Data management and analysis methods. In *Handbook of qualitative research* (2nd ed.). Sage.

Ryan, G. W., & Bernard, H. R. (2003). Techniques to identify themes. *Field Methods, 15*, 85–109.

Silverman, D. (2011). *Interpreting qualitative data: A guide to the principles of qualitative research*. SAGE.

Stone, P. J., Dunphy, D. C., Smith, M. S., & Ogilvie, D. M. (1966). *The general inquirer: A computer approach to content analysis*. Cambridge, MA: MIT Press.

The Joint Comission. (2007). *What did the doctor say?Improving health literacy to protect patient safety*. Joint Comission.

WHO. (2009). *Background note: regional preparatory meeting on promoting health literacy*. WHO.

WHO. (2017). *Strategic communication framework for effective communication.* World Health Organization.

WHO. (2019). Improving health through health literacy. *Journal of The Who Regional Office For Europe Public Health - Panorama, 5*(2-3), 123-329.

WHO. (2019). Panorama. *Journal of The Who Regional Office For Europe*, *5*(2-3).

WHO. (2019). *9th Health conference on health promotion*. Retrieved on 19 october 2019: https://www.who.int/healthpromotion/conferences/9gchp/health-literacy/en/

WHO. (2020). *Coronavirus*. Retrieved on 24 march 2020 https://www.who.int/health-topics/coronavirus#tab=tab_1

Woolf, S. H., Grol, R., Hutchinson, A., Eccles, M., & Grimshaw, J. (1999). Potential benefits, limitations, and harms of clinical guidelines. *British Medical Journal*, *318*(7182), 527–530. doi:10.1136/bmj.318.7182.527 PMID:10024268

World Health Organization. (1998). *Health Promotion Glossary*. WHO.

World Health Report. (2002). *Reducing risks, promoting healthy life*. Geneva: World Health Organization.

APPENDIX: COMPARISON BETWEEN THE "P" DAY (PANDEMIC) SPEECH ON 12 MARCH 2020, AND THE DAY AFTER MADE BY THE WHO DIRECTOR-GENERAL ON 13 MARCH 2020. (SOURCE: WHO WEBSITE)

WHO Director-General's opening remarks at the Mission briefing on COVID-19 - 12 March 2020

12 March 2020

Excellencies, dear colleagues and friends,

First of all, I would like to say good morning.

As you know, yesterday I said that that the global COVID-19 outbreak can now be described as a pandemic.

This is not a decision we took lightly.

We have made this assessment for two main reasons: first, because of the speed and scale of transmission. Almost 125,000 cases have now been reported to WHO, from 118 countries and territories. In the past two weeks, the number of cases reported outside China has increased almost 13-fold, and the number of affected countries has almost tripled.

The second reason is that despite our frequent warnings, we are deeply concerned that some countries are not approaching this threat with the level of political commitment needed to control it.

Let me be clear: describing this as a pandemic does not mean that countries should give up.

The idea that countries should shift from containment to mitigation is wrong and dangerous.

On the contrary, we have to double down.

This is a controllable pandemic.

Countries that decide to give up on fundamental public health measures may end up with a larger problem, and a heavier burden on the health system that requires more severe measures to control.

All countries must strike a fine balance between protecting health, preventing economic and social disruption, and respecting human rights.

We urge all countries to take a comprehensive approach tailored to their circumstances – with containment as the central pillar.

We are calling on countries to take a four-pronged strategy:

First, prepare and be ready.

There are still 77 countries and territories with no reported cases, and 55 countries and territories that have reported 10 cases or less.

And all countries with cases have unaffected areas. You have an opportunity to keep it that way. Prepare your people and your health facilities.

Second, detect, prevent and treat.

You can't fight a virus if you don't know where it is. That means robust surveillance to find, isolate, test and treat every case, to break the chains of transmission.

Third, reduce and suppress.

To save lives we must reduce transmission.

That means finding and isolating as many cases as possible and quarantining their closest contacts.

Even if you cannot stop transmission, you can slow it down and protect health facilities, old age homes and other vital areas – but only if you test all suspected cases.

And fourth, innovate and improve.

This is a new virus and a new situation. We're all learning, and we must all find new ways to prevent infections, save lives, and minimize impact.

All countries have lessons to share.

WHO is working day and night to support all countries.

We have shipped supplies of personal protective equipment to 57 countries, we're preparing to ship to a further 28, and we've shipped lab supplies to 120 countries.

We've published an R&D roadmap, with a set of core protocols for how studies should be done.

We've published a comprehensive package of technical guidance.

We've had more than 176,000 enrollments in our COVID training courses on OpenWHO.

We're working with the World Economic Forum and the International Chambers of Commerce to engage the private sector. We're also working with FIFA.

We're working with our colleagues across the UN system to support countries to develop their preparedness and response plans, according to the 8 pillars.

And more than 440 million U.S. dollars has now been pledged to **WHO's Strategic Preparedness and Response Plan**

We thank those countries that have contributed, especially those that have contributed fully flexible funds.

Because this is a dynamic situation, we need the greatest flexibility possible to provide the best support possible.

In the spirit of solidaryty, we ask countries not to earmark funds for this response.

Thank you all once again for your support and commitment.

As I keep saying, we're all in this together.

I thank you.

THE DAY AFTER

13 March 2020

Good afternoon everyone.

I want to start today by acknowledging that even though COVID-19 has captured the world's attention, there are still many other health issues people continue to face every single day, and that WHO is continuing to work on.

Babies are still being born. Essential surgery is continuing. People still need emergency care after road traffic crashes. People still need treatment for cancer, diabetes, HIV, malaria and many other diseases.

And for all of these, we need health workers.

Today I want to send a personal and sincere thank you to every health worker around the world – especially nurses and midwives, who we are celebrating this year through the International Year of the Nurse and the Midwife.

You do a heroic job. We know that this crisis is putting a huge burden on you and your families. We know you are stretched to the limit.

You have our admiration, our respect, and our commitment to doing everything we can to keep you safe and enable you to do your job.

More than 132,000 cases of COVID-19 have now been reported to WHO, from 123 countries and territories.

5,000 people have lost their lives, a tragic milestone.

Europe has now become the epicenter of the pandemic, with more reported cases and deaths than the rest of the world combined, apart from China.

More cases are now being reported every day than were reported in China at the height of its epidemic.

We're encouraged that many countries are now acting on the 8 pillars of WHO's Strategic Preparedness and Response Plan.

Most countries now have a national plan; most are taking a multi-sectoral approach and most have laboratory testing capacity.

WHO has evidence-based guidance that every country can use, according to each of the 8 pillars.

And we're continuing to support countries to prepare and respond.

We have shipped supplies of personal protective equipment to **56 countries, we're shipping to a further 28 countries,** and we've sent almost 1.5 million diagnostic tests to 120 countries.

Our message to countries continues to be: you must take a comprehensive approach. Not testing alone. Not contact tracing alone. Not quarantine alone. Not social distancing alone. Do it all.

Any country that looks at the experience of other countries with large epidemics and thinks **"that won't happen to us"** is making a deadly mistake. It can happen to any country.

The experience of China, the Republic of Korea, Singapore and others clearly demonstrates that aggressive testing and contact tracing, combined with social distancing measures and community mobilization, can prevent infections and save lives.

Japan is also demonstrating that a whole-of-government approach led by Prime Minister Abe himself, supported by in-depth investigation of clusters, is a critical step in reducing transmission.

WHO has clear advice for governments, businesses and individuals.

First, prepare and be ready.

Every person must know the signs and symptoms and how to protect themselves and others.

Every health worker should be able to recognize this disease, provide care and know what to do with their patients.

Every health facility should be ready to cope with large numbers of patients, and ensure the safety of staff and patients.

Second, detect, protect and treat.

You can't fight a virus if you don't know where it is. Find, isolate, test and treat every case, to break the chains of transmission.

Every case we find and treat limits the expansion of the disease.

Third, reduce transmission.

Do not just let this fire burn.

Isolate the sick and quarantine their contacts. In addition, measures that increase social distancing such as cancelling sporting events may help to reduce transmission. These measures, of course, should be based on local context and risk assessment, and should be time limited.

Even if you cannot stop transmission, you can slow it down and save lives.

And fourth, innovate and learn.

This is a new virus and a new situation. We're all learning, and we must all find new ways to prevent infections, save lives, and minimize impact. All countries have lessons to share.

There are simple, effective things we can all do to reduce the risk of infection for ourselves and those around us. Clean your hands regularly with an alcohol-based rub or soap and water. Cover your mouth and nose with your elbow if you cough or sneeze.

Stay home if you're sick. Avoid unnecessary travel and large social gatherings. Comply with the advice of your local or national health authority. Find and share reliable information.

And finally, you can give.

Together with the United Nations Foundation and the Swiss Philanthropy Foundation, WHO is today launching the COVID-19 Solidarity Response Fund, to enable individuals and organizations to contribute.

Until now, we have been relying mainly on governments to support the response.

We thank all those countries who have supported WHO's Strategic Preparedness and Response Plan, including Japan, which this week contributed US$46 million to WHO. [NOTE: This text has been corrected to $46 million. On 10 March, Japan announced an overall contribution to the global COVID-19 response of 15.5 billion yen.]

Now everyone can contribute.

Funds raised will be used to coordinate the response, to buy masks, gloves, gowns and goggles for health workers, to buy diagnostic tests, to improve surveillance, and to invest in research and development.

To give to the COVID-19 Solidarity Response Fund, go to who.int, and look for the orange "Donate" button at the top of the page.

We thank Google, Facebook and the individuals who have already contributed.

Every dollar donated is a dollar towards saving lives.

We're all in this together.

I thank you.

Related Readings

To continue IGI Global's long-standing tradition of advancing innovation through emerging research, please find below a compiled list of recommended IGI Global book chapters and journal articles in the areas of the fundamentals, models, and dimensions of health communication and literacy. These related readings will provide additional information and guidance to further enrich your knowledge and assist you with your own research.

Adam, C., Bailly, C., & Dugdale, J. (2018). Communication During Bushfires, Towards a Serious Game for a Serious Matter. *International Journal of Information Systems for Crisis Response and Management*, *10*(2), 79–105. doi:10.4018/IJISCRAM.2018040104

Akanksha, E. (2021). Principles and Applications of Narrowband IoT. In S. K. Routray & S. Mohanty (Eds.), *Principles and Applications of Narrowband Internet of Things (NBIoT)* (pp. 46–85). IGI Global. doi:10.4018/978-1-7998-4775-5.ch003

Akhtar, S. (2018). Increasing Health Literacy to Improve Clinical Trial Recruitment. In V. E. Papalois & M. Theodosopoulou (Eds.), *Optimizing Health Literacy for Improved Clinical Practices* (pp. 94–108). IGI Global. doi:10.4018/978-1-5225-4074-8.ch006

Akyüz, A. (2019). Corporate Scandals Involving Social Media. In H. Dinçer & S. Yüksel (Eds.), *Handbook of Research on Global Issues in Financial Communication and Investment Decision Making* (pp. 442–456). IGI Global. doi:10.4018/978-1-5225-9265-5.ch020

Al-Jenaibi, B. (2019). Building Organizations Image. In M. Habib (Ed.), *Handbook of Research on the Evolution of IT and the Rise of E-Society* (pp. 89–107). IGI Global. doi:10.4018/978-1-5225-7214-5.ch005

Al-Jenaibi, B. (2019). Reputation Management Techniques and E-Collaboration. In E. C. Idemudia (Ed.), *Handbook of Research on Technology Integration in the Global World* (pp. 64–86). IGI Global. doi:10.4018/978-1-5225-6367-9.ch004

Alagu, A., & Thanuskodi, S. (2020). Information Literacy Skills Among Students of Higher Education Institutions With Special Reference to Tamil Nadu. In S. Thanuskodi (Ed.), *Challenges and Opportunities of Open Educational Resources Management* (pp. 40–62). IGI Global. doi:10.4018/978-1-7998-3559-2.ch003

Albuquerque, C. (2019). The Contribution of Technologies to Promote Healthy Aging and Prevent Frailty in Elderly People. In C. Albuquerque (Ed.), *Emerging Trends and Innovations in Privacy and Health Information Management* (pp. 142–168). IGI Global. doi:10.4018/978-1-5225-8470-4.ch006

Ali, S., Batool, A., Tariq, A., Bhat, A. H., Qureshi, A., Teli, B. B., Qasim, I., Kumar, S., Gangadharan, A., Kumar, R., & Prasad, B. V. (2021). Nutrition and Cancer. In S. Kumar, M. A. Rizvi, & S. Verma (Eds.), *Handbook of Research on Advancements in Cancer Therapeutics* (pp. 570–586). IGI Global. doi:10.4018/978-1-7998-6530-8.ch021

Anderson, M., Tucker, D., Miller, F. G., Vaz, K., Anderson-Jackson, L., & McGrowder, D. (2020). Quality of Life and Well-Being of Breast Cancer Patients. In S. Padmanaban & C. Subudhi (Eds.), *Psycho-Social Perspectives on Mental Health and Well-Being* (pp. 67–94). IGI Global. doi:10.4018/978-1-7998-1185-5.ch004

Andrade, J. G., & Ferreira, N. J. (2021). Communication Crisis Management of the Public Security Policy. In L. Oliveira, F. Tajariol, & L. B. Gonçalves (Eds.), *Digital Services in Crisis, Disaster, and Emergency Situations* (pp. 199–220). IGI Global. doi:10.4018/978-1-7998-6705-0.ch009

Areskoug Josefsson, K., Nordin, A., & Kjellström, S. (2021). Trust and Self-Efficacy as Enablers and Products of Co-Production in Health and Welfare Services. In A. O. Thomassen & J. B. Jensen (Eds.), *Processual Perspectives on the Co-Production Turn in Public Sector Organizations* (pp. 42–58). IGI Global. doi:10.4018/978-1-7998-4975-9.ch003

Backholm, K., Högväg, J., Lindholm, J., Knutsen, J., & Westvang, E. (2018). Promoting Situation Awareness. *International Journal of Information Systems for Crisis Response and Management, 10*(1), 38–56. doi:10.4018/IJISCRAM.2018010103

Bajaj, S., & Manchanda, S. (2019). Nutraceutical and Functional Foods in Cancer Management and Therapy. In R. K. Keservani, A. K. Sharma, & R. K. Kesharwani (Eds.), *Nutraceutical and Functional Foods in Disease Prevention* (pp. 341–390). IGI Global. doi:10.4018/978-1-5225-3267-5.ch012

Bar-Lev, S., & Beimel, D. (2020). Common-Sense Epidemiology in the Age of Electronic Patient Records (EPR). In R. W. McHaney, I. Reychev, J. Azuri, M. E. McHaney, & R. Moshonov (Eds.), *Impacts of Information Technology on Patient Care and Empowerment* (pp. 343–364). IGI Global. doi:10.4018/978-1-7998-0047-7.ch017

Barhoi, D., Giri, S., Upadhaya, P., & Nath Barbhuiya, S. (2021). Chemopreventive and Therapeutic Potential of Phytopharmaceuticals Against Oral Cancer. In S. Kumar, M. A. Rizvi, & S. Verma (Eds.), *Handbook of Research on Advancements in Cancer Therapeutics* (pp. 541–569). IGI Global. doi:10.4018/978-1-7998-6530-8.ch020

Bartlett, J. C. (2020). Information Literacy and Science Misinformation. In K. Dalkir & R. Katz (Eds.), *Navigating Fake News, Alternative Facts, and Misinformation in a Post-Truth World* (pp. 1–17). IGI Global. doi:10.4018/978-1-7998-2543-2.ch001

Beaunoyer, E., & Guitton, M. J. (2018). Effective Use of Virtual Communities for Health-Purposes in the Elderly. In C. El Morr (Ed.), *Novel Applications of Virtual Communities in Healthcare Settings* (pp. 127–146). IGI Global. doi:10.4018/978-1-5225-2958-3.ch005

Bilal, R., Khan, B. M., & Young, R. (2018). Breast Cancer Detection and Diagnosis. In I. El Naqa (Ed.), *Emerging Developments and Practices in Oncology* (pp. 1–27). IGI Global. doi:10.4018/978-1-5225-3085-5.ch001

Boateng, J. K. (2019). Education, Social Capital, Physical, and Psychological Access to Healthcare Among Female Migrants in Informal Settlements in Accra City, Ghana. In I. Biao (Ed.), *Learning Cities, Town Planning, and the Creation of Livelihoods* (pp. 205–232). IGI Global. doi:10.4018/978-1-5225-8134-5.ch012

Bozkurt, S. (2020). Re-Establishing the School in the Light of Information Technology. In M. Durnali (Ed.), *Utilizing Technology, Knowledge, and Smart Systems in Educational Administration and Leadership* (pp. 184–202). IGI Global. doi:10.4018/978-1-7998-1408-5.ch010

Brand, J. D., & Pohl, G. M. (2021). Model/Anti-Model Advocacy Responses to Hospitality Industry Sexual Harassment. In Encyclopedia of Organizational Knowledge, Administration, and Technology (pp. 1736-1748). IGI Global. http://doi:10.4018/978-1-7998-3473-1.ch119

Capolupo, N., & Piscopo, G. (2020). Communicating Natural Calamity. In S. M. Loureiro & H. R. Kaufmann (Eds.), *Exploring the Power of Electronic Word-of-Mouth in the Services Industry* (pp. 352–363). IGI Global. doi:10.4018/978-1-5225-8575-6.ch019

Cardoso, P., Peçaibes, V., Giesteira, B., & Castro, L. C. (2021). Positive Play. In R. Alexandre Peixoto de Queirós & A. J. Marques (Eds.), *Handbook of Research on Solving Modern Healthcare Challenges With Gamification* (pp. 154–185). IGI Global. doi:10.4018/978-1-7998-7472-0.ch010

Carvalho, C. L., & Barbosa, B. (2021). Communication During a Pandemic. In L. Oliveira, F. Tajariol, & L. B. Gonçalves (Eds.), *Digital Services in Crisis, Disaster, and Emergency Situations* (pp. 282–303). IGI Global. doi:10.4018/978-1-7998-6705-0.ch013

Chatterjee, A., Sarkar, S., Rong, M., & Chatterjee, D. (2021). Artificial Neural Network in Operation Management Regarding Communication Issue. In Encyclopedia of Organizational Knowledge, Administration, and Technology (pp. 2303-2320). IGI Global. http://doi:10.4018/978-1-7998-3473-1.ch159

Clack, L., & Nagi, B. (2020). Examination of the Impact of Patient Engagement Tools on Patient Satisfaction. *International Journal of Patient-Centered Healthcare*, *10*(1), 37–46. doi:10.4018/IJPCH.2020010103

Cmeciu, C. (2021). Keep Calm and Get Informed. In L. Oliveira, F. Tajariol, & L. B. Gonçalves (Eds.), *Digital Services in Crisis, Disaster, and Emergency Situations* (pp. 246–267). IGI Global. doi:10.4018/978-1-7998-6705-0.ch011

Dandotiya, B. (2019). Health Effects of Air Pollution in Urban Environment. In A. Karmaoui (Ed.), *Climate Change and Its Impact on Ecosystem Services and Biodiversity in Arid and Semi-Arid Zones* (pp. 96–115). IGI Global. doi:10.4018/978-1-5225-7387-6.ch006 di San Marco, E. C., Vegni, E., & Borghi, L. (2019). Chronic Illnesses, Vulnerability, and Uncertainty. *International Journal of Patient-Centered Healthcare, 9*(1), 50–63. doi:10.4018/IJPCH.2019010104

Dinç Aydemir, S. (2021). Shifting Our Lenses to Behavioral Finance Paradigm. In A. Bejaoui (Ed.), *Corporate Leadership and Its Role in Shaping Organizational Culture and Performance* (pp. 174–202). IGI Global. doi:10.4018/978-1-5225-8266-3.ch009

Dinçer, H., Yüksel, S., Gökalp, Y., & Eti, S. (2021). SERVQUAL-Based Evaluation of Service Quality in Turkish Health Industry With Fuzzy Logic. In P. Manolitzas, C. Zopounidis, M. Talias, E. Grigoroudis, & N. Matsatsinis (Eds.), *Interdisciplinary Perspectives on Operations Management and Service Evaluation* (pp. 213–233). IGI Global. doi:10.4018/978-1-7998-5442-5.ch011

Dinçer, H., Yüksel, S., Yazici, M., & Pınarbaşı, F. (2019). Assessing Corporate Social Responsibilities in the Banking Sector. In H. Dinçer & S. Yüksel (Eds.), *Handbook of Research on Global Issues in Financial Communication and Investment Decision Making* (pp. 1–27). IGI Global. doi:10.4018/978-1-5225-9265-5.ch001

Domdouzis, K. (2018). Artificial-Intelligence-Based Service-Oriented Architectures (SOAs) for Crisis Management. In M. Habib (Ed.), *Handbook of Research on Investigations in Artificial Life Research and Development* (pp. 79–95). IGI Global. doi:10.4018/978-1-5225-5396-0.ch005

Edoh, T. O. (2019). Internet-of-Things-Enabled Pre-Screening for Diseases. In T. Edoh, P. Pawar, & S. Mohammad (Eds.), *Pre-Screening Systems for Early Disease Prediction, Detection, and Prevention* (pp. 1–49). IGI Global. doi:10.4018/978-1-5225-7131-5.ch001

El Hiba, O., Laaradia, M. A., Azzaoui, F., Brahim, M. A., Bitar, A., Chatoui, H., Kiai, H., Rais, H., Sellami, S., & El Kherchi, O. (2019). Prostate Cancer and Environmental Exposure. In K. Kahime, M. El Hidan, O. El Hiba, D. Sereno, & L. Bounoua (Eds.), *Handbook of Research on Global Environmental Changes and Human Health* (pp. 130–151). IGI Global. doi:10.4018/978-1-5225-7775-1.ch008

Ellison, S. R., & Dhuse, J. (2019). Using Competency-Based Learning to Improve Clinical Skills. In Optimizing Medical Education With Instructional Technology (pp. 108-147). IGI Global. doi:10.4018/978-1-5225-6289-4.ch007

Epure, M., & Mihăeş, L. C. (2019). Integrated Marketing Communication and the Ethics of Advertising. In M. Epure & L. C. Mihăeş (Eds.), *The Role of Language and Symbols in Promotional Strategies and Marketing Schemes* (pp. 1–27). IGI Global. doi:10.4018/978-1-5225-5778-4.ch001

Fakhri, K. U., Alotaibi, B. S., Kumar, S., Kumar, U., Sonkar, S. C., Mathur, A., Kazim, Z., Perwez, A., Yasin, D., Zeya, B., Ahmad, F. J., & Rizvi, M. M. (2021). Phytopharmaceuticals in Cancer Treatment. In S. Kumar, M. A. Rizvi, & S. Verma (Eds.), *Handbook of Research on Advancements in Cancer Therapeutics* (pp. 639–668). IGI Global. doi:10.4018/978-1-7998-6530-8.ch025

Faria, M. C. (2020). Health Promotion and Wellness in Aging. In C. Fonseca, M. J. Lopes, D. Mendes, F. Mendes, & J. García-Alonso (Eds.), *Handbook of Research on Health Systems and Organizations for an Aging Society* (pp. 12–28). IGI Global. doi:10.4018/978-1-5225-9818-3.ch002

Faris, M. A., & Ghazzawi, H. (2020). Health-Improving and Disease-Preventing Potential of Camel Milk Against Chronic Diseases and Autism. In O. A. Alhaj, B. Faye, & R. P. Agrawal (Eds.), *Handbook of Research on Health and Environmental Benefits of Camel Products* (pp. 155–184). IGI Global. doi:10.4018/978-1-7998-1604-1.ch008

Fernández-Avelino, J., Alor-Hernández, G., Paredes-Valverde, M. A., & Sánchez-Morales, L. N. (2021). Developing Chatbots for Supporting Health Self-Management. In R. A. Pazos-Rangel, R. Florencia-Juarez, M. A. Paredes-Valverde, & G. Rivera (Eds.), *Handbook of Research on Natural Language Processing and Smart Service Systems* (pp. 135–156). IGI Global. doi:10.4018/978-1-7998-4730-4.ch006

Fogel, J., & Herzog, R. (2020). Direct-to-Consumer Prescription Medication Advertisements and Use of Different Types of Media. *Journal of Electronic Commerce in Organizations, 18*(4), 51–72. doi:10.4018/JECO.2020100103

Frank, A. L. (2020). The Role of Humanities in Medical Education. In R. Gotian, Y. Kang, & J. Safdieh (Eds.), *Handbook of Research on the Efficacy of Training Programs and Systems in Medical Education* (pp. 148–155). IGI Global. doi:10.4018/978-1-7998-1468-9.ch008

Gahtori, R., & Paliwal, A. (2021). Role of Herbal Medicine/Phyto-Therapy in Cancer Prevention by Inhibiting Epithelial-Mesenchymal Transition (EMT) Pathways. In A. Hussain & S. Behl (Eds.), *Treating Endocrine and Metabolic Disorders With Herbal Medicines* (pp. 215–234). IGI Global. doi:10.4018/978-1-7998-4808-0.ch009

Galli, B. J. (2020). Effective Strategies for Communication Management in a Project Management Environment. *International Journal of Applied Logistics*, *10*(2), 86–92. doi:10.4018/IJAL.2020070105

Galli, B. J. (2020). The Relationship and Impact of Communication on Change Management. *International Journal of Responsible Leadership and Ethical Decision-Making*, *2*(2), 1–16. doi:10.4018/IJRLEDM.2020070101

Gigauri, I. (2021). Corporate Social Responsibility and COVID-19 Pandemic Crisis. *International Journal of Sustainable Entrepreneurship and Corporate Social Responsibility*, *6*(1), 30–47. doi:10.4018/IJSECSR.2021010103

Golt, S. G. (2019). Crisis Communication and Management. In S. E. Daly (Ed.), *Assessing and Averting the Prevalence of Mass Violence* (pp. 194–208). IGI Global. doi:10.4018/978-1-5225-5670-1.ch008

Gonçalves, L., & Oliveira, L. (2021). Forest Fire Scenarios in Digital Platforms. In L. Oliveira, F. Tajariol, & L. B. Gonçalves (Eds.), *Digital Services in Crisis, Disaster, and Emergency Situations* (pp. 149–176). IGI Global. doi:10.4018/978-1-7998-6705-0.ch007

Gonzalez-Usach, R., Yacchirema, D., Julian, M., & Palau, C. E. (2019). Interoperability in IoT. In Handbook of Research on Big Data and the IoT (pp. 149-173). IGI Global. doi:10.4018/978-1-5225-7432-3.ch009

Goswami, S., Mahanta, K., Goswami, S., Jigdung, T., & Devi, T. P. (2018). Ageing and Cancer. In B. V. Prasad & S. Akbar (Eds.), *Handbook of Research on Geriatric Health, Treatment, and Care* (pp. 206–235). IGI Global. doi:10.4018/978-1-5225-3480-8.ch012

Grünberg, L. R. (2021). In Need for More Tailored Feminist Stories in a Time of Crisis. In R. Ciolăneanu & R. Marinescu (Eds.), *Handbook of Research on Translating Myth and Reality in Women Imagery Across Disciplines* (pp. 1–23). IGI Global. doi:10.4018/978-1-7998-6458-5.ch001

Günçavdı, G. (2020). What Do Teachers Need to Become a Peace Educator? In S. Polat & G. Günçavdı (Eds.), *Empowering Multiculturalism and Peacebuilding in Schools* (pp. 179–197). IGI Global. doi:10.4018/978-1-7998-2827-3.ch008

Hafeez, Z. B., Fakhri, K. U., Zafaryab, M., & Rizvi, M. M. (2021). Functional Mechanisms of Green Tea Polyphenols and Their Molecular Targets in Prevention of Multiple Cancers. In S. Kumar, M. A. Rizvi, & S. Verma (Eds.), *Handbook of Research on Advancements in Cancer Therapeutics* (pp. 587–605). IGI Global. doi:10.4018/978-1-7998-6530-8.ch022

Halatsi, M., Bilirakis, E., Petousis, S., Vavoulidis, E., & Dinas, K. (2021). Co-Testing. In K. Dinas, S. Petousis, M. Kalder, & G. Mavromatidis (Eds.), *Handbook of Research on Oncological and Endoscopical Dilemmas in Modern Gynecological Clinical Practice* (pp. 104–120). IGI Global. doi:10.4018/978-1-7998-4213-2.ch008

Hamid, S. B., & Hamid, A. F. (2019). Roles of Nutraceuticals and Functional Food in Prevention of Cardiovascular Disease. In R. K. Keservani, A. K. Sharma, & R. K. Kesharwani (Eds.), *Nutraceutical and Functional Foods in Disease Prevention* (pp. 126–165). IGI Global. doi:10.4018/978-1-5225-3267-5.ch005

Handwerk, S. E., & Handwerk, K. (2019). Teenage Pregnancy. In D. Akella (Ed.), *Socio-Cultural Influences on Teenage Pregnancy and Contemporary Prevention Measures* (pp. 1–32). IGI Global. doi:10.4018/978-1-5225-6108-8.ch001

Hofer, G. (2020). Investigating Expressions of Pain and Emotion in Authentic Interpreted Medical Consultations. In I. Souza & E. E. Fragkou (Eds.), *Handbook of Research on Medical Interpreting* (pp. 136–164). IGI Global. doi:10.4018/978-1-5225-9308-9.ch006

Humphrey, S., Ngo, T., & Wang, T. (2021). Digital Storytelling and Teachers' Disciplinary Multiliteracies. In L. Haas & J. Tussey (Eds.), *Connecting Disciplinary Literacy and Digital Storytelling in K-12 Education* (pp. 59–84). IGI Global. doi:10.4018/978-1-7998-5770-9.ch004

Inthiran, A., Alhashmi, S. M., & Ahmed, P. K. (2018). Health Searching Behaviour of Citizens From Countries in the Middle East and North African Region. *International Journal of E-Health and Medical Communications*, *9*(2), 59–73. doi:10.4018/IJEHMC.2018040104

Ippoliti, E., Casale, A., Calvano, M., & Guadagnoli, F. (2019). Giving Form to Absence. In C. Inglese & A. Ippolito (Eds.), *Analysis, Conservation, and Restoration of Tangible and Intangible Cultural Heritage* (pp. 329–365). IGI Global. doi:10.4018/978-1-5225-6936-7.ch014

Jacob, R., & Rani, D. (2020). Do Pregnant Women Using Smartphones Care About Their Privacy? *International Journal of Information Communication Technologies and Human Development, 12*(4), 19–36. doi:10.4018/IJICTHD.2020100102

Jewitt-Harris, J. A., & Ready, A. R. (2018). Health Literacy in the Development of Kidney Transplantation Programs in Low- and Middle-Income Countries. In V. E. Papalois & M. Theodosopoulou (Eds.), *Optimizing Health Literacy for Improved Clinical Practices* (pp. 228–241). IGI Global. doi:10.4018/978-1-5225-4074-8.ch013

Just, B., & Seo, K. K. (2020). Creating a Computer Simulation with Ill-Structured Problems for Physical Therapists in the Acute Care Setting. In Y. Qian (Ed.), *Teaching, Learning, and Leading With Computer Simulations* (pp. 104–127). IGI Global. doi:10.4018/978-1-7998-0004-0.ch004

Kalkavan, H., & Ersin, I. (2019). Determination of Factors Affecting the South East Asian Crisis of 1997 Probit-Logit Panel Regression. In H. Dinçer & S. Yüksel (Eds.), *Handbook of Research on Global Issues in Financial Communication and Investment Decision Making* (pp. 148–167). IGI Global. doi:10.4018/978-1-5225-9265-5.ch008

Kallis, R. B., & Meluch, A. L. (2021). Workplace Cyberbullying and Online Harassment as an Organizational Threat. In L. Ramos Salazar (Ed.), *Handbook of Research on Cyberbullying and Online Harassment in the Workplace* (pp. 176–196). IGI Global. doi:10.4018/978-1-7998-4912-4.ch009

Kaloudas, D., & Penchovsky, R. (2018). Plant-Derived Compounds and Their Potential Role in Drug Development. *International Journal of Biomedical and Clinical Engineering, 7*(1), 53–66. doi:10.4018/IJBCE.2018010104

Kara, A., & Ant, H. (2018). Strategical Reputation Management in PR. In A. Erdemir (Ed.), *Reputation Management Techniques in Public Relations* (pp. 56–78). IGI Global. doi:10.4018/978-1-5225-3619-2.ch004

Kasemsap, K. (2018). An Overview of Global Health Initiatives and Practices. In V. E. Papalois & M. Theodosopoulou (Eds.), *Optimizing Health Literacy for Improved Clinical Practices* (pp. 198–209). IGI Global. doi:10.4018/978-1-5225-4074-8.ch011

Kasemsap, K. (2018). Nutrition and Functional Foods. In A. Verma, K. Srivastava, S. Singh, & H. Singh (Eds.), *Nutraceuticals and Innovative Food Products for Healthy Living and Preventive Care* (pp. 158–175). IGI Global. doi:10.4018/978-1-5225-2970-5.ch007

Kasemsap, K. (2018). Public Relations, Organizational Communication, and Crisis Management. In A. Erdemir (Ed.), *Reputation Management Techniques in Public Relations* (pp. 1–15). IGI Global. doi:10.4018/978-1-5225-3619-2.ch001

Kaufhold, M., Riebe, T., Reuter, C., Hester, J., Jeske, D., Knüver, L., & Richert, V. (2018). Business Continuity Management in Micro Enterprises: Perception, Strategies, and Use of ICT. *International Journal of Information Systems for Crisis Response and Management, 10*(1), 1–19. doi:10.4018/IJISCRAM.2018010101

Kedhari Sundaram, M., Silas, S., & Hussain, A. (2021). Combinational Therapy Using Chemotherapeutic Agents and Dietary Bioactive Compounds. In A. Hussain & S. Behl (Eds.), *Treating Endocrine and Metabolic Disorders With Herbal Medicines* (pp. 188–214). IGI Global. doi:10.4018/978-1-7998-4808-0.ch008

Keil, L. J., & Jerome, A. M. (2019). Strategic Communication in Crisis. In A. Normore, M. Javidi, & L. Long (Eds.), *Handbook of Research on Strategic Communication, Leadership, and Conflict Management in Modern Organizations* (pp. 315–337). IGI Global. doi:10.4018/978-1-5225-8516-9.ch016

Kerr, S. E. (2019). Emergency Management and Communication Improvements. In G. A. Crews (Ed.), *Handbook of Research on School Violence in American K-12 Education* (pp. 474–493). IGI Global. doi:10.4018/978-1-5225-6246-7.ch024

Kharmoum, N., Retal, S., Rhazali, Y., Ziti, S., & Omary, F. (2021). A Disciplined Method to Generate UML2 Communication Diagrams Automatically From the Business Value Model. In Y. Rhazali (Ed.), *Advancements in Model-Driven Architecture in Software Engineering* (pp. 218–237). IGI Global. doi:10.4018/978-1-7998-3661-2.ch012

Koca, G., & Eğilmez, Ö. (2021). Structural Modeling and Analysis of Barriers Encountered in Gamification Applications in Health. In R. Alexandre Peixoto de Queirós & A. J. Marques (Eds.), *Handbook of Research on Solving Modern Healthcare Challenges With Gamification* (pp. 34–53). IGI Global. doi:10.4018/978-1-7998-7472-0.ch003

Kökalan, Ö. (2018). Corporate Reputation Management in Times of Crisis. In A. Erdemir (Ed.), *Reputation Management Techniques in Public Relations* (pp. 79–91). IGI Global. doi:10.4018/978-1-5225-3619-2.ch005

Kostić, S. C., & Šarenac, J. G. (2020). "New Normal" Strategic Communication. In A. Özbebek Tunç & P. Aslan (Eds.), *Business Management and Communication Perspectives in Industry 4.0* (pp. 71–92). IGI Global. doi:10.4018/978-1-5225-9416-1.ch005

Kostyuchenko, Y. V., Pushkar, V., Malysheva, O., & Yuschenko, M. (2020). On the Behavior-Based Risk Communication Models in Crisis Management and Social Risks Minimization. *International Journal of Cyber Warfare & Terrorism, 10*(2), 27–45. doi:10.4018/IJCWT.2020040102

Kotsanis, Y. (2018). Models of Competences for the Real and Digital World. In K. Koutsopoulos, K. Doukas, & Y. Kotsanis (Eds.), *Handbook of Research on Educational Design and Cloud Computing in Modern Classroom Settings* (pp. 52–80). IGI Global. doi:10.4018/978-1-5225-3053-4.ch004

Kouroubali, A., Koumakis, L., Kondylakis, H., & Katehakis, D. G. (2019). An Integrated Approach Towards Developing Quality Mobile Health Apps for Cancer. In A. Moumtzoglou (Ed.), *Mobile Health Applications for Quality Healthcare Delivery* (pp. 46–71). IGI Global. doi:10.4018/978-1-5225-8021-8.ch003

Kouroubali, A., Koumakis, L., Kondylakis, H., & Katehakis, D. G. (2020). Smart Healthcare Apps for Quality Cancer Patient Support. *International Journal of Big Data and Analytics in Healthcare, 5*(1), 28–48. doi:10.4018/IJBDAH.2020010103

Krueger, J. M. (2018). Backward Planning, Forward Motion. In Changing the Scope of Library Instruction in the Digital Age (pp. 60-84). IGI Global. http://doi:10.4018/978-1-5225-2802-9.ch003

Kumar, A. A. (2020). Healthcare Reform. In Evaluating Challenges and Opportunities for Healthcare Reform (pp. 144-166). IGI Global. doi:10.4018/978-1-7998-2949-2.ch007

Kumar, R., & Rizvi, S. I. (2019). The Protective Role of Nutraceuticals and Functional Food in Hyperlipidemia. In R. K. Keservani, A. K. Sharma, & R. K. Kesharwani (Eds.), *Nutraceutical and Functional Foods in Disease Prevention* (pp. 233–254). IGI Global. doi:10.4018/978-1-5225-3267-5.ch008

Kumar, S. V., Akashe, S., & Kim, H. (2020). Feasible Challenges and Applications of IoT in Healthcare. In C. Chakraborty (Ed.), *Smart Medical Data Sensing and IoT Systems Design in Healthcare* (pp. 178–200). IGI Global. doi:10.4018/978-1-7998-0261-7.ch008

Kuşay, Y. (2019). Digital Storytelling as a Part of Participatory Culture in Communication and Public Relation Practices. In R. Yılmaz, M. N. Erdem, & F. Resuloğlu (Eds.), *Handbook of Research on Transmedia Storytelling and Narrative Strategies* (pp. 271–291). IGI Global. doi:10.4018/978-1-5225-5357-1.ch014

Lafer, E. M., McCuiston, M., & Swanson, A. (2021). Yoga Therapy. In S. Telles & R. K. Gupta (Eds.), *Handbook of Research on Evidence-Based Perspectives on the Psychophysiology of Yoga and Its Applications* (pp. 159–178). IGI Global. doi:10.4018/978-1-7998-3254-6.ch010

Langaro, D., Loureiro, S. M., & Soares, A. (2020). When Consumers' Complaints Fall Into Public Domain. In S. M. Loureiro & H. R. Kaufmann (Eds.), *Exploring the Power of Electronic Word-of-Mouth in the Services Industry* (pp. 124–137). IGI Global. doi:10.4018/978-1-5225-8575-6.ch008

Lejbkowicz, I. (2020). Web-Based Information for Patients and Providers. In R. W. McHaney, I. Reychev, J. Azuri, M. E. McHaney, & R. Moshonov (Eds.), *Impacts of Information Technology on Patient Care and Empowerment* (pp. 19–33). IGI Global. doi:10.4018/978-1-7998-0047-7.ch002

Lindholm, J., Backholm, K., & Högväg, J. (2021). Information Overload! In L. Oliveira, F. Tajariol, & L. B. Gonçalves (Eds.), *Digital Services in Crisis, Disaster, and Emergency Situations* (pp. 50–76). IGI Global. doi:10.4018/978-1-7998-6705-0.ch003

Mackintosh, S. E., & Katsaros, E. (2020). Building Interprofessional Competencies Into Medical Education and Assessment. In Building a Patient-Centered Interprofessional Education Program (pp. 84-112). IGI Global. http://doi:10.4018/978-1-7998-3066-5.ch005

Malanga, D. F., & Chigona, W. (2018). Mobile Health Initiatives in Malawi. *International Journal of Privacy and Health Information Management*, *6*(1), 49–60. doi:10.4018/IJPHIM.2018010104

Malika, A. S., Hajar, K., Loubna, B., El Hiba, O., Rachida, M., Leila, B., Souad, S., & Hanane, R. S. (2019). Breast Cancer With Relevance for Heavy Metals, Mycotoxines, and Pesticides. In K. Kahime, M. El Hidan, O. El Hiba, D. Sereno, & L. Bounoua (Eds.), *Handbook of Research on Global Environmental Changes and Human Health* (pp. 152–192). IGI Global. doi:10.4018/978-1-5225-7775-1.ch009

Mareti, E., Margioula-Siarkou, C., Mavromatidis, G., & Guyon, F. (2021). High-Risk Patients for Gynaecological Cancer. In K. Dinas, S. Petousis, M. Kalder, & G. Mavromatidis (Eds.), *Handbook of Research on Oncological and Endoscopical Dilemmas in Modern Gynecological Clinical Practice* (pp. 49–63). IGI Global. doi:10.4018/978-1-7998-4213-2.ch004

Marsh, K., Saunders, A., & Zeuschner, C. (2018). The Health Impact of Eating Foods of Animal Origin. In D. Bogueva, D. Marinova, & T. Raphaely (Eds.), *Handbook of Research on Social Marketing and Its Influence on Animal Origin Food Product Consumption* (pp. 17–36). IGI Global. doi:10.4018/978-1-5225-4757-0.ch002

Marshall, P., & Marinova, D. (2019). Health Benefits of Eating More Plant Foods and Less Meat. In D. Bogueva, D. Marinova, T. Raphaely, & K. Schmidinger (Eds.), *Environmental, Health, and Business Opportunities in the New Meat Alternatives Market* (pp. 38–61). IGI Global. doi:10.4018/978-1-5225-7350-0.ch003

Mayo-Cubero, M. (2021). Social Media and Digital Information Sources in News Coverage of Crisis, Disaster, and Emergency Situations. In L. Oliveira, F. Tajariol, & L. B. Gonçalves (Eds.), *Digital Services in Crisis, Disaster, and Emergency Situations* (pp. 268–281). IGI Global. doi:10.4018/978-1-7998-6705-0.ch012

Mbaka, C. A. (2020). The Language Challenge of Diabetes Information and Education in Nigeria's Multi-Lingual Setting. In K. O. Oyesomi & A. Salawu (Eds.), *Emerging Trends in Indigenous Language Media, Communication, Gender, and Health* (pp. 263–275). IGI Global. doi:10.4018/978-1-7998-2091-8.ch014

McGrowder, D. A., Miller, F. G., Brown, J. G., Wilson-Clarke, C., & Anderson-Jackson, L. (2021). The Role of E-Health Interventions in Improving Clinical Outcomes and Overall Health for Prostate Cancer Patients. In D. Yadav, A. Bansal, M. Bhatia, M. Hooda, & J. Morato (Eds.), *Diagnostic Applications of Health Intelligence and Surveillance Systems* (pp. 144–171). IGI Global. doi:10.4018/978-1-7998-6527-8.ch007

Mcnamara, S., & Pan, C. (2020). Adapted Physical Education in the Special Education Process. In A. Singh, M. Viner, & C. J. Yeh (Eds.), *Special Education Design and Development Tools for School Rehabilitation Professionals* (pp. 61–85). IGI Global. doi:10.4018/978-1-7998-1431-3.ch004

Medhekar, A. (2019). Role, Rules, and Regulations for Global Medical Tourism Facilitators. In M. Chand Dhiman & V. Chauhan (Eds.), *Handbook of Research on International Travel Agency and Tour Operation Management* (pp. 81–100). IGI Global. doi:10.4018/978-1-5225-8434-6.ch006

Mirabolghasemi, M., Iahad, N. A., & Ramayah, T. (2019). Influential Factors in Breast Cancer Patients' Performance Using Malaysian Social Network Support Groups. *International Journal of Healthcare Information Systems and Informatics, 14*(4), 73–90. doi:10.4018/IJHISI.2019100105

Mkrttchian, V., Vertakova, Y., Gamidullaeva, L. A., Gaidarenko, L., & Ivanov, M. (2019). Avatar-Based Management Techniques for Breaking Down Language and Cultural Barriers in Modern Russian Corporations. In Breaking Down Language and Cultural Barriers Through Contemporary Global Marketing Strategies (pp. 79-101). IGI Global. doi:10.4018/978-1-5225-6980-0.ch005

Moeller, C. L. (2018). Sharing Your Personal Medical Experience Online. In S. Sekalala & B. C. Niezgoda (Eds.), *Global Perspectives on Health Communication in the Age of Social Media* (pp. 185–209). IGI Global. doi:10.4018/978-1-5225-3716-8.ch007

Mohamed, H. S. (2017). The Effects of Utilizing Social Media Tools During Crisis from Public Relations Practitioners' Views in the UAE. *International Journal of Online Marketing*, *7*(4), 21–38. doi:10.4018/IJOM.2017100102

Nădrag, L., & Buzarna-Tihenea, A. G. (2018). The Role of Communication in Business Decision Making. In I. Oncioiu (Ed.), *Ethics and Decision-Making for Sustainable Business Practices* (pp. 164–186). IGI Global. doi:10.4018/978-1-5225-3773-1.ch010

Naeim, A., Xie, Z., Johansen, L., Wenger, N. S., Elashoff, D., Petruse, A., & Rahbar, G. (2020). Using Tablets to Collect Breast Cancer Risk Information in an Underserved Population. *International Journal of E-Health and Medical Communications*, *11*(4), 90–104. doi:10.4018/IJEHMC.20201001.oa1

Nanda, S. (2019). *Psycho-Social Health*. IGI Global. doi:10.4018/978-1-5225-7384-5.ch003

Naqvi, N. C., Wong-Goodrich, S. J., Martinage, A., Gordon, S. L., DeCuffa, J. A., & Collins, M. (2020). Increasing Knowledge of Autism Spectrum Disorders Among Urban Special Educators in Tanzania. *International Journal of Teacher Education and Professional Development*, *3*(2), 1–18. doi:10.4018/IJTEPD.2020070101

Natalia, B. (2019). Skills Development With Educational Software. In E. A. Railean (Ed.), *Handbook of Research on Ecosystem-Based Theoretical Models of Learning and Communication* (pp. 139–153). IGI Global. doi:10.4018/978-1-5225-7853-6.ch008

Nikiforou-Lialiampidou, M., Moga, M., Kalder, M., Pratilas, G., & Dinas, K. (2021). Chemoprevention in Breast Cancer. In K. Dinas, S. Petousis, M. Kalder, & G. Mavromatidis (Eds.), *Handbook of Research on Oncological and Endoscopical Dilemmas in Modern Gynecological Clinical Practice* (pp. 338–354). IGI Global. doi:10.4018/978-1-7998-4213-2.ch023

Niskanen, T. (2019). A Sociotechnical Systems Approach Applying a Novel Taxonomy to a Survey for the Assessment of Safety Performance. In A. Realyvásquez, A. A. Maldonado-Macías, & K. C. Arredondo (Eds.), *Advanced Macroergonomics and Sociotechnical Approaches for Optimal Organizational Performance* (pp. 71–98). IGI Global. doi:10.4018/978-1-5225-7192-6.ch004

Noor, S., Guo, Y., Shah, S. H., Nawaz, M. S., & Butt, A. S. (2020). Research Synthesis and Thematic Analysis of Twitter Through Bibliometric Analysis. *International Journal on Semantic Web and Information Systems, 16*(3), 88–109. doi:10.4018/IJSWIS.2020070106

Nwogwugwu, D. I. (2021). Evaluation of Research Trends in Social Media Crisis Communication. In L. Oliveira, F. Tajariol, & L. B. Gonçalves (Eds.), *Digital Services in Crisis, Disaster, and Emergency Situations* (pp. 177–198). IGI Global. doi:10.4018/978-1-7998-6705-0.ch008

Nyambane, R. O. (2021). Effect of Electronic Media Sources on Cervical Cancer Awareness Among Women in Kenya. In A. O. Akwala, J. K. Ngetich, & A. W. Theuri (Eds.), *Dialectical Perspectives on Media, Health, and Culture in Modern Africa* (pp. 39–58). IGI Global. doi:10.4018/978-1-5225-8091-1.ch003

Ogunyombo, O. E., & Bello, S. (2020). Exploring the Use of Indigenous Languages in Antenatal Care Sessions Among Mothers in Lagos State. In K. O. Oyesomi & A. Salawu (Eds.), *Emerging Trends in Indigenous Language Media, Communication, Gender, and Health* (pp. 19–44). IGI Global. doi:10.4018/978-1-7998-2091-8.ch002

Oh, S. K., Hong, S., & Park, H. S. (2020). The Tipping Point. *International Journal of Social Media and Online Communities, 12*(1), 23–39. doi:10.4018/IJSMOC.2020010103

Okada, A., Ishida, Y., & Yamauchi, N. (2018). In Prosperity Prepare for Adversity. In Innovative Perspectives on Public Administration in the Digital Age (pp. 42-64). IGI Global. doi:10.4018/978-1-5225-5966-5.ch003

Okasha, N. (2020). Using Health Psychology to Inspire Entrepreneurial Innovation in Dubai. In H. C. Webb & H. A. Al Numairy (Eds.), *Entrepreneurial Innovation and Economic Development in Dubai and Comparisons to Its Sister Cities* (pp. 198–222). IGI Global. doi:10.4018/978-1-5225-9377-5.ch010

Pai, R. R., & Alathur, S. (2019). Predicting Mobile Health Technology Acceptance by the Indian Rural Community. *International Journal of Electronic Government Research, 15*(4), 37–62. doi:10.4018/IJEGR.2019100103

Palanisamy, R., Taskin, N., & Verville, J. (2021). Factors Influencing Interprofessional Collaboration in Healthcare Environment. In J. Zhao (Ed.), *Collaborative Convergence and Virtual Teamwork for Organizational Transformation* (pp. 60–104). IGI Global. doi:10.4018/978-1-7998-4891-2.ch004

Pandey, J. R., Jha, A., Mukherjee, S. K., & Saha, S. K. (2019). An Empirical Note on Comparative Perceptions of Indian Patients and Physicians in Direct-to-Consumer Promotion of Pharmaceutical Products. In P. Ordoñez de Pablos (Ed.), *Dynamic Perspectives on Globalization and Sustainable Business in Asia* (pp. 128–153). IGI Global. doi:10.4018/978-1-5225-7095-0.ch009

Papanikolaou, A., Liberis, A., & Vatopoulou, A. (2021). Surgical Prevention in Ovarian Cancer. In K. Dinas, S. Petousis, M. Kalder, & G. Mavromatidis (Eds.), *Handbook of Research on Oncological and Endoscopical Dilemmas in Modern Gynecological Clinical Practice* (pp. 194–206). IGI Global. doi:10.4018/978-1-7998-4213-2.ch014

Parnell, T. A. (2018). Weaving Health Literacy Strategies Throughout the Fabric of Healthcare Organizations. In V. E. Papalois & M. Theodosopoulou (Eds.), *Optimizing Health Literacy for Improved Clinical Practices* (pp. 17–31). IGI Global. doi:10.4018/978-1-5225-4074-8.ch002

Pathak, S. (2019). Disaster Crisis Communication Innovations. *International Journal of Disaster Response and Emergency Management, 2*(2), 1–16. doi:10.4018/IJDREM.2019070101

Paul, A. (2019). The Relationship Between Nigerian University Students' Body Literacy Level and Their Awareness of Embodied Learning. In V. Wang (Ed.), *Handbook of Research on Transdisciplinary Knowledge Generation* (pp. 296–310). IGI Global. doi:10.4018/978-1-5225-9531-1.ch021

Pereira, M. C., Rebehy, P. C., Faleiros, F., & Galvao, M. C. (2019). Social Innovation to Achieve Global Health. In L. C. Carvalho & P. Isaías (Eds.), *Handbook of Research on Entrepreneurship and Marketing for Global Reach in the Digital Economy* (pp. 522–537). IGI Global. doi:10.4018/978-1-5225-6307-5.ch022

Petersen, L., Fallou, L., Reilly, P., & Serafinelli, E. (2017). European Expectations of Disaster Information provided by Critical Infrastructure Operators. *International Journal of Information Systems for Crisis Response and Management, 9*(4), 23–48. doi:10.4018/IJISCRAM.2017100102

Petousis, S., Margioula-Siarkou, C., Margioula-Siarkou, G., Guyon, F., & Mavromatidis, G. (2021). Screening Tests for Gynaecological Cancer. In K. Dinas, S. Petousis, M. Kalder, & G. Mavromatidis (Eds.), *Handbook of Research on Oncological and Endoscopical Dilemmas in Modern Gynecological Clinical Practice* (pp. 32–48). IGI Global. doi:10.4018/978-1-7998-4213-2.ch003

Premi, M., & Bansal, V. (2021). Nutraceuticals for Management of Metabolic Disorders. In A. Hussain & S. Behl (Eds.), *Treating Endocrine and Metabolic Disorders With Herbal Medicines* (pp. 298–320). IGI Global. doi:10.4018/978-1-7998-4808-0.ch013

Prybutok, G., Ta, A. V., Liu, X., & Prybutok, V. (2020). An Integrated Structural Equation Model of eHealth Behavioral Intention. *International Journal of Healthcare Information Systems and Informatics, 15*(1), 20–39. doi:10.4018/IJHISI.2020010102

Pyle, A. S. (2019). Fixing the SIC. In A. Normore, M. Javidi, & L. Long (Eds.), *Handbook of Research on Strategic Communication, Leadership, and Conflict Management in Modern Organizations* (pp. 1–16). IGI Global. doi:10.4018/978-1-5225-8516-9.ch001

Queiroz-Franklin, M. (2020). An Overview of Medical Interpreting in Brazil. In I. Souza & E. E. Fragkou (Eds.), *Handbook of Research on Medical Interpreting* (pp. 80–97). IGI Global. doi:10.4018/978-1-5225-9308-9.ch004

Ra, S. (2018). Intercultural Communication Challenge. In O. I. Seel (Ed.), *Redefining Translation and Interpretation in Cultural Evolution* (pp. 258–273). IGI Global. doi:10.4018/978-1-5225-2832-6.ch014

Rata, L., Birnaz, N., & Nadejda, B. (2019). Ecological Approach to Learning and Communication. In E. A. Railean (Ed.), *Handbook of Research on Ecosystem-Based Theoretical Models of Learning and Communication* (pp. 167–183). IGI Global. doi:10.4018/978-1-5225-7853-6.ch010

Reis, A. M., & Soares, B. (2021). The Brand NHS. In New Techniques for Brand Management in the Healthcare Sector (pp. 142-160). IGI Global. http://doi:10.4018/978-1-7998-3034-4.ch009

Reychav, I., McHaney, R. W., Zhu, L., & Moshonov, R. (2020). Patient-Centered Empowerment Through Evidence-Based Engagement in Sensitive Clinical Settings. In R. W. McHaney, I. Reychev, J. Azuri, M. E. McHaney, & R. Moshonov (Eds.), *Impacts of Information Technology on Patient Care and Empowerment* (pp. 155–175). IGI Global. doi:10.4018/978-1-7998-0047-7.ch009

Richards, D. (2021). Cultivating Health Policy Changemakers Through Communication Training and Digital Media Education. In L. S. Byrd (Ed.), *Cultivating Entrepreneurial Changemakers Through Digital Media Education* (pp. 165–170). IGI Global. doi:10.4018/978-1-7998-5808-9.ch011

Rocha, N. P., Rodrigues dos Santos, M., Cerqueira, M., & Queirós, A. (2019). Mobile Health to Support Ageing in Place. *International Journal of E-Health and Medical Communications*, *10*(3), 1–21. doi:10.4018/IJEHMC.2019070101

Rosiek-Kryszewska, A., & Rosiek, A. (2018). The Involvement of the Patient and his Perspective Evaluation of the Quality of Healthcare. In A. Rosiek-Kryszewska & K. Leksowski (Eds.), *Healthcare Administration for Patient Safety and Engagement* (pp. 121–144). IGI Global. doi:10.4018/978-1-5225-3946-9.ch007

Ruffin, T. R. (2018). Reflections and Understanding of Quality Management in Healthcare. In V. E. Papalois & M. Theodosopoulou (Eds.), *Optimizing Health Literacy for Improved Clinical Practices* (pp. 153–174). IGI Global. doi:10.4018/978-1-5225-4074-8.ch009

Ryynänen, S., & Vasari, P. (2019). Using the Reflective Strategy and the Game Theory Perspective During the Patient Complaint Process. *International Journal of Innovation in the Digital Economy*, *10*(3), 53–63. doi:10.4018/IJIDE.2019070105

Sabourin, R., & Ahmed, R. (2020). Empathizing With the Criminally Insane. *International Journal of Cyber Behavior, Psychology and Learning*, *10*(1), 54–73. doi:10.4018/IJCBPL.2020010105

Sanderson, E. E. (2021). Fostering Community Agents Through Health Communication. In L. S. Byrd (Ed.), *Cultivating Entrepreneurial Changemakers Through Digital Media Education* (pp. 156–164). IGI Global. doi:10.4018/978-1-7998-5808-9.ch010

Sasso, A. (2020). In Through the Looking Glass. In I. Souza & E. E. Fragkou (Eds.), *Handbook of Research on Medical Interpreting* (pp. 397–420). IGI Global. doi:10.4018/978-1-5225-9308-9.ch017

Schilling, D. L., Sharp, K., & Waldman, R. (2020). Moving From Vertical to Horizontal. In Building a Patient-Centered Interprofessional Education Program (pp. 35-45). IGI Global. doi:10.4018/978-1-7998-3066-5.ch002

Sezgin, M., & Bayoğlu, F. (2020). Comparison of Public Relations Education at Undergraduate and Graduate Levels in Turkey and EU Member States. In Y. Bayar (Ed.), *Handbook of Research on Social and Economic Development in the European Union* (pp. 510–541). IGI Global. doi:10.4018/978-1-7998-1188-6.ch030

Singh, P., Khan, S. A., & Goyal, P. K. (2021). Evaluation of Topology-Based Routing Protocols for Dissemination of Emergency Messages in Urban Vehicular Traffic Scenarios in India. In R. S. Rao, N. Singh, O. Kaiwartya, & S. Das (Eds.), *Cloud-Based Big Data Analytics in Vehicular Ad-Hoc Networks* (pp. 46–74). IGI Global. doi:10.4018/978-1-7998-2764-1.ch003

Soczywko, J., & Rutkowska, D. (2018). The Patient/Provider Relationship in Emergency Medicine. In A. Rosiek-Kryszewska & K. Leksowski (Eds.), *Healthcare Administration for Patient Safety and Engagement* (pp. 74–105). IGI Global. doi:10.4018/978-1-5225-3946-9.ch005

Souza, T. de V. I. E. (2020). The Medical Interpreter Mediation Role. In Handbook of Research on Medical Interpreting (pp. 99-135). IGI Global. http://doi:10.4018/978-1-5225-9308-9.ch005

Spalletta, M., Fanara, D., & De Rosa, P. (2021). Setting the Aware Agenda of the COVID-19 Health Emergency. In L. Oliveira, F. Tajariol, & L. B. Gonçalves (Eds.), *Digital Services in Crisis, Disaster, and Emergency Situations* (pp. 221–245). IGI Global. doi:10.4018/978-1-7998-6705-0.ch010

Stieglitz, S., Mirbabaie, M., & Fromm, J. (2017). Understanding Sense-Making on Social Media During Crises. *International Journal of Information Systems for Crisis Response and Management*, *9*(4), 49–69. doi:10.4018/IJISCRAM.2017100103

Tari, I. (2020). Media Business Literacy in the Digital Age. In N. O. Taskiran (Ed.), *Handbook of Research on Multidisciplinary Approaches to Literacy in the Digital Age* (pp. 105–129). IGI Global. doi:10.4018/978-1-7998-1534-1.ch007

Tavares, J., Santinha, G., Gonçalves, L. J., & Forte, T. (2021). Using Digital Tools to Improve Policy Making and Citizens' Decisions in Healthcare. In L. Oliveira, A. Amaro, & A. Melro (Eds.), *Handbook of Research on Cultural Heritage and Its Impact on Territory Innovation and Development* (pp. 99–113). IGI Global. doi:10.4018/978-1-7998-6701-2.ch006

Teixeira-Santos, L., Bobrowicz-Campos, E., Ventura, F., Parola, V., Coelho, A., Almeida, M. D., Gil, I., Moreno-Casbas, M. T., & Apóstolo, J. (2020). Technology as a Pathway for Older People to Engage in Activities Promoting Successful Ageing. In D. Mendes, C. Fonseca, M. J. Lopes, J. García-Alonso, & J. M. Murillo (Eds.), *Exploring the Role of ICTs in Healthy Aging* (pp. 68–94). IGI Global. doi:10.4018/978-1-7998-1937-0.ch005

Tekin, K. (2018). Issue Management in the Digital World. In A. Erdemir (Ed.), *Reputation Management Techniques in Public Relations* (pp. 204–221). IGI Global. doi:10.4018/978-1-5225-3619-2.ch011

Thanh Tung, B. (2021). Natural Product Compounds for Breast Cancer Treatment. In S. Kumar, M. A. Rizvi, & S. Verma (Eds.), *Handbook of Research on Advancements in Cancer Therapeutics* (pp. 606–626). IGI Global. doi:10.4018/978-1-7998-6530-8.ch023

Theuri, A. W. (2021). The Influence of Intercultural Communication for Immigrant Traders in Kenyan Informal Urban Markets. In A. O. Akwala, J. K. Ngetich, & A. W. Theuri (Eds.), *Dialectical Perspectives on Media, Health, and Culture in Modern Africa* (pp. 165–183). IGI Global. doi:10.4018/978-1-5225-8091-1.ch010

Tsene, L., & Briana, M. (2019). CSR Wave. In A. Antonaras & P. Dekoulou (Eds.), *Cases on Corporate Social Responsibility and Contemporary Issues in Organizations* (pp. 299–312). IGI Global. doi:10.4018/978-1-5225-7715-7.ch017

Turarbekova, L. (2020). Educational Approaches and Strategies in the Knowledge Society. In G. Tazhina & J. Parker (Eds.), *Toward Sustainability Through Digital Technologies and Practices in the Eurasian Region* (pp. 132–151). IGI Global. doi:10.4018/978-1-7998-2551-7.ch008

Türkmenoğlu, M. A. (2018). Putting Humanity Before Brand Reputation in the Context of Turkey. In A. Erdemir (Ed.), *Reputation Management Techniques in Public Relations* (pp. 339–357). IGI Global. doi:10.4018/978-1-5225-3619-2.ch017

Vaz de Almeida, C., & Belim, C. (2021). Health Professionals' Communication Competences as a Light on the Patient Pathway. *International Journal of Applied Research on Public Health Management*, *6*(1), 14–29. doi:10.4018/IJARPHM.2021010102

Vosnakis, C., Pratilas, G., & Mavromatidis, G. (2021). Short and Long-Term Follow-Up of Women After Treatment for Primary Gynecological and Breast Cancer. In K. Dinas, S. Petousis, M. Kalder, & G. Mavromatidis (Eds.), *Handbook of Research on Oncological and Endoscopical Dilemmas in Modern Gynecological Clinical Practice* (pp. 64–81). IGI Global. doi:10.4018/978-1-7998-4213-2.ch005

Waldman, S. D., Waldman, C. W., Waldman, R. A., & Abuabara, J. O. (2020). How to Use Technology and Telehealth to Enhance the Interprofessional Community of Practice. In Building a Patient-Centered Interprofessional Education Program (pp. 113-119). IGI Global. http://doi:10.4018/978-1-7998-3066-5.ch006

Wickramasinghe, N. (2020). Minority Health and Wellness. In N. Wickramasinghe (Ed.), *Handbook of Research on Optimizing Healthcare Management Techniques* (pp. 116–126). IGI Global. doi:10.4018/978-1-7998-1371-2.ch008

Xochelli, A., Stamatopoulos, K., & Karamanidou, C. (2019). Patient Involvement in Health Care. Different Terms Same Concept? *International Journal of Reliable and Quality E-Healthcare*, *8*(1), 1–10. doi:10.4018/IJRQEH.2019010101

Yaseen, S. G., & Al Omoush, K. S. (2020). Mobile Crowdsourcing Technology Acceptance and Engagement in Crisis Management. *International Journal of Technology and Human Interaction*, *16*(3), 1–23. doi:10.4018/IJTHI.2020070101

Yeo, Y., & Sohn, C. (2021). Intention-Behavior Gap in the Use of Personal Health Records (PHRs). *International Journal of E-Adoption*, *13*(1), 18–35. doi:10.4018/IJEA.2021010102

Zammar, N. (2021). Crisis Communication in the Age of Social Media and the Case of Dairy Khoury. In Encyclopedia of Organizational Knowledge, Administration, and Technology (pp. 2181-2196). IGI Global. doi:10.4018/978-1-7998-3473-1.ch151

Ziadlou, D. (2020). Digital Transformation Leadership for Smart Healthcare Organizations. In K. Sandhu (Ed.), *Opportunities and Challenges in Digital Healthcare Innovation* (pp. 72–96). IGI Global. doi:10.4018/978-1-7998-3274-4.ch005

Zizka, L. (2020). Reflection and SoTL. In R. C. Plews & M. L. Amos (Eds.), *Evidence-Based Faculty Development Through the Scholarship of Teaching and Learning (SoTL)* (pp. 96–120). IGI Global. doi:10.4018/978-1-7998-2212-7.ch006

About the Authors

Celia Belim is an assistant professor at the School of Social and Political Sciences, University of Lisbon (ISCSP-ULisboa), lecturing on Communication Sciences (CC)'s scientific area since 2000. Currently, she is the executive coordinator of the graduate degree of the referred scientific area. She has a PhD on CC. She coordinates projects, such as *Communicate health* and *Agendas and communication*. Since 2000, she has participated in several conferences, and publishes in her fields of interest, such as health communication, having published, by invitation from Rowman & Littlefield Publishers. She has received five academic awards.

Cristina Vaz de Almeida is a researcher (PhD), specialist in health literacy (HL) and director of a post-graduate studies on Health Literacy at the Higher Institute of Applied Psychology (ISPA) since 2012. She has a permanent intervention as a lecturer and key-note speaker in HL for training health professionals, at national and international level. Since 2007, she has participated in Portuguese social projects. She has been working for more than 19 years at Lisbon Holy House of Mercy-Santa Casa da Misericórdia de Lisboa (SCML). She is coordinator and co-author of several books, articles and chapters of Health Literacy, Health Communication and Marketing Communication.

Index

I

K

M

N

P

Q

R

S

T

V

www.ingramcontent.com/pod-product-compliance
Lightning Source LLC
LaVergne TN
LVHW081523300926
849161LV00006B/1277